HIKE LIST

* See hike descriptions for important updates

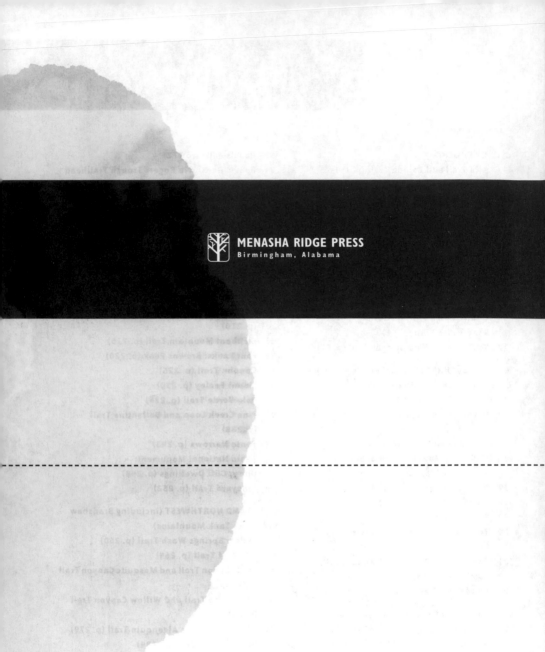

MENASHA RIDGE PRESS
Birmingham, Alabama

60 HIKES WITHIN 60 MILES

PHOENIX

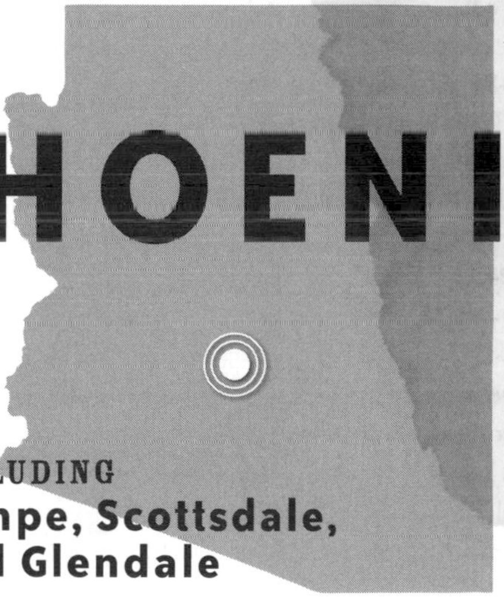

INCLUDING
**Tempe, Scottsdale,
and Glendale**

SECOND EDITION

CHARLES LIU

Copyright © 2009 Charles Liu
All rights reserved
Printed in the United States of America
Published by Menasha Ridge Press
Distributed by Publishers Group West
Second edition, fourth printing 2011

Library of Congress Cataloging-in-Publication Data

Liu, Charles, 1968 June 27–
    60 Hikes within 60 miles, Phoenix : including Tempe, Scottsdale, and Glendale / Charles Liu.—2nd ed.
      p. cm.
    ISBN 13: 978-0-89732-688-9 (alk. paper)
    ISBN 10: 0-89732-688-1 (alk. paper)
    1. Hiking—Arizona—Phoenix Region—Guidebooks. 2. Phoenix Region (Ariz.)—Guidebooks. I. Title. II. Title: Sixty hikes within 60 miles, Phoenix. II.

    GV199.42.A72P485 2009
    796.5109791'73—dc22   2008046161

Cover design by Steveco International and Scott McGrew
Tex design by Steveco International
Cover photo Charles Liu
Text photos by Charles Liu
Maps by Jennie Zehmer, Scott McGrew, and Charles Liu

Menasha Ridge Press
P.O. Box 43673
Birmingham, AL 35243
www.menasharidge.com

IN MEMORY OF CHRIS NICHOLAS (1970–2007), A FELLOW HIKER, FRIEND, AND LOVING HUSBAND AND FATHER.   —CHARLES LIU

TABLE OF
CONTENTS

* See hike descriptions for important updates

ACKNOWLEDGMENTS

When presented with the prospect of tackling this project, I felt justifiably elated for such an incredible opportunity and yet equally concerned about the monumental task at hand. Metropolitan Phoenix is the fifth-largest city in the country, and there are hundreds of trails around it. To render adequate coverage and to choose the 60 best trails turned out to be more challenging than I had imagined. Thankfully, over the years I have developed an extensive network of avid hiking friends who are always willing to offer sage advice, trail companionship, and other assistance. Many have contributed to this book in a direct or subtle manner, and some have even done so unknowingly. For their help, I'm sincerely grateful.

The following individuals have contributed in specific ways. I would like to acknowledge them here in alphabetical order. Please forgive any accidental omissions.

Lisa Cozzetti provided valuable guidance on South Mountain National Trail and the Boulder Canyon Trail to LaBarge Canyon.

John Daleiden suggested combining Mormon Trail with the Hidden Valley Loop as an alternative to the popular National–Mormon Loop. He also assisted in plotting an enjoyable route around Hayden Butte, also known as A-Mountain, and Tempe Town Lake.

Pat Donahue recommended Fish Creek for its superb scenery.

Amy Kemper assisted with fact checking and research for the second edition.

Skip and Zenda Treaster brought Circlestone to my attention and gave fascinating insights on this remote archaeological treasure.

The following groups of people also contributed significantly.

A special recognition goes to members of Take-A-Hike and CharlesHike for tagging along on my often torturous hiking excursions and for volunteering as photo subjects on these trips.

I also owe a debt of gratitude to Dr. David Pheanis, John Daleiden, and Jim Garvey for writing letters of recommendation.

I'd like to thank Russell Helms and the Menasha Ridge Press staff for entrusting me with this book and for providing seasoned advice and guidance.

Many thanks go to Webmasters around the Phoenix area for publishing hike information, photos, and other related data. Some notable sources of valuable data include the Arizona Republic, HikeArizona.com, City of Phoenix, City of Tempe, City of Scottsdale, City of Glendale, Maricopa County, Arizona State Parks, U.S. Bureau of Land Management, U.S.D.A. Forest Service, and the National Park Service.

Last but not least, I'd like to acknowledge my family, Mary Liu, Shaung Liu, and Jana Langseth-Liu, for offering support in many ways during the yearlong effort.

This book is dedicated to Arizona hikers and to those who work tirelessly to maintain and improve trails in the vicinity.

—CHARLES LIU

FOREWORD

Welcome to Menasha Ridge Press's *60 Hikes within 60 Miles,* a series designed to provide hikers with the information they need to find and hike the very best trails surrounding metropolitan areas typically underserved by outdoor guidebooks.

Our strategy was simple: First, find a hiker who knows the area and loves to hike. Second, ask that person to spend a year researching the most popular and very best trails around. And third, have that person describe each trail in terms of difficulty, scenery, condition, elevation change, and all other categories of information that are important to hikers. "Pretend you've just completed a hike and met up with other hikers at the trailhead," we told each author. "Imagine their questions; be clear in your answers."

An experienced hiker and writer, Charles Liu has selected 60 of the best hikes in and around the Phoenix metropolitan area. From city parks and preserves that highlight the diverse Sonoran desert landscape to rugged Central Arizona mountains and forests, Liu provides hikers (and walkers) with a great variety of hikes—and all within roughly 60 miles of Phoenix.

You'll get more out of this book if you take a moment to read the introduction explaining how to read the trail listings. The "Topographic Maps" section will help you understand how useful topos are on a hike and will also tell you where to get them. And though this is a "where-to," not a "how-to" guide, readers who have not hiked extensively will find the introduction of particular value.

As much for the opportunity to free the spirit as well as to free the body, let these hikes elevate you above the urban hurry.

All the best,
The Editors at Menasha Ridge Press

ABOUT THE AUTHOR

CHARLES LIU

Charles Liu immigrated to the United
States from China in 1980 and settled in a
suburb of Phoenix with his extended family. Spending his formative years attend-
ing Arizona State University, Liu grew
increasingly fond of the Grand Canyon
State's diverse outdoor offerings. Hiking
quickly became his passion; in particular
he adopted a keen preference for challeng-
ing day hikes and alpine mountaineering.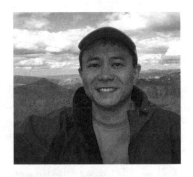
An avid outdoorsman and an active member of several hiking
clubs and creator of his own hiking group, Liu has led countless
hikes over the years, including annual treks to the depths of the
Grand Canyon and to the 12,633-foot summit of Humphreys
Peak, Arizona's highest point.

An engineer by trade, Liu spends much of his spare time
hiking, photographing, and writing about trails in and around
Phoenix. He can often be found racing up Camelback Mountain
after work, relieving stress from a high-tech career, or traips-
ing through the Superstition Wilderness on weekends. Aptly
nicknamed "Mad Hiker," Liu finds fulfillment in tough hiking
challenges. He has recently conquered Mount Whitney in California, Mount Rainier in Washington, and most of Colorado's
54 "fourteeners." Liu's extensive hiking experience, attention to
detail, and passion for hiking make him an ideal trail guide for
the *60 Hikes* series.

To contact the author with comments or suggestions you can
email him at **madhiker@gmail.com** or visit **www.madhiker
.org/6060**.

PREFACE

An acquaintance once questioned my hiking hobby: "So you like to wander around in the desert?" After chuckling at her sardonic observation, I had to explain that my obsession with hiking went far beyond the physical act of walking through the scenery. To me, hiking satisfies many mental, physical, and spiritual needs. This versatile activity is a means to elevate one's intellect as well as the heart rate. It forges a bond between man and nature, instills confidence and increases awareness, promotes health and relieves stress, challenges the body, and sharpens the mind. Striking a balance between exercise and travel, hiking can take you to amazing places, where breathtaking vistas, deep canyons, emerald forests, open deserts, tranquil streams, and alpine mountaintops reward those who venture away from the comforts of their air-conditioned homes. Requiring very little up-front investment, hiking is perhaps the perfect hobby, suitable for all ages and any level of physical fitness. It's certainly much more than a walk in the desert!

Of course, I didn't always feel this way about hiking. Indeed, I spent many years living in the Grand Canyon State, oblivious to the wonders that lay in my backyard, before I began exploring the outdoors on foot. I'm embarrassed to admit that what really spurred me into action and kicked off a lifelong pursuit was a fit of hormone-driven teenage angst. Looking to burn off some frustration from "girl problems," I decided on a whim that climbing a mountain would do the trick and make me feel better. I had remembered some friends talking about hiking Piestewa Peak, which was known as Squaw Peak at the time, so I whipped my car around and headed toward the famous Phoenix landmark.

My inaugural hike began on a perfect autumn afternoon. I remembered that it was a cool and breezy day with a clear sky and some lingering clouds—an ideal setting for hiking. I found the trailhead and arrived wearing casual sport sandals, the wrong choice of footwear for the effort, but I didn't care. Charging uphill

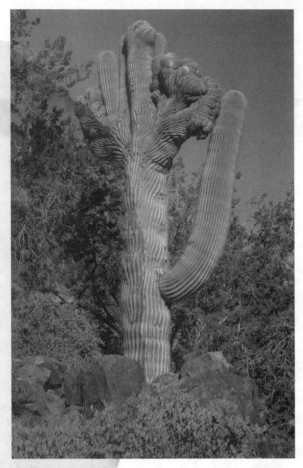

A rare crested saguaro stands above the Cave Creek Trail.

at full throttle, I quickly felt my chest constricting, my legs burning from lactic-acid buildup, and my heart pounding in my throat. Despite the cool breeze, sweat was beading on my forehead and running down my face. That's when I realized that I hadn't brought any water. "What a rookie mistake!" I thought to myself as I labored to catch my breath.

I made it to the summit that day on sheer bravado of youth, and the physical exertion provided a complete catharsis for my woes. By the time I reached the top, I felt winded and spent, yet content. While resting on the rocky summit and admiring a panoramic view of the city some 1,200 feet below me, a perfect Arizona sunset began to play out its colorful drama in the western sky. Wow! I caught myself gasping out loud at the beauty of the moment. Some other hikers next to me also echoed their awe. Later that night, as I limped down the mountain in the dark with quivering legs and a parched tongue, I made a mental promise to hike again, and soon.

In general, it takes more than one perfect hike to christen a hiker, and I was no exception to the rule. Over the next few years, I stayed mostly within city limits and occasionally hiked around the islands of mountain preserves. Camelback Mountain became my favorite destination, and for good reason. It was the perfect in-town hike for my tastes. I loved the scenic red rocks, the challenging slope, the friendly fellow hikers, and of course the gorgeous sunsets from the summit. I looked forward to going there after work, to stretch my legs after a day of cubicle imprisonment, and to visit familiar faces on the mountain. Yes, I had slowly but surely begun the metamorphosis into a hiker. Camelback Mountain served as both trainer and proving ground, whipping me into shape and allowing me to test new techniques and gear. I had even developed a custom rating system for hikes, using the Echo Canyon Trail as a standard unit of measure. The transformation was nearly complete.

Then in the summer of 1995, my experiences on a trip to the Grand Canyon not only validated my self-proclaimed moniker "Mad Hiker" but accentuated hiking as my defining characteristic. A few friends and I gathered for a trip into the depths of the Grand Canyon, arguably the greatest place on Earth to hike. We ignored all posted warnings and rangers' advice and decided to hike down to the Colorado River and back in one day, a colossal death march of 17 miles with a mile of elevation gain. The challenge was irresistible.

I had visited the Grand Canyon numerous times before but had never stepped foot below the rim. The all-day trek proved more grueling than we could have imagined, but it was also an exhilarating thrill ride played in slow motion. I realized that day while walking through the Canyon's grandiose splendor, examining the scenery up close, and admiring hidden perspectives unseen from rim-side overlooks that hiking allows me to participate in nature and to witness places that are otherwise unreachable. At the end of a torturous day, peering back into the Canyon and retracing our steps with my eyes, I felt an overwhelming sense of joy, pride, and wonder. Despite aching muscles and blistered feet, I longed for more. I was addicted, head-over-heels in love with hiking.

Over the past decade, I have sought out increasingly challenging hikes and finally began to explore in earnest the wonders in my backyard. My reach stretched beyond city limits, extended to the rest of Arizona, and eventually broadened to the highest peaks in the western states. Hiking became a more serious endeavor because I made an extra effort to research each destination, its history, and what I might find along the way. I learned about the intricate ecosystems that make up the Sonoran Desert. I memorized the names of plants and wildflowers, of birds and butterflies, and even of snakes and lizards. I watched in amazement as the most delicate blossoms sprang from the prickliest plants. The more I learned, the more I felt in tune with my surroundings and the more I enjoyed each hike. Every hike became an opportunity to expand my understanding of the world, and I grew eager to share that newfound knowledge. This book is the vessel through which I shall attempt to share the treasures that exist just outside our doors, to help everyone discover what the Phoenix area has to offer.

Visitors from out of town sometimes tell me that before arriving in Arizona, they had imagined it to be a giant sand dune, much like movie scenes of the Sahara Desert. Nothing could be further from the truth. Arizonans are blessed with a wide range of climate zones, supporting rich variations in flora and fauna. If you take the time to study it closely, you'll find the desert teeming with life and buzzing with activity. With ample mountainous terrain nearby and 325 days of sunshine a year, the aptly named "Valley of the Sun" is ideally suited for outdoor activity.

The City of Phoenix spans a staggering 517 square miles and houses more than 1.5 million people, making it the fifth-largest city in the United States. Within its boundaries, Phoenix has three major mountain preserves where dozens of trails cater to the daily exerciser or the weekend warrior. South Mountain covers the entire southern border of Phoenix, while Piestewa Peak anchors a series of mountains on the northern end of town. Camelback Mountain stands alone and dominates the central

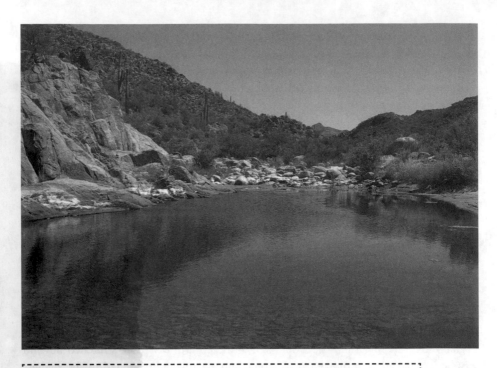

A tranquil pool mirrors the sky along Boulder Canyon Trail in the Superstition Wilderness.

Phoenix skyline. Residents flock to these popular destinations to witness stunning views, to socialize, and to get a workout.

Phoenix's suburbs also boast their share of parks, greenbelts, and preserves to serve more than 4 million residents in the metropolitan area. Nearly every suburb offers trails to explore—some more than others. The City of Scottsdale and the McDowell Sonoran Conservancy in particular have made significant strides in conservation by purchasing state trust land in the McDowell mountain range and turning it into a preserve. New trails, trailheads, and access areas entice longtime Valley residents and newbies alike. The second edition of this book explores some new McDowell trails. More are on their way in coming years, so check back soon.

While a wide assortment of terrain exists in the Phoenix metropolitan area, the rest of Arizona offers hikers even greater choices. Beyond the Valley of the Sun, a ring of rugged mountains awaits exploration. County and state parks provide excellent facilities and convenient access to the foothills trails on the fringes of the city. Tonto National Forest and Prescott National Forest encompass several key wilderness areas and hundreds of trails just a short drive from town, transporting hikers into a world that they might not expect to find near Phoenix—one of lush forests, quiet meadows, trickling mountain streams, and thrilling summits. This book also covers hikes in three national monuments: Sonoran Desert, Agua Fria, and Tonto. Finally, a series of dams provides the strict water management necessary for desert living. The resultant lakes behind the dams also offer scenic settings for hiking and water-related recreation.

This book attempts to address the needs of every hiker. Whether you are a complete newbie without a pair of hiking shoes to your name or a seasoned veteran with hundreds of hikes under your belt, you'll find something worthwhile between these covers. My hope is that the information provided here will help guide you through your own discovery process and help you enrich your hiking experience. Perhaps you will learn of a new trail, pick up a tip to improve your technique, or find the inspiration to reach a higher summit. Perhaps these pages will even pique your interest in enhancing your hiking skills with elements of climbing, mountaineering, or canyoneering. The possibilities are endless, and this book is merely a beginning. Happy hiking!

HIKING RECOMMENDATIONS

1 TO 3 MILES

4 TO 6 MILES

7 TO 9 MILES

MORE THAN 9 MILES

FLAT HIKES

FLAT HIKES (continued)

STEEP HIKES

HIKES WITH SWIMMING HOLES

HIKES NEAR STREAMS OR LAKES

HIGH-ALTITUDE HIKES

HIKES WITH SCRAMBLING OR CLIMBING

MULTIUSE TRAILS

TRAILS WITH RUINS

TRAILS WITH RUINS (*continued*)

BEST FOR CHILDREN

BEST FOR DOGS

BEST FOR SOLITUDE

BEST FOR WILDLIFE WATCHING

BEST FOR WILDFLOWERS

BEST FOR REGULAR WORKOUTS

BEST FOR REGULAR WORKOUTS (*continued*)

BEST SCENIC HIKES

BEST FOR RUNNERS

INTRODUCTION

Welcome to *60 Hikes within 60 Miles: Phoenix*. If you're new to hiking or even if you're a seasoned trail-smith, take a few minutes to read the following introduction. We explain how this book is organized and how to use it.

HIKE DESCRIPTIONS

Each hike contains eight key items: a locator map, an "In Brief" description of the trail, a KEY AT-A-GLANCE INFORMATION box, directions to the trail, a trail map, an elevation profile, a trail description, and a description of nearby activities. Combined, the maps and information provide a clear method to assess each trail from the comfort of your favorite reading chair.

IN BRIEF

A "taste of the trail." Think of this section as a snapshot focused on the historical landmarks, beautiful vistas, and other sights you may encounter on the trail.

KEY AT-A-GLANCE INFORMATION

The information in the key at-a-glance boxes gives you a quick idea of the specifics of each hike. There are 15 basic elements covered.

LENGTH The length of the trail from start to finish. There may be options to shorten or extend the hikes, but the mileage corresponds to the described hike. Consult the hike description to help decide how to customize the hike for your ability or time constraints.

ELEVATION GAIN The difference between minimum elevation and maximum elevation during the hike. Ups and downs on the trail may add significantly to the amount of effort required.

CONFIGURATION A description of what the trail might look like from overhead. Trails can be loops, out-and-backs (trails on which one enters and leaves along the same path), figure eights, or balloons.

1

DIFFICULTY   The degree of effort an average hiker should expect on a given hike. For simplicity, difficulty is described as "easy," "moderate," or "difficult."

SCENERY   A summary of the overall environs of the hike and what to expect in terms of plant life, wildlife, streams, and historic buildings.

EXPOSURE   A quick check of how much sun you can expect on your shoulders during the hike. Descriptors used are self-explanatory and include terms such as shady, exposed, and sunny.

TRAFFIC   Indicates how busy the trail might be on an average day and if you might be able to find solitude out there. Trail traffic, of course, varies from day to day and season to season.

SURFACE   A description of the trail surface, be it paved, rocky, dirt, or a mixture of materials.

HIKING TIME   The length of time it takes to hike the trail. Most of the estimates in this book reflect an average speed of 2 miles per hour. Difficult terrain and scrambling can add significantly to the amount of time required.

WATER REQUIREMENT   The recommended amount of water one needs to take along for each hike. Having enough water is paramount when hiking in the desert. The required amount of fluid will increase with ambient temperature and pace.

ACCESS   A notation of hours of service and fees or permits needed to access the trail (if any).

MAPS   Which maps are the best, or easiest, for this hike, and where to get them.

FACILITIES   What to expect in terms of restrooms, water, and other amenities available at the trailhead or nearby.

DOGS   Whether four-legged hiking buddies are allowed on the trail.

SPECIAL COMMENTS   These comments cover little extra details that don't fit into any of the above categories. Here you'll find information on trail-hiking options and facts, or tips on how to get the most out of your hike.

DIRECTIONS TO THE TRAIL

The detailed directions given for each hike will lead you to its trailhead. If you use GPS technology, the UTM and latitude/longitude coordinates provided allow you to navigate directly to the trailhead.

TRAIL DESCRIPTIONS

The trail description is the heart of each hike. Here the author provides a summary of the trail's essence and highlights any special sights along the hike. Ultimately, the hike description will help you choose which hikes are best for you.

NEARBY ACTIVITIES

Look here for information on nearby trails, other activities, or points of interest.

WEATHER

Phoenix is notorious for its blistering summer heat. With the mercury routinely exceeding 110 degrees, Phoenicians often joke that they live next door to the devil. Peak temperatures occur from late June to mid-July before seasonal monsoons— annual weather disturbances that cause regular thunderstorms—bring some measure of relief. The scorching Arizona sun and oppressive heat can make outdoor activities miserable and often downright dangerous.

Seasoned Phoenix residents have developed strategies to cope with their extreme climate. Relatively low humidity causes temperatures to drop significantly at night. Therefore, veteran desert hikers take full advantage of cool early mornings and late evenings. They religiously apply sunblock and hydrate well before a hike. Many seek outings to higher elevations and near streams on the hottest days.

Excluding its merciless summers, Phoenix boasts mild and pleasant weather, especially in winter. Measurable snow occurs only once every 20 years in Phoenix. As a matter of fact, locals have coined the term "snowbirds" for the seasonal influx of winter visitors attempting to escape frigid conditions elsewhere in the country. Perpetually low humidity blesses Arizona with ample sunshine and accounts for its magnificent sunsets.

AVERAGE DAILY TEMPERATURES AND RAINFALL BY MONTH

	JAN	FEB	MAR	APR	MAY	JUN
High	65	69	74	83	92	102
Low	43	47	51	58	66	75
Mean	54	58	62	70	79	88
Low	0.83	0.77	1.07	0.25	0.16	0.09

	JUL	AUG	SEP	OCT	NOV	DEC
High	104	102	97	86	73	65
Low	81	80	75	63	50	44
Mean	94	92	86	75	62	54
Low	0.99	0.94	0.75	0.79	0.73	0.92

Phoenix receives an average of only seven inches of rain per year, making it one of the driest regions in the country. However, desert storms can be sudden and violent. Flash floods, blinding dust storms, and rapidly changing temperatures can wreak havoc on anyone unprepared for monsoon conditions, which typically invade the Valley of the Sun from mid-July through mid-September. Winter rains are somewhat milder and occur between December and March, bringing life and color to desert plants that are poised to respond. Early spring is the most colorful time of the year, when wildflowers blanket hillsides with splashes of gold, and fragrant citrus blossoms perfume the air.

The Sonoran Desert can be exquisitely beautiful but also unforgiving to those who are unprepared for its harsh realities. To hike safely in a desert environment requires knowledge and preparation. Having common sense doesn't hurt either. Bring plenty of water, apply ample sunblock, and always tell someone where you are going. Wilderness areas near Phoenix feature rugged and remote mountains that reach elevations in excess of 7,000 feet. Temperature extremes, sudden storms, and intense solar radiation occur at these altitudes. Whether visiting desert foothills in town or exploring remote mountain trails, hikers need to be aware of their environment and its risks and to come prepared with proper clothing and gear.

ALLOCATING TIME

On flat or lightly undulating terrain, the author averages 3.5 miles per hour when hiking. That speed drops in direct proportion to the steepness of a path. Navigation of obstacles such as brush and boulders, off-trail exploration of flora and fauna, photography, and rest stops also extend a hike. Give yourself plenty of time. Few people enjoy rushing through a hike, and fewer still take pleasure in scrambling down a rocky chute after dark. Remember, too, that your pace naturally slackens over the back half of a long trek.

MAPS

The maps in this book have been produced with great care and, used with the hiking directions, will direct you to the trail and help you stay on course. However, you will find superior detail and valuable information in the United States Geological Survey's (USGS) 7.5–minute series topographic maps. Topo maps are available online in many locations, including **http://terraserver-usa.com** and **http://maps.google.com** (click "terrain"). You can view and print topos of the entire United States there and view aerial photographs of the same area. The downside to topos is that most of them are outdated, having been created 20 to 30 years ago. But they still provide excellent topographic detail.

If you're new to hiking, you might be wondering, "What's a topographic map?" In short, a topo indicates not only linear distance but elevation, using contour lines. Contour lines spread across the map like dozens of intricate spiderwebs. Each line represents a particular elevation, and at the base of each topo, a contour's interval designation is given. If the contour interval is 200 feet, then the height difference between each contour line is 200 feet. Follow five contour lines up on the same map, and the elevation has increased by 1,000 feet.

Let's assume that the 7.5–minute series topo reads "Contour Interval 40 feet," that the short trail we'll be hiking is two inches in length on the map, and that it crosses five contour lines from beginning to end. What do we know? Well, because the linear scale of this series is 2,000 feet to the inch (roughly two and three-quarters inches representing one mile), we know our trail is approximately four-fifths of a mile long (2 inches are 4,000 feet). We also know we'll be climbing or descending 200 vertical feet (five contour lines are 40 feet each) over that distance. The elevation designations written on occasional contour lines will tell us if we're heading up or down.

In addition to outdoor shops and bike shops, major universities and some public libraries have topos; you might try photocopying the ones you need to avoid buying them. If you want your own and can't find them locally, visit the United States Geological Survey Web site at **http://topomaps.usgs.gov.**

GLOBAL POSITIONING SYSTEM (GPS)
TRAILHEAD COORDINATES

To collect accurate map data, the author hiked each trail with a handheld GPS unit (Garmin eTrex Legend). Data collected was then downloaded and plotted onto a digital USGS topo map. In addition to rendering a highly accurate trail outline, this book also includes the GPS coordinates for each trailhead in two different coordinate systems. For readers who own a GPS unit, whether handheld or onboard a vehicle, the GPS coordinates provided on the first page of each hike may be entered into the GPS unit to locate trailheads with precision. More accurately known as Universal Transverse Mercator (UTM) coordinates, the first set of given GPS coordinates index a specific map location using a grid method. The survey datum used to arrive at the UTM coordinates is NAD27 CONUS. Just make sure your GPS unit is set to navigate using the UTM system in conjunction with NAD27 datum. For added convenience, the second edition of this book also gives trailhead coordinates in latitude and longitude for those who prefer to navigate using that geographic coordinate system. Typically, handheld GPS units use the WGS84 datum by default, so the latitude and longitude coordinates are specified using WGS84.

Most trailheads, which begin in parking areas, can be reached by car. However, some hikes still require a short walk from a parking area to reach the trailhead. A handheld GPS unit may be useful for navigation beyond the driving directions. That said, however, readers can easily access all trailheads and find the routes described in this book by using the directions given, the overview map, and the trail map, which shows at least one major road leading into the area. For those who enjoy using the latest GPS technology, the necessary data have been provided. A brief explanation of the geographic coordinate systems follows.

UTM COORDINATES—ZONE, EASTING, AND NORTHING

Three numbers labeled zone, easting, and northing appear within the trailhead coordinates box on the first page of each hike; for example, the Camelback Mountain Summit Trail hike on page 26 includes the following data:

> **UTM Zone (NAD27)** 12S
> **Easting** 0409661
> **Northing** 3709315

The zone number (12) refers to one of the 60 longitudinal (vertical) zones of a map using the UTM projection. Each zone is 6 degrees wide. The zone letter (S) refers to one of the 20 latitudinal (horizontal) zones that span from 80° South to 84° North.

The easting number (0409661) references in meters how far east the point is from the zero value for eastings, which runs north–south through Greenwich, England. Increasing easting coordinates on a topo map or on your GPS screen indicate you are moving east. Decreasing easting coordinates indicate you are moving west. Since lines of longitude converge at the poles, they are not parallel like lines of latitude. This means that the distance between full easting coordinates is 1,000 meters near the equator but becomes smaller as you travel farther north or south. The difference is small enough to be ignored until you reach the polar regions.

In the northern hemisphere the northing number (3709315) references in meters how far you are from the equator. Above the equator, northing coordinates increase by 1,000 meters between each parallel line of latitude (east–west lines). On a topo map or GPS receiver, increasing northing numbers indicate you are traveling north.

In the southern hemisphere, the northing number references how far you are from a latitude line that is 10 million meters south of the equator. Below the equator northing coordinates decrease by 1,000 meters between each line of latitude. On a topo map, decreasing northing coordinates indicate you are traveling south.

Remember that whenever you use UTM coordinates, the GPS should be set up to use the NAD27 CONUS datum. If you don't make this setting on your GPS unit, the coordinates given in the book will differ greatly from what your GPS unit measures while standing at the trailhead.

LATITUDE AND LONGITUDE

A more commonly used coordinate system specifies each point on the globe with a pair of angular measurements—latitude and longitude. Similar to X-Y coordinates that specify points on a two-dimensional plane, the latitude and longitude coordinates specify a point on our spherical planet. These coordinates are also given in the trail-head coordinates box.

Latitude is specified in degrees and measures the north-south angular distance between a point on the map and the Earth's equatorial plane, which divides the Earth into a northern hemisphere and a southern hemisphere. A point on the equator has latitude 0, while the North Pole has latitude 90 degrees. Points of equal latitude trace out concentric circles called parallels. The 38th Parallel became a well-known latitude during the Korean War. Since the United States lies in the northern hemisphere, latitudes for points within the United States will be some number between 0 and 90.

Longitude is also specified in degrees and measures the east-west angular distance between a point on the map and an arbitrary reference point—the Royal Observatory at Greenwich in England—designated as having 0 longitude. Points of equal longitude form meridians and run vertically from the North Pole to the South Pole. The 0-degree longitudinal line is also known as the Prime Meridian. Longitude values increase as you move away horizontally from the Prime Meridian. Everything to the east of the Prime Meridian is in the eastern hemisphere, and everything to its west is in the western hemisphere. For arbitrary reasons, points in the western hemisphere are given a negative longitude. So 111 degrees west is the same thing as -111 degrees longitude. The longitudinal line at 180 degrees—points farthest from the Prime Meridian—also serves (roughly) as the International Date Line.

Since longitude and latitude are angular coordinates, they are sometimes noted in degrees (denoted by °), minutes ('), and even seconds (") for better readability. A typical GPS unit comes from the factory set to display latitude/longitude coordinates in degrees and minutes. Therefore, all latitude/longitude coordinates are specified in degrees and minutes in this book. Make sure your GPS unit is set to use the WGS84 datum when using latitude/longitude coordinates. Again, WGS84 is a typical default setting on many GPS units.

For the same example given above, the trailhead for Camelback Mountain Summit Trail has the following latitude/longitude coordinates:

Latitude N33°31.283'
Longitude W111°58.410'

These coordinates specify a point in the northern hemisphere, 33 degrees and 31.283 minutes north of the Equator, and in the western hemisphere, 111 degrees and 58.410 minutes west of the Prime Meridian.

TRAIL ETIQUETTE

Following are some suggestions to improve not only your hiking experience but the environment for those who follow you. Whether you're on a city, county, state, or national park trail, always remember that great care and resources have gone into creating these trails. Treat the trail, wildlife, and fellow hikers with respect.

1. **Hike on designated trails only. Respect trail and road closures (ask if not sure), avoid trespassing on private land, and obtain all required permits and authorization. Also, leave gates as you find them or as marked. Note that some of the trails in this book include sections off the main trails. Clear directions are provided.**

2. **Leave only footprints. Be sure to pack out what you pack in. No one likes to see the trash someone else has left behind.**

3. **Never spook animals. An unannounced approach, a sudden movement, or a loud noise startles most animals. A surprised snake or skunk can be dangerous to you, others, and themselves.**

4. **Plan ahead. Know your equipment, your ability, and the area in which you are hiking—and prepare accordingly. Be self-sufficient at all times; carry necessary supplies for changes in the weather or other conditions. A well-executed trip is a satisfaction to you and to others.**

5. **Be courteous to other hikers, bikers, or equestrians you meet on the trails. It is customary to yield to equestrians, hikers going uphill, and faster hikers.**

WATER

"How much is enough? One bottle? Two? Three?! But think of all that extra weight!" Well, one simple physiological fact should convince you to err on the side of excess when it comes to deciding how much water to pack: A hiker working hard in 90-degree heat needs approximately ten quarts of fluid every day. That's two and a half gallons—12 large water bottles or 16 small ones. In other words, pack along one or two bottles even for short hikes.

Around Phoenix, water sources are scarce at best, and hikers must be prepared to take along all the water they need on a hike. Look in the Key At-A-Glance Information for the minimum recommended amount of water for each hike. Keep in mind that high ambient temperatures and physiological differences among individuals may require you to drink more than the recommended amount.

There are a few perennial streams near Phoenix, and serious backpackers hit the trail prepared to purify water found along the route. This method, while less dangerous than drinking untreated water, comes with risks. Purifiers with ceramic filters are the safest but also the most expensive. Many hikers pack along the slightly distasteful tetraglycine-hydroperiodide tablets (sold under the names Potable Aqua, Coughlan's, and others).

Probably the most common waterborne "bug" that hikers face is giardia, which may not affect you until one to four weeks after ingestion. It will have you passing noxious rotten-egg gas, vomiting, shivering, and living in the bathroom. There are other parasites to worry about, including E. coli and cryptosporidium (these are harder to kill than giardia).

For most people, the pleasures of hiking make carrying water a relatively minor price to pay to remain healthy. If you're tempted to drink "found water," do so only if you understand the risks involved. Better yet, hydrate prior to your hike, carry (and drink) six to ten ounces of water for every mile you plan to hike, and hydrate after the hike.

FIRST-AID KIT

A typical kit may contain more items than seem necessary. These are just the basics:

Ace bandages or Spenco joint wraps

Antibiotic ointment (Neosporin or the generic equivalent)

Aspirin, ibuprofen, or acetaminophen

Band-Aids

Benadryl or the generic equivalent— diphenhydramine (an antihistamine, in case of allergic reactions)

Butterfly-closure bandages

Comb and tweezers (for removing stray cactus needles from your skin)

Emergency poncho

Epinephrine in a prefilled syringe (for those known to have severe allergic reactions to such things as bee stings)

Gauze (one roll)

Gauze compress pads (a half dozen 4 inch x 4 inch)

Hydrogen peroxide or iodine

Insect repellent

LED flashlight or headlamp

Matches or pocket lighter

Mirror for signaling passing aircraft

Moleskin/Spenco "Second Skin"

Pocketknife or multipurpose tool

Snakebite kit

Sunblock

Water-purification tablets or water filter (on longer hikes)

Whistle (more effective in signaling rescuers than your voice)

SNAKES AND GILA MONSTERS

The mere mention of snakes strikes fear in the hearts of some hikers. Hike enough in the desert and you are bound to meet a snake. It's the price desert dwellers pay for a relative dearth of nagging insects, ticks, and poison ivy. However, snakes pose less risk than most people imagine, and they certainly need not keep you from enjoying a hike. Knowing their habitat, understanding their behavior, and respecting their territory are the keys to minimizing risks associated with a snake encounter.

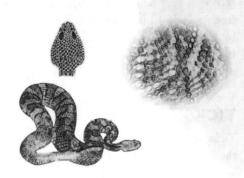

Rattlesnakes, named for the noisy rattles at the tips of their tails, are the most common snakes found in deserts and mountains near Phoenix. They belong to a group of venomous snakes called pit vipers—pit because they have concave heat-sensing glands on the sides of their faces and viper because they have venom-conducting fangs. There are over a dozen species of Arizona rattlesnakes, many of which are protected by law. Western diamondbacks are the largest and most common, and the nearly identical Mojave rattlers are the most dangerous. You'd do well to avoid both. True to their name, diamondbacks are usually brown in color with speckled dark-brown diamond-shaped blotches on their backs. Alternating black and white stripes line their tail just below the rattle. Mojave rattlers share the diamondbacks' blotchy pattern and black and white tail stripes, but the white stripes are notably wider than the black ones. Mojave rattlers sometimes show a greenish tint. These dangerous snakes carry a potent neurotoxin that is ten times more powerful than the hemotoxins of other rattlesnakes. Since the Mojave rattler is so close in appearance to a diamondback, it is very difficult to tell them apart, especially during a stressful snake encounter.

Armed with deadly venom, heat-sensing glands, and effective camouflage, rattlesnakes are efficient predators and thrive on small rodents. Fortunately, they are not aggressive by nature and rarely attack humans, unless sufficiently provoked. Most snakebites occur when an inattentive hiker steps on a snake or when a foolish person plays with one out of curiosity. Always give rattlesnakes plenty of space and never approach one on purpose.

Rattlesnakes prefer warmth but not searing heat. They are most active during spring and around dusk. Their favorite hangouts are among rock crevices, tall brush, and under shady branches. Vigilantly watch your step while hiking, and peer over any rock outcroppings before using them as handholds. Rattlesnakes do not like company. When you get too close for comfort, they will let you know by coiling into a defensive posture and emitting a loud rattle that you will likely remember for a long time. Heed their warning. Back up slowly and give them ample space. More often than not, they will back down and seek shelter under a nearby rock. If a snake obstinately obstructs the trail, find a way around it. Never aggravate snakes by poking them or throwing rocks at them. If you often hike with a dog, keep the pet on a close leash. Dogs often chase snakes, and that can lead to trouble for you and your hiking buddy.

Gila monsters are the largest lizards in the country and one of only two venomous lizards in the world. They are native to the Southwest and can be found in the mountains near Phoenix. Bulky and awkward-looking, they grow to two feet in length and have bright and distinctive brown, pink, yellow, and black markings. Staying out of sight most of their lives, Gila monsters rarely make a public appearance. They move slowly and pose little threat to hikers. However, those who molest these animals may receive a very painful and tenacious bite, from which it may be nearly impossible to free yourself. Unlike snakes, Gila monsters don't have fangs. They deliver their venom by gripping the victim within the jaws and letting the poison seep into the wound. If you happen upon a Gila monster on a hike, count yourself lucky and take some pictures, but do not attempt to touch or otherwise pester it.

TICKS

Ticks are not often found in the deserts around Phoenix. However, they do exist in the higher elevations, around streams, and in lush forested areas. Among local varieties of ticks, brown dog ticks and Rocky Mountain wood ticks are most common. You can use several strategies to reduce your chance of ticks getting under your skin. Some people choose to wear light-colored clothing, so ticks can be spotted before they make it to the skin. Insect repellent containing DEET is an effective deterrent. Most importantly, though, be sure to inspect yourself at the end of a hike. During your post-hike shower, take a moment to do a more complete body check. For ticks that are already embedded, removal with tweezers is best.

POISON IVY

Thankfully, poison ivy isn't as common near Phoenix as it is in most other places in the country. However, these itch-causing plants do grow near perennial streams and ponds. Recognizing and avoiding poison ivy, oak, and sumac are the most effective ways to prevent the painful, itchy rashes associated with these plants. Poison ivy occurs as a vine or groundcover, 3 leaflets to a leaf; poison oak occurs as either a vine or shrub, also with 3 leaflets; and poison sumac flourishes in swampland, each leaf having 7 to 13 leaflets. Urushiol, the oil in the sap of these plants, is responsible for the rash. Within 14 hours of exposure, raised lines and/or blisters will appear on the affected area, accompanied by a terrible itch. Refrain from scratching because bacteria under your fingernails can cause an infection. Wash and dry the rash thoroughly, applying a calamine lotion to help dry out the rash. If itching or blistering is severe, seek medical attention. If you do come into contact with one of these plants, remember that oil-contaminated clothes, pets, or hiking gear can easily cause an irritating rash on you or someone else, so wash not only any exposed parts of your body but also clothes, gear, and pets if applicable.

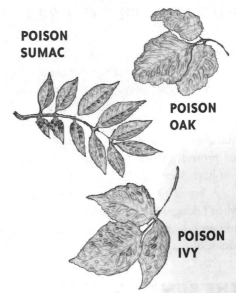

POISON SUMAC

POISON OAK

POISON IVY

MOSQUITOES

While not a common occurrence, individuals can become infected with the West Nile virus from the bite of an infected mosquito. Culex mosquitoes, the primary varieties that transmit West Nile virus to humans, thrive in urban rather than wilderness areas. They lay their eggs in stagnant water and can breed in any standing water that remains for more than five days. Most people infected with West Nile virus have no symptoms of illness, but some may become ill, usually 3 to 15 days after being bitten.

The Phoenix area has proven to be one of the riskiest for West Nile virus because of an abundance of stagnant swimming pools in the city. Most at risk are the elderly and those with weakened immune systems. Though the risk of infection is relatively low, hikers should consider taking measures to prevent mosquito bites. Remedies include using insect repellent and wearing clothes that completely cover the arms and legs.

SUN

The Valley of the Sun lives up to its name. Sunburn is a serious threat to hikers around Phoenix. High-altitude hikes exacerbate the risk of overexposure. Aside from the obvious pain and suffering and unsightly peeling associated with prolonged sun exposure, sunburn can be extremely harmful to the skin. Arizona unfortunately reigns in the category of skin cancer occurrence in the country. To avoid looking like a lobster at the end of your hike, apply sunblock with a minimum SPF rating of 30 before setting out. Reapply the sunblock every few hours to all exposed areas of your body. Don't forget your ears, nose, and the back of your neck. Wear a wide-brim hat and long shirts and pants for ultimate protection.

HIKING WITH CHILDREN

No one is too young for a hike in the woods or through a city park. Be careful, though. If you have an infant, flat and short trails are probably best. Toddlers who have not quite mastered walking can still tag along, riding on an adult's back in a child carrier. Use common sense to judge a child's capacity to hike a particular trail, and always expect that the child will tire quickly and need to be carried.

When packing for the hike, remember the child's needs as well as your own. Make sure children are adequately clothed for the weather, have proper shoes, and are protected from the sun with sunblock. Kids also dehydrate quickly, so make sure you have plenty of fluids for everyone.

A list of hike recommendations for children is provided on page XX. Finally, when hiking with children, remember the trip will be a compromise. A child's energy and enthusiasm alternate between bursts of speed and long stops to examine bugs, sticks, dirt, and other attractions.

THE BUSINESS HIKER

Whether you're in the Phoenix area on business or are a resident, these 60 hikes offer perfect quick getaways from the busy demands of commerce. The City of Phoenix is home to some of the best urban parks and mountain preserves in the United States. Instead of eating inside, you can pack a lunch and head out to picnic along the Indian Bend Wash Greenbelt or on Tempe Town Lake. Jumpstart your day with a power hike up Piestewa Peak, or wind down from a stress-filled meeting by watching the sunset from atop Camelback Mountain. You can also plan ahead and take a small group of your business comrades on a nearby hike in South Mountain or to the Wind Cave in Usery Park.

THE WINTER VISITOR

Phoenix may be hot during summer, but its mild winters draw seasonal visitors by the thousands. Family reunions, weddings, and holiday vacations seem to happen more often here between November and April than at other times of the year. Many people spend nearly half a year living in Phoenix and the rest of the time in their hometowns.

While the rest of the country shivers under a blanket of snow and ice, Phoenicians enjoy their best hiking weather. Instead of writhing in discomfort after overindulging in Thanksgiving turkey, try burning it off with a family outing to Pinnacle Peak. A Christmas vacation to Phoenix just wouldn't be complete without hiking up Camelback Mountain in shorts and a Santa hat. You can even call your snowbound midwestern friends from the summit to brag about the weather. Early spring in Phoenix is the best time to attempt longer hikes in the wilderness areas near town. When conditions are ripe, wildflower displays can be absolutely stunning in the Superstitions and the White Tanks. No matter how you end up in Phoenix in winter, be sure to take advantage of its superb hiking opportunities.

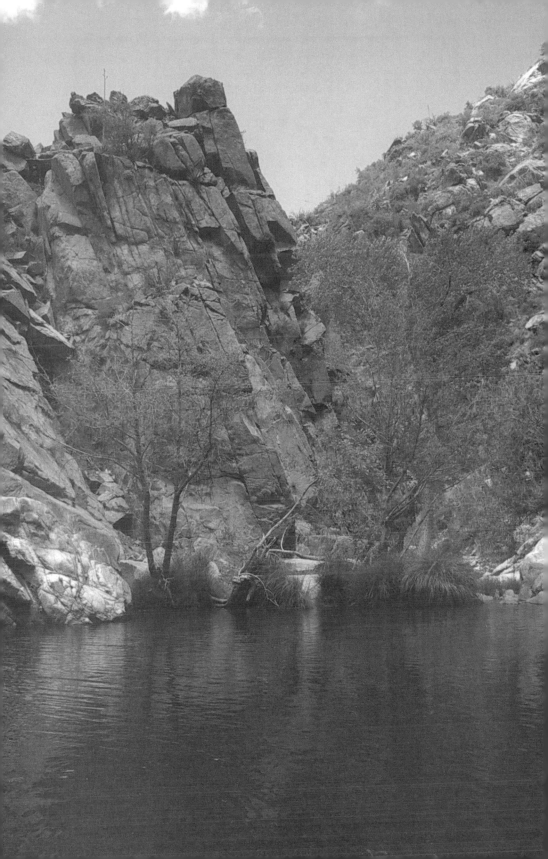

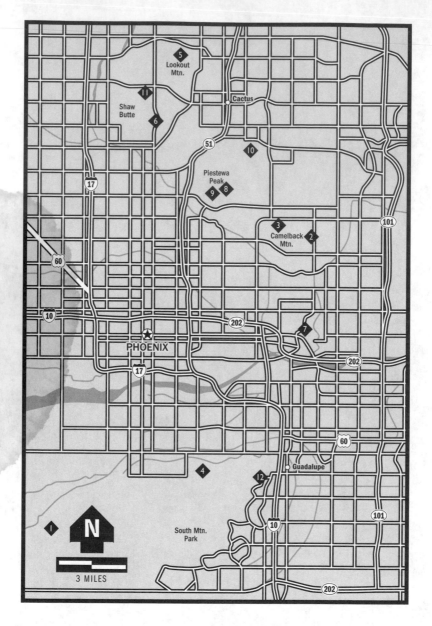

CITY OF PHOENIX

01 ALTA TRAIL AND BAJADA TRAIL

KEY AT-A-GLANCE INFORMATION

LENGTH: 8.5 Miles

ELEVATION GAIN: 1,200 feet

CONFIGURATION: Loop

DIFFICULTY: Alta Trail: difficult; Bajada Trail: easy

SCENERY: City panorama, South Mountain Park, Sierra Estrella, desert

EXPOSURE: Limited shade, mostly exposed

TRAFFIC: Light

TRAIL SURFACE: Crushed rock, gravel, packed dirt

HIKING TIME: 4 hours

WATER REQUIREMENT: 2.5 quarts

SEASON: Year-round; hot in summer

ACCESS: Trails open sunrise–sunset, park open 5 a.m.–10 p.m.; free parking

MAPS: USGS Lone Butte and Laveen, park map on trailhead plaques and available from visitor center

FACILITIES: None at trailhead. Visitor center, restrooms, picnic areas, riding stables, and go-cart racecourse available inside park

DOGS: Yes, leashed at all times

COMMENTS: Not as crowded as the trails on the eastern end of South Mountain. For more information, visit http://phoenix.gov/parks/hikesoth.html.

GPS Trailhead Coordinates

UTM Zone   12S

Easting   0393577

Northing   3688294

Latitude   N33°19.819'

Longitude   W111°8.650'

IN BRIEF

Fewer fellow hikers and a complete lack of mountain bikers make the Alta Trail inviting to those who prefer to hike undisturbed in South Mountain Park. Alta Trail is the most challenging trail in the park. The Bajada Trail and the tail end of the National Trail complete an enjoyable loop.

DESCRIPTION

There are three mountain ranges within the 16,000-acre confines of South Mountain Park, the largest municipal park in the country. The Ma Ha Tuak Range, the most unpronounceable of the three, is also the least visited mountain range. Located away from the busiest sections of South Mountain Park, the Ma Ha Tuak Range offers hikers a challenging trek sans the crowds and mountain bikers. Alta is the only trail in the Ma Ha Tuak Range. As its name suggests, the Alta Trail along Ma Ha Tuak's spine gains 1,200 feet in elevation, the most in South Mountain Park. However, some of the best views of the Phoenix skyline await those who accept this challenge.

Directions

Travel south on Central Avenue until it terminates at South Mountain Park. Once inside the park, follow the main road to the junction of Summit Road and San Juan Road. Follow San Juan Road 4 miles until it ends at the San Juan Lookout.

This loop hike can also be accessed via the Alta–Bajada junction on San Juan Road. Limited parking is available here.

San Juan Road is currently accessible by car only one weekend per month due to recent fire damage. Check the City of Phoenix Parks Web site for latest road information.

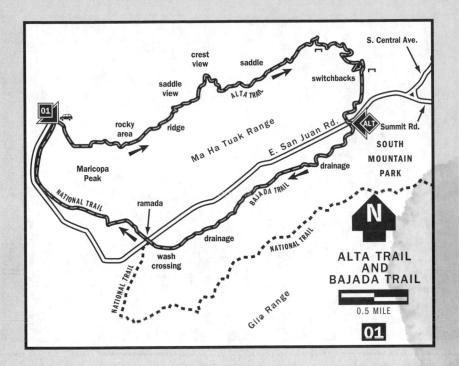

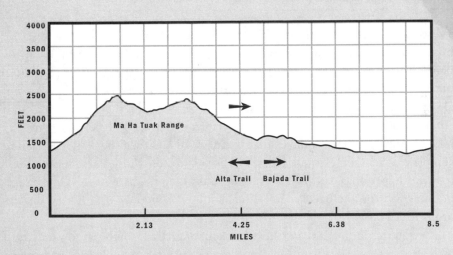

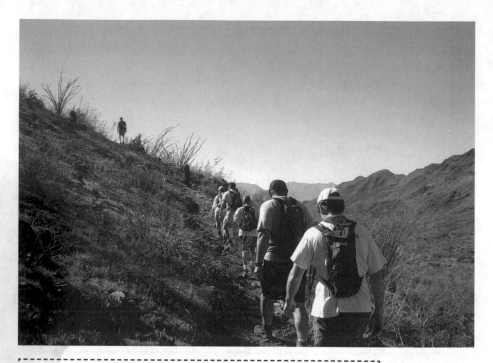

Members of Take-A-Hike Arizona tackle the Bajada Trail in South Mountain Park.

South Mountain Park boasts a superb network of trails that begs creative hikers to define their own loops. A popular loop includes the Alta Trail, the Bajada Trail, and the tail end of the National Trail. The Alta Trail runs from the San Juan Lookout at the extreme northwestern corner of the park to a point along San Juan Road, which traverses the valley between the Ma Ha Tuak and Gila mountain ranges. Hikers can either arrange a car shuttle for a one-way hike on Alta Trail or take the gentler Bajada Trail and then the National Trail to complete a pleasant 8.5-mile loop. The Bajada Trail, whose name means slope in Spanish, parallels San Juan Road and runs along the base of the Gila Range. Looping back on the Bajada Trail offers a mild warmdown after hiking the rigorous Alta Trail.

Begin this loop at the San Juan Lookout and climb southeast toward Maricopa Peak. The well-defined Alta Trail immediately ascends a hefty slope among desert grasses and palo verde trees, with views of southwestern Phoenix in the distance. At 0.4 miles, the trail bends north and provides a little respite from your laborious task. Soon, the pace picks up again as the trail rounds a corner and resumes its uphill trend. You are now walking up the flank of a narrow upper basin on the northern side of the mountain. Similar to most mountains in the Sonoran Desert, the northern slopes host more trees and shrubs such as the brittlebush, creosotes, and smaller cacti, while the drier southern slopes cater to the needs of giant saguaros and teddy bear chollas.

Steeper switchbacks greet you near 0.6 miles. Choose your steps carefully because the trail becomes a bit rocky and loose. Large boulders here provide some cool shade in early mornings and late afternoons. Continue ascending a fairly steep grade along the northern flank of the Ma Ha Tuak Range to an ocotillo-studded ridge crest at 1.1 miles. If you need a break here, turn to admire the Sierra Estrella mountain range behind you to the west, most of southwestern Phoenix, and the White Tank Mountains to the northwest. A bit farther along the trail, top out on the summit ridge where you have an open view to the south as well. The Gila River Indian Reservation and the interior valley of South Mountain Park are visible from this vantage point.

Forge ahead along the trail as it continues to ascend switchbacks toward the tallest point of the hike. At 1.5 miles, reach a prominent saddle at 2,460 feet of elevation where an awesome view of Phoenix presents itself. This saddle is a great spot to take a breather. In addition to the tall buildings of downtown Phoenix along Central Avenue and the crowded metropolis, you can spot pointy Piestewa Peak, the sleeping camel of Camelback Mountain, and numerous mountains to the northeast.

Even though you have just conquered the highest point on the hike, much work remains because the trail bobs up and down along the ridgeline. Past the high saddle point, the Alta Trail descends a series of switchbacks and drops 220 feet in elevation to a patch of rough terrain. Then, the cruel ascent resumes as the trail traverses the side of a steep hill toward the east, with the antenna array on top of Mount Suppoa barely visible directly ahead. When you reach the top of the ridge again at 2.5 miles, a narrow saddle offers an unobstructed view into the interior of South Mountain Park. Continue northeast near the top of the ridge, crossing over to the southern side of the hill at 2.8 miles.

Your climb finally ends at a 2,390-foot saddle, regaining most of the lost elevation from the highest point on the hike. From here, you enjoy a great view of Four Peaks off in the distance and the relaxing feeling that all the elevation gain is now behind you. The Alta Trail begins to descend gently at first but then steeply via a series of switchbacks through fields of teddy bear cholla, fishhook barrel cactus, and some elephant trees. As you descend, look for several rock benches built under chollas, and look across the valley for an abandoned mine on the northern side of the Gila Range.

Once the trail drops down to the valley floor between the Ma Ha Tuak and Gila ranges, it flattens out and becomes much easier to negotiate. Hike southwestward with the Sierra Estrella mountains directly ahead of you until the Alta Trail terminates on San Juan Road at a small parking lot where the Bajada Trail begins. You have just covered the most challenging 4.6 miles in South Mountain Park.

To loop back to the San Juan Lookout, head out on the Bajada Trail from the parking lot and climb up to the skirt of the Gila Range. Even though the slope of this climb pales in comparison to the Alta Trail, the short ascent will still make your muscles strain and take notice. Fortunately, the Bajada Trail

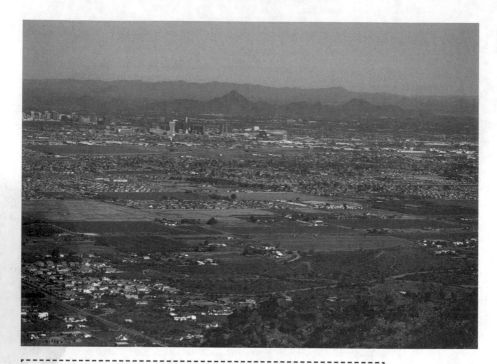

Panoramic view of Downtown Phoenix from the Alta Trail in South Mountain Park.

soon levels out and traces a path parallel to the road and along the base of the mountain.

The Bajada Trail stays mostly level and takes you through classic Sonoran Desert scenery. The gentle stroll along the Bajada Trail contrasts sharply with the huffing-and-puffing difficulty of the Alta Trail. At 5.3 and 6.5 miles, cross a couple of drainages on the side of the hill, and then cross the main dry wash on the valley floor. Just before reaching San Juan Road again, the Bajada Trail terminates at a junction with the National Trail.

The last section of this loop hike follows the westernmost part of the National Trail. Much like the Bajada Trail, the final 1.5 miles of the National Trail remains relatively flat. Cross San Juan Road and continue along the National Trail as it skirts the western end of the Ma Ha Tuak Range. The trail asymptotically approaches San Juan Road and ends at the San Juan Lookout where the loop began.

NEARBY ACTIVITIES

South Mountain hosts many hiking and biking trails including National (page 40), Desert Classic, Mormon (page 31), Ranger, and Telegraph Pass (page 109). Many other recreational activities such as picnicking and horseback riding are also available. The Environmental Education Center, located near the Central Avenue entrance, has a superb visitor center, complete with a three-dimensional model of the entire park.

CAMELBACK MOUNTAIN: CHOLLA TRAIL 02

IN BRIEF

Camelback Mountain is the tallest point in the city of Phoenix. From the 2,704-foot summit of Camelback, hikers command an impressive 360-degree panorama of the city and surrounding mountain ranges. The Cholla Trail offers hikers an easier, albeit longer, way to reach the top of Camelback Mountain than does the popular Summit (Echo Canyon) Trail (page 26). Fans of cityscape can appreciate the Cholla Trail for its open views along the way.

DESCRIPTION

When people say, "I'm hiking Camelback Mountain," they usually mean they are climbing up the Summit (Echo Canyon) Trail on the northwestern end of the mountain and the head of the sleeping camel shape for which the mountain was named. The Summit Trail, with its cliffs of red sandstone and huge boulders, does offer a very scenic experience of Camelback Mountain. However, the Summit Trail is also steep and sometimes overcrowded. A less crowded and somewhat easier way to summit Camelback Mountain is to hike up the Cholla Trail from the mountain's gentler eastern end. Nearly 2 miles in length, the Cholla Trail

KEY AT-A-GLANCE INFORMATION

LENGTH: 3.8 miles

ELEVATION GAIN: 1,331 feet

CONFIGURATION: Out-and-back (if you choose the optional one-way hike down Summit Trail, subtract 0.8 miles)

DIFFICULTY: Moderate

SCENERY: Desert, city panorama

EXPOSURE: Late-afternoon shade, otherwise exposed

TRAFFIC: Heavy

TRAIL SURFACE: Packed dirt, gravel, stair-steps, some scrambling

HIKING TIME: 2 hours

WATER REQUIREMENT: 1–1.5 quarts

SEASON: Year-round; hot in summer

ACCESS: Open sunrise to sunset; free but limited parking

MAPS: USGS Paradise Valley

FACILITIES: None

DOGS: Yes, leashed at all times

COMMENTS: No parking available at the Cholla Trailhead. Park in designated spots along the western side of Invergordon Road or along the southern side of Jackrabbit Road. For more information, visit http://phoenix.gov/parks/hikecmlb.html.

Directions

From Loop 202: Exit onto 44th Street and drive north 3.5 miles to Camelback Road. Turn east on Camelback Road and continue 2.7 miles to Invergordon Road. Turn north on Invergordon Road, drive 0.7 miles, and park in marked spots on the western side of the street.

From Loop 101: Exit onto Chaparral Road, and drive west 3.2 miles until it Ts into Invergordon Road. Turn north on Invergordon and park on the western side of the street.

GPS Trailhead Coordinates

UTM Zone 12S

Easting   0411979

Northing   3708425

Latitude   N33°30.813'

Longitude   W111°56.907'

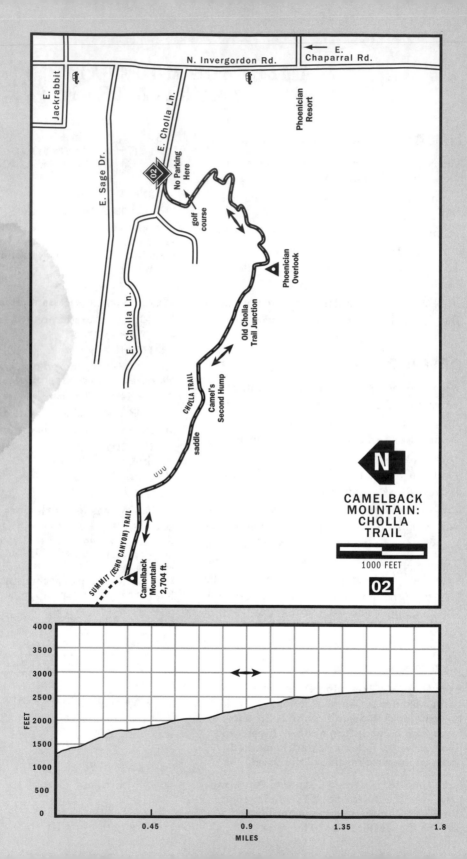

E. Chaparral Rd.

N. Invergordon Rd.

E. Jackrabbit

E. Sage Dr.

E. Cholla Ln.

E. Cholla Ln.

02

No Parking Here

golf course

Phoenician Resort

Phoenician Overlook

Old Cholla Trail Junction

CHOLLA TRAIL

Camel's Second Hump

saddle

SUMMIT (ECHO CANYON) TRAIL

Camelback Mountain 2,704 ft.

N

CAMELBACK MOUNTAIN: CHOLLA TRAIL

1000 FEET

02

FEET

4000
3500
3000
2500
2000
1500
1000
500
0

0.45   0.9   1.35   1.8

MILES

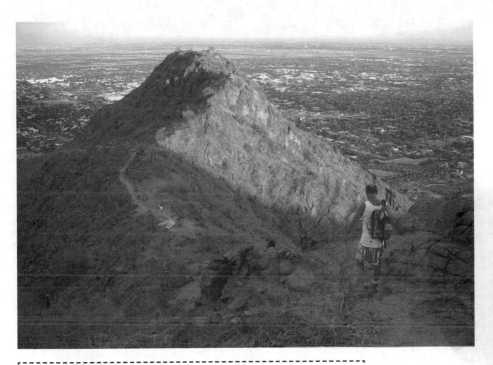

A hiker descends at sunset from Camelback Mountain along the Cholla Trail.

meanders up the spine of the sleeping camel and gives those not endowed with legs of steel a pleasant route to experience the wonders of this mountain. Fans of city views will also appreciate Cholla because it delivers ample wide-open vistas.

The Cholla Trail is not without its own challenges though, the first of which is to find desirable parking. In the late 1990s, residents near the original Cholla Trailhead petitioned the city to reroute the Cholla Trail because of noise and vandalism. As a result, you can no longer park near the trailhead on Cholla Lane, for which the trail was named. Instead, you must park in designated spots along the western side of Invergordon Road or along the southern side of Jackrabbit Road. The first half mile of your hike, therefore, is spent reaching the trailhead by walking along Invergordon Road and turning west up Cholla Lane. Stay on the southern side of Cholla Lane where a gravel trail ascends gently. Take this opportunity to warm up your leg muscles and to gawk at the opulent mansions along the street.

About 0.5 miles from your car and at the end of a white fence along the Phoenician Resort golf course, an obvious plaque marks the official trailhead for the Cholla Trail. Your journey up Camelback Mountain begins here. The first section of trail rounds the edge of the golf course. Watch out for low-flying golf balls! As you climb, the trail bends back toward the southeast and then levels out. From this flat stretch, you can survey the scenery. To your left lies a palm-lined putting green flanked by white sand traps. Look up toward the horizon,

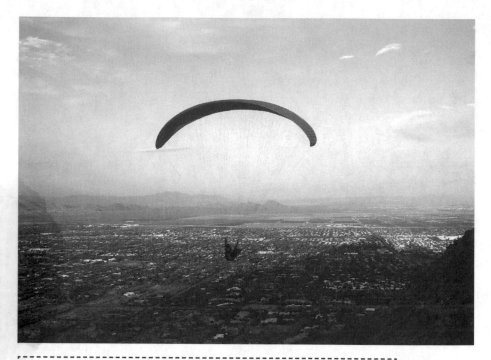

A parachuter takes off on a sunset ride from the Cholla Trail on Camelback Mountain.

and you'll see the McDowell Mountains to the northeast. Straight ahead in the distance, the unmistakable shape of Four Peaks graces the horizon.

At the end of the straightaway, the Cholla Trail ascends via switchbacks. Now skirting the eastern flank of the mountain, work your way up to the ridge along the sleeping camel's spine. The trail becomes a bit more difficult to negotiate as smooth gravel and neat steps give way to rougher terrain. At 0.25 miles and 0.5 miles from the trailhead (0.75 miles and 1 mile from your car), wide overlooks provide open views of the East Valley and the Phoenician Resort.

The trail alternates between climbing switchbacks and gentle straights for a while as you ascend the hill, passing creosote bushes, palo verde trees, various cacti, and ocotillo plants. The trail bends northwest and takes you up along the northern side of the camel's lower hump. At about 0.7 miles from the trailhead, you'll come to a small metal railing along the side of the trail and a sign that reads Area Closed. This is where the original Cholla Trail meets the current one. If you look carefully, you can just see the faint remnants of the old trail snaking downhill toward an empty cul-de-sac, the original parking area for the Cholla Trail.

Continue climbing uphill until you reach a prominent saddle point at 1 mile from the trailhead. Take a breather here and enjoy the views to either side. You need the extra strength because the remainder of the Cholla Trail presents more of a challenge than what you have encountered so far. The trail takes you steeply up the ridge over boulders and slippery gravel-covered slopes. In some spots, such as the small rock face at 1.1 mile from the trailhead, you may have to scramble up using your hands. Rest assured though: this trail is not a technical route. Just be careful. If you become unsure of the trail's direction, look for blue paint dots to guide you.

Continue to climb until you reach the summit ridge where you can clearly see the top. Hike the top of this ridge toward the summit. At about 1.25 miles from the trailhead, you'll climb through a notch in a large boulder. After this point, you'll see the rocky crest of the ridge jutting up directly in front of you like a shark's dorsal fin. You can follow the main trail as it drops down to skirt the ridge to its left, or if you feel a bit adventurous, tackle the ridge straight on. Look for a lone tree directly in front of the rocky ridge crest, and use a conveniently extended branch to hoist yourself up and to the right. This seemingly unlikely turn is actually a split in the trail. If you follow it to the right side of the ridge crest, you'll have 10 feet of exposed traverse to start your adrenaline flowing. The two routes meet up again about 100 feet farther along the trail, and the rest of the climb is obvious.

The 2,704-foot summit of Camelback Mountain is one of my favorite places in Phoenix. From this central vista point, you can see for miles in all directions. As your lungs recover from the climb, take a moment to explore the wide summit. Beautifully landscaped resorts, golf courses, and mansions dot the base of Camelback. A ring of mountains surrounds the sprawling metropolis of the fifth-largest city in the United States. If you are not afraid of heights, go to the northeastern side of the summit and peer over the sheer cliff there. You might find some brave souls rappelling down or parasailing off the cliff. If you are lucky, a beautiful desert sunset will reward your travails, and there's no better place in Phoenix to watch it than from right here.

Return the same way you came for a 3.8-mile round-trip hike. Alternatively, you may choose to shorten your hike by 0.8 miles and descend down the more scenic Summit (Echo Canyon) Trail. This option requires that you have a ride waiting in Echo Canyon Park. Biking or jogging around the mountain are other enjoyable possibilities.

NEARBY ACTIVITIES

Many upscale resorts and spas such as the Phoenician and Camelback Inn surround Camelback Mountain. The Indian Bend Wash Greenbelt (page 85), a system of parks, golf courses, bike paths, and lakes, lies 4 miles to the east along Hayden Road. Piestewa Peak (pages 48 and 52), another popular urban hiking destination, sits 4 miles away to the northwest. The smaller Mummy Mountain is located directly north of Camelback Mountain.

03 CAMELBACK MOUNTAIN: SUMMIT (ECHO CANYON) TRAIL

KEY AT-A-GLANCE INFORMATION

LENGTH: 2.2 miles

ELEVATION GAIN: 1,264 feet

CONFIGURATION: Out-and-back (an optional one-way hike down the Cholla Trail is 1.4 miles plus 0.5 miles to the parking area for the Cholla Trail)

DIFFICULTY: Difficult

SCENERY: Desert, sandstone cliffs, city panorama

EXPOSURE: Partial early-morning and late-afternoon shade, otherwise exposed

TRAFFIC: Heavy

TRAIL SURFACE: Rocky, stair-steps, boulders, handrail-assisted steep sections

HIKING TIME: 1.5 hours

WATER REQUIREMENT: 1–1.5 quarts

SEASON: Year-round; hot in summer

ACCESS: Open sunrise to sunset; free but very limited parking

MAPS: USGS Paradise Valley, trailhead plaque

FACILITIES: Portable toilets and water

DOGS: Yes, leashed at all times

COMMENTS: Parking is extremely limited at Echo Canyon Park. For more information, visit http://phoenix.gov/parks/hikecmlb.html.

GPS Trailhead Coordinates

UTM Zone   12S

Easting   0409661

Northing   3709315

Latitude   N33°31.283'

Longitude   W111°58.410'

IN BRIEF

Perhaps the best in-town hike in Phoenix, Camelback Mountain offers a central location, a rigorous climb of 1,264 feet to its summit, rugged sandstone cliffs, a 360-degree panoramic view from the top, and the chance to see a perfect sunset. Whether you're a resident or visitor, this hike is a must-do.

DESCRIPTION

Named for its double-hump shape, Camelback Mountain resembles a giant sleeping camel in the middle of metropolitan Phoenix. Like an oasis of wilderness in a sea of housing developments and shopping centers, Camelback is a welcome respite from the hustle and bustle of urban life. There are two trails to the summit of Camelback Mountain. The popular Summit Trail, which is more commonly known as Echo Canyon Trail, runs up the western side, and the slightly easier Cholla Trail scales Camelback Mountain's gentler eastern ridge.

The Summit Trail starts at the end of a small parking lot inside Echo Canyon Park. A drinking fountain, shaded benches, and portable toilets give hikers one last chance to prepare for the challenge ahead. The 1,264-foot

Directions

From Loop 202: Exit onto 44th Street and drive north 4.5 miles. Follow 44th Street as it bends eastward into McDonald Drive. As McDonald Drive bends north into Tatum Boulevard, turn east onto McDonald Drive, and then immediately turn south onto Echo Canyon Parkway. Parking is available inside Echo Canyon Park or along Echo Canyon Parkway.

From Loop 101: Exit onto McDonald Drive and drive west 5 miles to Echo Canyon Parkway.

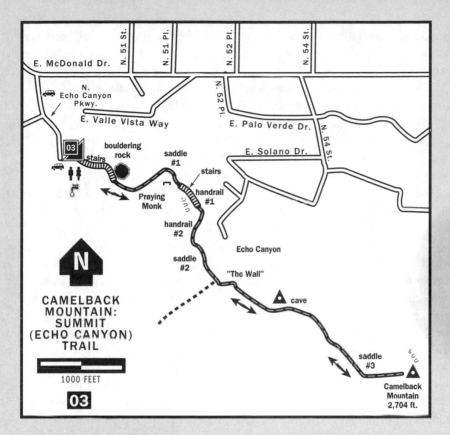

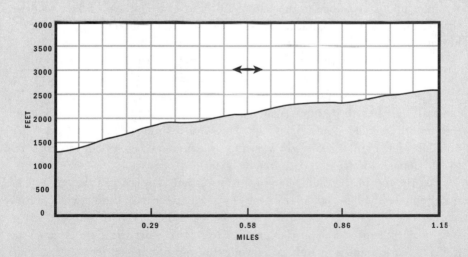

climb to its summit is just over a mile in length but can humble all but the most accomplished athletes, so remember to take the hike at your own pace to avoid exhaustion. During summer, when the temperature soars above 100 degrees, consider splashing water on your clothing before starting the hike to keep cool. You will likely be completely dry again before reaching the summit.

Almost immediately, the trail climbs steeply up Echo Canyon in stadium-like steps. In February and March wildflowers dot the landscape along this section. Purple lupines, yellow brittlebush, and Mexican gold poppies stand in stark contrast against green grasses and red rocks. About 0.1 mile into the hike, the trail wraps around a large rock where many local climbers hone their bouldering skills. As you round this rock, the city fades away and the beauty of Echo Canyon engulfs you. Sheer cliffs and red sandstone formations reminiscent of Sedona frame your field of view. These rocks make up the sleeping camel's head, which is relatively young compared to the metamorphic rock that comprises the rest of Camelback Mountain. At 0.2 miles, you top out on a small saddle where two cement benches greet you. Take a quick breather here to enjoy the view. The town of Paradise Valley lies straight ahead, and you can turn around to see the parking lot, already 250 feet below you. Above and to the right looms a famous rock formation known as the Praying Monk. Though it may not look like it from this vantage point, this formation actually resembles a person kneeling in prayer at the base of Camelback Mountain when seen from the East Valley.

Continue your hike by following the obvious trail to the right, sandwiched between formidable cliffs and a chain-link fence shielding houses below from falling rocks and wandering hikers. After the stairs, approach a handrail-assisted scramble up a steep slope in the shadows of a towering precipice. Don't worry; this part looks scarier than it really is. When eventually descending this section, however, remember that it may be easier to lower yourself down backward while facing uphill. One more handrail-assisted climb up some boulders, and you are done with the camel's head at about 0.5 miles. From here, you are on your own. There are no more steps or rails to guide you. Traverse a small flat stretch in the trail; just before it climbs again the trail forks. The left fork takes you up the smooth rock face some locals call "The Wall," while the right fork runs up a boulder-strewn gully. Bear right here and take the boulders unless you are sure-footed enough to tackle a 45-degree incline.

At the top of the gully, enjoy your first open view toward the south. The trail bends to the left and climbs relatively gently to a small saddle where a rock marker reads "3/4." If you are adventurous, leave the trail here and turn left to visit the best-kept secret on Camelback Mountain. Skirt the right edge of the hill on your left and be careful with your footing. About 100 feet later, a small shallow cave presents itself. From the cave opening, you can rest and enjoy a secluded view of Paradise Valley's many mansions and golf courses. Remember to duck when leaving the cave and returning to the trail.

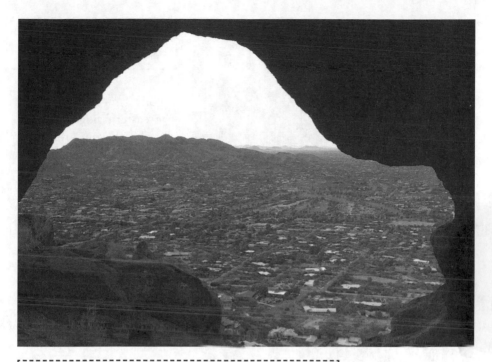

Gazing at Paradise Valley from a hidden cave on the Echo Canyon Trail.

What comes next is a long, steep section of boulder hopping. Just keep your head down and work your way slowly up this beast. If you need to take a break, do so at about 0.9 miles, where you have a view of a castle-like home to your right nestled into the mountainside. Right about here, the trail makes a nearly 90-degree bend to the left. On the way down, however, this little bend is not obvious, so make a mental note of where the trail is. By now your lungs and legs are probably burning, and you might be wondering when you are ever going to reach the top. Be aware that you cannot see the summit from here. The top of this steep section is a false peak, though it isn't far from the true summit. The trail bends one last time to the left and ascends the final 0.1 mile to the 2,704-foot peak of Camelback Mountain.

The wide summit of Camelback can easily accommodate a large crowd and usually has one. Everyone from sweaty trail runners to camera-toting tourists is enjoying the view from the highest point in Phoenix. Who can blame them? From here, you command a sweeping 360-degree panorama of the Phoenix area. Take a well-deserved rest, and see if you can find the following landmarks in a clockwise survey of the landscape: the Phoenician Resort at the base of the mountain to the southeast, South Mountain, Sky Harbor International Airport, downtown Phoenix and Chase Field (formerly Bank One Ballpark), Piestewa Peak, McDowell Mountains, Four Peaks, Superstition Mountains, and the

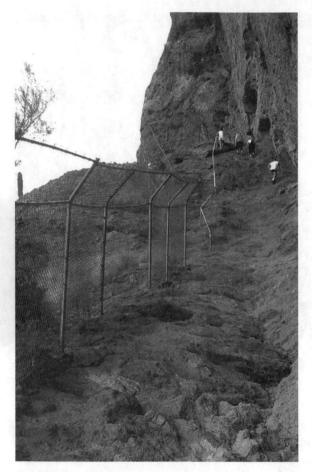

Hikers ascend a handrail-assisted section of Echo Canyon Trail under a sheer cliff.

Cholla Trail running down the eastern ridge of Camelback. If you are lucky enough to hike Camelback at the right time on a partly cloudy day, you might also experience an amazing display of color. Nothing beats the silhouette of a saguaro cactus or an ocotillo plant against a brilliant Arizona sunset. Warning: Avoid dawdling because hiking down in near darkness can be treacherous.

After you have soaked up the scenery, return the way you came. Alternatively, you may descend the 1.4-mile Cholla Trail down the eastern ridge of Camelback Mountain. This option requires a car shuttle to Invergordon Road, the parking area for the Cholla Trail. The truly ambitious day hiker can attempt a "double crossing," descending the Cholla Trail and then coming back up. Insane as it may seem, many locals make this double crossing a daily routine. Cross trainers sometimes jog the additional 3 miles from the Cholla Trailhead back to Echo Canyon Park.

NEARBY ACTIVITIES

Many upscale resorts and spas such as the Phoenician and Camelback Inn surround Camelback Mountain. The Indian Bend Wash Greenbelt (page 85), a system of parks, golf courses, bike paths, and lakes, lies 4 miles to the east along Hayden Road. Piestewa Peak (pages 48 and 52), another popular urban hiking destination, sits 4 miles away to the northwest. The smaller Mummy Mountain is located directly north of Camelback Mountain.

HIDDEN VALLEY TRAIL VIA MORMON TRAIL 04

IN BRIEF

Hidden Valley Trail is the hidden gem of South Mountain that traverses an enclave of wilderness where all signs of the city disappear. Perched atop the Guadalupe Range, this quiet half-mile trail boasts some of the most scenic rock formations in the region, including a natural rock tunnel and Fat Man's Pass.

DESCRIPTION

South Mountain contains over 16,000 acres of desert and mountain preserves, spanning almost the entire southern boundary of Phoenix. It is the largest municipal park in the country. Since 1924, visitors have enjoyed these mountains for their rustic beauty. The Civilian Conservation Corps built numerous trails, roads, picnic facilities, and lookouts in the park. Today, more than 3 million visitors come here annually to enjoy splendid hiking, mountain biking, sightseeing, and various other recreational activities. Though the population of Phoenix and visitor traffic to South Mountain have skyrocketed in recent decades, one part of South Mountain remains relatively untouched by the constant influx of people: Hidden Valley.

The half mile long Hidden Valley Trail takes hikers through this stretch of charming wilderness, which lies atop the Guadalupe Range and holds the most scenic rock formations in the entire park. Two such formations, a

KEY AT-A-GLANCE INFORMATION

LENGTH: 3.9 miles
ELEVATION GAIN: 775 feet
CONFIGURATION: Balloon
DIFFICULTY: Moderate, a little easy scrambling
SCENERY: Desert, city views, Hidden Valley, Fat Man's Pass, unique rock formations
EXPOSURE: Completely open, very little shade
TRAFFIC: Moderate
TRAIL SURFACE: Gravel, crushed rock, packed dirt, smooth bedrock
HIKING TIME: 2 hours
WATER REQUIREMENT: 2 quarts
SEASON: Year-round; hot in summer
ACCESS: Open 5:30 a.m.–7:30 p.m.; free parking
MAPS: USGS Lone Butte, park map posted on plaques at trailheads
FACILITIES: Drinking water and shaded ramada, no toilet
DOGS: Yes, leashed at all times
COMMENTS: This is the shortest route to visit Hidden Valley in South Mountain Park. For more information, visit http://phoenix. gov/parks/hikesoth.html.

Directions

Exit Interstate 10 at Baseline Road and drive west 3.7 miles to 24th Street. Turn south onto 24th Street and follow it until it ends at Valley View Drive. Turn left to find the trailhead parking lot on Valley View Drive.

GPS Trailhead Coordinates

UTM Zone 12S
Easting 0404148
Northing 3692184
Latitude N33°21.983'
Longitude W112°1.862'

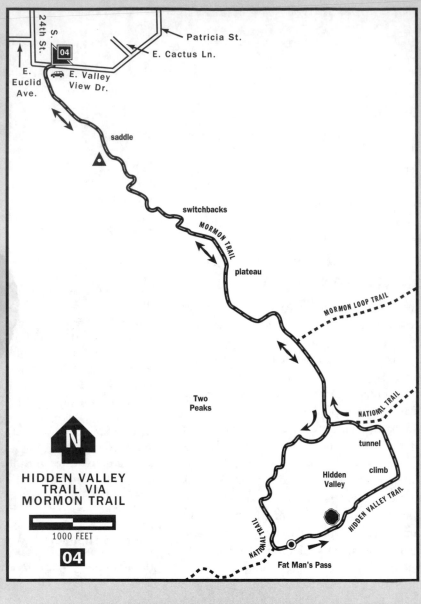

S. 24th St.

04

Patricia St.

E. Cactus Ln.

E. Euclid Ave.

E. Valley View Dr.

saddle

switchbacks

MORMON TRAIL

plateau

MORMON LOOP TRAIL

Two Peaks

NATIONAL TRAIL

tunnel

climb

Hidden Valley

HIDDEN VALLEY TRAIL

NATIONAL TRAIL

Fat Man's Pass

N

HIDDEN VALLEY
TRAIL VIA
MORMON TRAIL

1000 FEET

04

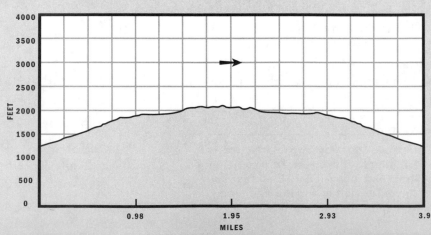

FEET

4000
3500
3000
2500
2000
1500
1000
500
0

0.98   1.95   2.93   3.9

MILES

A hiker prepares to squeeze through Fat Man's Pass, a narrow passage on the Hidden Valley Trail.

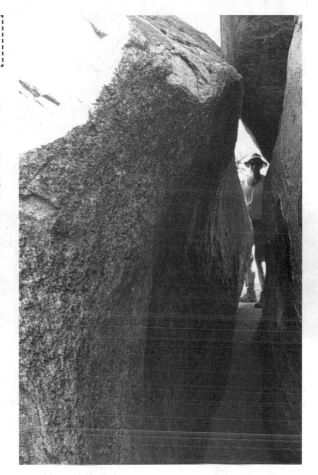

natural rock tunnel and Fat Man's Pass, act as sentinels posted at the ends of the trail to guard the entrances into Hidden Valley. Once you're inside, all signs of the city vanish, along with most of the traffic and noise on the busy National Trail (page 40). The tranquil valley further entices you with sandy wash beds and beautiful granite boulders and rocks unlike those found elsewhere on South Mountain.

The Hidden Valley Trail is really just a detour along the National Trail, forming a small loop beginning at 2.6 miles on National's 15-mile course. The easiest way to reach Hidden Valley is to hike up the Mormon Trail, which intersects this loop on the National Trail side. The resulting Mormon–National–Hidden Valley balloon is one of the most enjoyable short hikes on South Mountain. This circuit presents a desirable alternative to the often overcrowded National–Mormon Loop that is accessible from the eastern end of South Mountain.

Park in a small lot on 24th Street and Valley View Drive. Begin by ascending the hill at the western end of the parking area up to the ridge where a trailhead plaque displays park information and a map. The Mormon Trail heads southeast atop the ridge and begins a moderate climb up South Mountain. Along the trail, you'll find familiar desert plants such as creosote bushes, palo verde trees, and saguaro cacti. At 0.3 miles, top out on a small saddle where you can turn and survey the parking lot below and the housing developments encroaching on the base of the mountain. From here, you can also see downtown Phoenix, Piestewa Peak, Camelback Mountain, McDowell Mountains, and the red sandstone buttes in Papago Park.

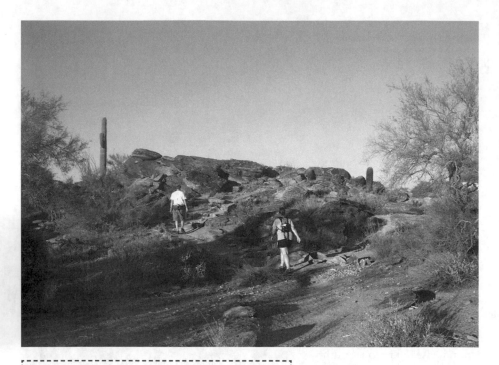

Hikers enjoy the late afternoon sun along the Mormon Trail.

Continue following the Mormon Trail as it snakes uphill. The trail gets progressively more difficult, and at 0.6 miles switchbacks carry you up a fairly steep section. Power through this section because it is the only moderately difficult ascent on this hike. The slope soon gives way to a high flat basin at 0.9 miles and an elevation of 1,900 feet. The Mormon Loop Trail joins in from the left at 1.1 mile. This trail parallels the National Trail and takes you to Pima Canyon Park at the eastern end of South Mountain. Continue straight on the Mormon Trail until it ends and Ts into the National Trail at a signed junction 1.4 miles into the hike.

At this point you can go either way. I prefer to go up first and do the loop in a counterclockwise direction because route finding in Hidden Valley is a bit easier when going from west to east. Turn right onto the National Trail and watch for speedy mountain bikers. National Trail meanders and climbs gently for 0.4 miles until it crests at 2,100 feet before dropping down slightly. At this point, look for trail marker number 13 at the Hidden Valley Trail junction. Turn left and leave the National Trail here. A few feet later, Fat Man's Pass comes into view.

This misnamed wonder is one of the most popular features on South Mountain. A thin crack measuring nearly 25 feet long and only nine inches wide at one point, Fat Man's Pass tempts kids and adults alike. Walls of the crack have been worn smooth by thousands of sweaty torsos squeezing through it over the years. Take off your pack and shuffle through sideways. Don't forget to suck in that gut! If you are claustrophobic or are carrying a few extra holiday pounds, simply go over the boulders instead of through the crack. Kids will also enjoy sliding down a naturally smooth rock just to the right of the entrance to Fat Man's Pass.

On the other side of Fat Man's Pass, walk along a sandy dry wash dotted with riparian brush. At 2 miles from the trailhead, a cluster of large boulders blocks the path. You can either squeeze under or climb over them and then jump down a few feet into a large open bowl. Turn to admire the scenic rocks through which you came before continuing along the sandy wash bottom. At 2.2 miles, a natural granite wall challenges you to climb or jump down five feet or so. Be careful with your footing on the smooth and slippery rock.

The trail turns north soon after the rock wall and arrives at the other striking feature along the Hidden Valley Trail, a natural rock tunnel formed by overlapping boulders. Look through the 30-foot-long tunnel and you can see its worn walls shimmer in the light from the other side. Watch your head as you walk through this wide tunnel. On the other side of the tunnel, look for some petroglyphs etched into the rock by the Hohokams who inhabited this area hundreds of years ago.

Hidden Valley Trail rejoins the National Trail at 2.4 miles from the Mormon Trailhead. Turn left onto National Trail here, and hike 0.2 miles to the Mormon Trail junction. Turn right and descend via the Mormon Trail with the skyline of Phoenix in front of you.

NEARBY ACTIVITIES

South Mountain Park boasts many hiking and biking trails, including Alta (page 16), Desert Classic, National (page 40), Ranger, and Telegraph Pass (page 109). Many other recreational activities such as picnicking and go-cart racing are also available. The Environmental Education Center, located near the Central Avenue entrance, has a superb visitor center, complete with historical exhibits and a three-dimensional model of the entire park. Dobbins Lookout and Buena Vista, both of which are accessible by car, offer superb views of Phoenix by day and the city lights by night.

05   LOOKOUT MOUNTAIN

KEY AT-A-GLANCE INFORMATION

LENGTH: Summit Trail 1.1 mile (optional Circumference Trail, add 2.6 miles)

ELEVATION GAIN: 500 feet

CONFIGURATION: Out-and-back (optional loop)

DIFFICULTY: Summit Trail, moderate; Circumference Trail, easy

SCENERY: Lookout Mountain, city panorama, desert

EXPOSURE: Completely exposed

TRAFFIC: Light to moderate

TRAIL SURFACE: Crushed rock, gravel, scree

HIKING TIME: 1 hour (optional loop, add 1.5 hours)

WATER REQUIREMENT: 1 quart (optional loop, add 1 quart)

SEASON: Year-round; hot in summer

ACCESS: Sunrise to sunset; free parking; alternate trailhead: 5:30 a.m.–10 p.m.

MAPS: USGS Sunnyslope, trailhead plaque

FACILITIES: Water only. Alternate trailhead: restrooms, picnic area, tennis courts, playground

DOGS: Yes, leashed at all times

COMMENTS: For more information, visit http://phoenix.gov/PARKS/hikelook.html, or call (602) 495-5540.

GPS Trailhead Coordinates

UTM Zone   12S

Easting   0402834

Northing   3721100

Latitude   N33°37.623'

Longitude   W112°2.897'

IN BRIEF

Lookout Mountain stands at the northern edge of the Phoenix Mountains Preserve and offers hikers a short but challenging climb to a 360-degree panoramic view from the summit. The longer and easier Circumference Trail winds around Lookout Mountain's base for a more leisurely hike.

DESCRIPTION

At 2,054 feet in elevation, Lookout Mountain's summit ranks among the highest peaks within the Phoenix city limits and provides choice views of the city below and of downtown. Located on Phoenix Mountains Preserve's northern edge, this rocky outpost also eludes the crowds that frequently swarm more popular trails within the preserve, such as Piestewa Peak Summit Trail (page 52). Lookout Mountain Summit Trail 150 measures only 0.6 miles, but it packs a respectable 500-foot elevation gain along a rocky path to the top. The milder and longer Circumference Trail 308 offers more leisurely hikers a chance to enjoy the scenery while minimizing the steep hills. These trails are short enough that you can easily hike both of them within a few hours.

Directions

Main Trailhead: **Take SR 51 to Bell Road. Exit onto Bell Road and drive west 2.6 miles to 16th Street. Turn south onto 16th Street and follow it 0.9 miles to the small parking lot next to the water tank.**

Lookout Mountain Park: **Take SR 51 to Cactus Road. Exit onto Cactus Road and drive west 1.6 miles to Cave Creek Road. Follow Cave Creek Road north 1 mile to Sharon Drive. Turn west onto Sharon Drive and continue 0.5 miles. Then turn north onto 18th Street and proceed 0.5 miles to Lookout Mountain Park.**

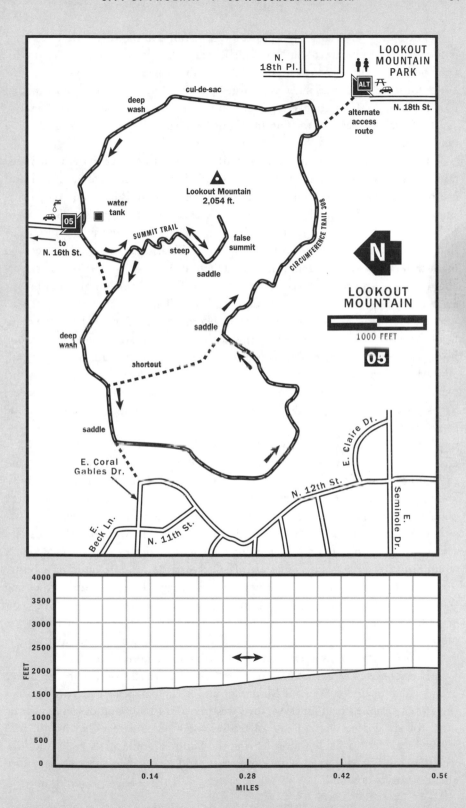

The main trailhead for both the Summit Trail and the Circumference Trail is located on 16th Street south of Bell Road. In addition, Lookout Mountain Park on the southeastern corner of the mountain provides an alternate trailhead and additional amenities such as a larger parking lot, a restroom, and shaded picnic areas. A short connecting trail links the park with the Circumference Trail. However, access to the Summit Trail from the park requires a hike to the main trailhead.

I'll start this hike from the main trailhead next to a large cylindrical water tank. Begin by hiking southwest along an obvious trail covered in gravel and crushed rock. Open desert terrain characterizes the foothills here, and only occasional creosote bushes and palo verde trees break the wide expanses. Cacti seem to be conspicuously absent from the landscape. There are many smaller use trails that branch out from the main trail, making navigation a hassle. However, the main trail is fairly easy to follow if you stay left at the first few forks. Brown rectangular posts also mark the correct route. At 0.1 mile, the Summit Trail breaks away from the Circumference Trail and heads uphill at the end of a wide turn.

Gentle turns give way to switchbacks beginning at 0.2 miles from the trailhead. Loose rocks challenge your footing while steeper slopes demand more effort from your legs. There are some confusing forks along the ascent, but in general, you want to stay with the switchbacks and avoid any spur trails that go straight. Nearly half way up the mountain, the Summit Trail straightens and gets considerably steeper as it heads for the saddle between the main summit and a smaller one to the west. Climb the scree-covered trail to the prominent saddle point at 0.4 miles from the trailhead. The saddle has an elevation of 1,875 feet and already commands a fine view. From there, finish your climb by turning left uphill around the southern side of Lookout Mountain. There are some loose and rocky steps here, and you might have to duck under a palo verde tree. Once on the summit ridge, the going gets considerably easier, and you can make a beeline for the peak.

Lookout Mountain's flat summit is aptly named. It overlooks the vast city surrounding the mountain preserve. To the south, major peaks within Phoenix Mountains Preserve, such as Piestewa Peak, North Mountain, and Shaw Butte, form a wall framing the distant downtown buildings. Behind them lie the long flat ridges of South Mountain and the jagged Sierra Estrella peaks. The panoramic view encompasses nearly all major mountain ranges that surround the metropolitan Phoenix area, so take your time to soak it all in. Return via the same route to the Summit Trail and Circumference Trail junction.

If you have some extra time, consider tacking on the 2.6-mile Circumference Trail, which encircles Lookout Mountain and a smaller peak to its west. From the aforementioned trail junction, turn west onto Trail 308 and descend a gentle slope toward a deep wash. The trail crosses the wash and veers left uphill. At a marked trail fork 0.3 miles after leaving the Summit Trail, break right and hike west toward a saddle point. Cross over this saddle and then turn left at a fork about 30 yards downhill.

The Lookout Mountain Circumference Trail winds around desert foothills below the summit.

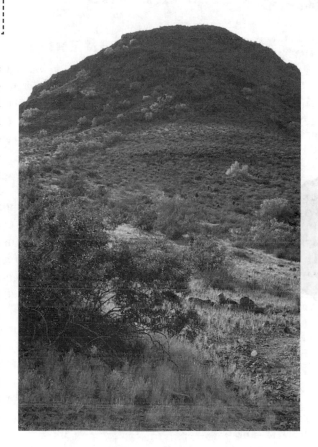

The trail parallels the preserve's western boundary and skirts the backyard fences of some homes in the area. Near the mountain's southwestern corner, embark on a moderate climb toward the east on loose rock. Roughly 1.4 miles after leaving the Summit Trail, reach a boulder-ridden saddle point between Lookout Mountain and its western sibling at 1,670 feet in elevation. Then, turn southeast and skirt the southern side of Lookout Mountain. There are many use trails that crisscross this area, so look for the brown posts to stay on the Circumference Trail.

At 1.9 miles after leaving the Summit Trail, look for a wide path that leads toward Lookout Mountain Park and the alternate trailhead. Follow the wide path southeast toward Lookout Mountain Park, but then leave the access trail by turning east. Another left turn takes you quite close to some backyards. Now sandwiched between Lookout Mountain and backyard fences, continue hiking north along Trail 308. The trail eventually curves around the eastern flank of Lookout Mountain and takes you back to the water tank and the main trailhead in 2.6 miles.

NEARBY ACTIVITIES

Phoenix Mountains Preserve contains many popular trails including Piestewa Peak (pages 48 and 52), Shaw Butte (page 62), and North Mountain (page 40). Shadow Mountain, located on the eastern side of Cave Creek Road and Sharon Drive, has no official trails. However, many use trails allow you to explore the mountain. On Central Avenue and the Arizona Canal, the Murphy Bridle Path offers a pleasantly shaded urban walk.

06 NORTH MOUNTAIN NATIONAL TRAIL

KEY AT-A-GLANCE INFORMATION

LENGTH: 1.6 miles

ELEVATION GAIN: 650 feet

CONFIGURATION: Out-and-back or loop (same distance)

DIFFICULTY: Moderate

SCENERY: City views, Phoenix Mountains Preserve, desert

EXPOSURE: Partial shade in mornings and late afternoons

TRAFFIC: Heavy

TRAIL SURFACE: Rock, gravel, pavement

HIKING TIME: 1 hour

WATER REQUIREMENT: 1 quart

SEASON: Year-round; hot in summer

ACCESS: Open 5 a.m.–11 p.m.; free parking

MAPS: USGS Sunnyslope

FACILITIES: Restroom, water, picnic areas, playground, ranger station

DOGS: Yes, leashed at all times

COMMENTS: Short but steep workout with panoramic views of the Phoenix Mountains Preserve. For more information, visit http://phoenix.gov/parks/hikenort.html, or call (602) 495-5540.

GPS Trailhead Coordinates

UTM Zone 12S

Easting 0401124

Northing 3716526

Latitude N33°35.139'

Longitude W112°3.973'

IN BRIEF

Centrally located, North Mountain provides Phoenix residents with an excellent hike for daily exercise. The North Mountain National Trail is short, steep, paved, and accessible nearly around the clock.

DESCRIPTION

North-central Phoenix residents are really fortunate to have the likes of North Mountain in their backyards. North Mountain National Trail 44 measures only 1.6 miles round-trip, and most of it is paved. A decent elevation gain of 650 feet induces a cardio workout, and the panoramic scenery from North Mountain's 2,104-foot summit indulges the senses. It's an ideal place for a quick workout anytime of the day and well into the night. Imagine how much money you can save on gym memberships by incorporating this trail into your daily routine!

Unlike other popular hikes such as Camelback Mountain (pages 21 and 26), Piestewa Peak (pages 48 and 52), and Shaw Butte (page

Directions

Exit SR 51 onto Northern Avenue and drive west 1.8 miles to Seventh Street. Turn north on Seventh Street and continue 2 miles to Peoria Avenue. Turn west at Peoria Avenue to enter North Mountain Park and then follow the one-way drive to the Maricopa picnic area at the northern end of the park. If the parking lot at Maricopa is full, use any of the other parking areas in the park.

A small alternate parking area is located outside North Mountain Park on Seventh Street, 0.5 miles north of Peoria. However, this parking lot is accessible only from the southbound lanes of Seventh Street.

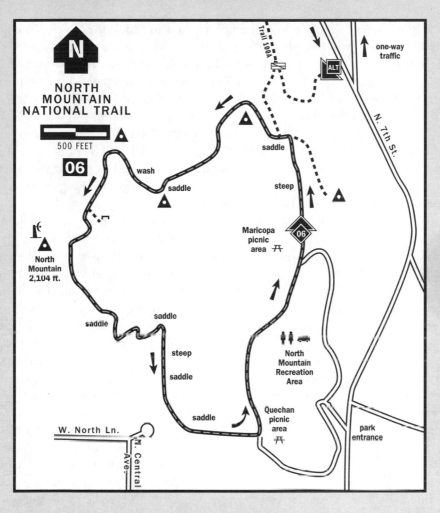

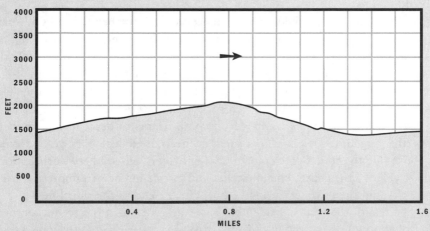

62), North Mountain seems to have ample parking to handle the crowds. Though the Maricopa picnic area where the trail begins has only a few spaces, there is a large parking lot in the center of North Mountain Park and other parking areas are sprinkled around the loop drive. There's even an alternate access point on Seventh Street outside the park. The recently constructed North Mountain Visitor Center just north of the park provides yet another option.

Most people hike to the summit and return along the paved service road, which is a fine route. However, North Mountain National Trail is actually a loop. The unpaved southern half of the trail sees much less traffic and offers open views toward the south. Those who prefer a rugged hiking experience appreciate the unpaved and steeper southern route.

Begin from the Maricopa picnic area at the park's northern end. The trail ascends a steep and rocky slope to a saddle at 0.15 miles where a spur trail takes off to the right toward some vista points. Turn left up a flight of stairs and then meet the paved service road, which allows service vehicles to reach the mountaintop antennas. You can see the alternate parking area at the base of the service road on Seventh Street. Looking down the service road, you can also see a gate. Trail 100A lies just beyond the gate and links North Mountain with trails near Shaw Butte and the new North Mountain Visitor Center.

Follow the steep service road uphill toward the summit. Along every bend in this road is an excellent view. The north-facing turns overlook the open basin below and Shaw Butte to the northwest. A saddle at 0.4 miles watches over North Mountain Park and the city to the south. Just below the antenna-studded summit, turn left into a vista point where a memorial bench beckons you to sit and take a break. From here, you actually look down upon the Pointe Tapatio Cliffs Resort and the Different Pointe of View Restaurant poised atop a hill across Seventh Street. Piestewa Peak, Four Peaks, and South Mountain are all within view. On a clear day you can even see Weaver's Needle in the Superstition Mountains.

North Mountain's true summit is fenced off, so the bench is a good turn-around point if you wish to stick to the pavement. However, consider taking the less-traveled southern route back down to North Mountain Park. Just below the summit, look for a brown post marking the spot where the trail leaves the road. Hike a short distance up to the ridgeline south of the summit. Walk the ridge toward the south on a trail of crushed rock with open views to both sides.

At 0.9 miles from the trailhead, the path begins to descend the southern tip of the ridgeline. Desert plants such as the triangle-leaf bursage and creosote bush line the trail. Some colorful flowers you might see here during spring include yellow brittlebush, blue phacelia, and purple lupine. An impressive view of the city and the downtown skyline opens at the end of the ridgeline.

The rest of the trail is a steep but short descent down the scenic southern slope of the mountain. Along the way, pass several saddles with good views, and a few sets of switchbacks. Turns are obvious and well marked. The trail

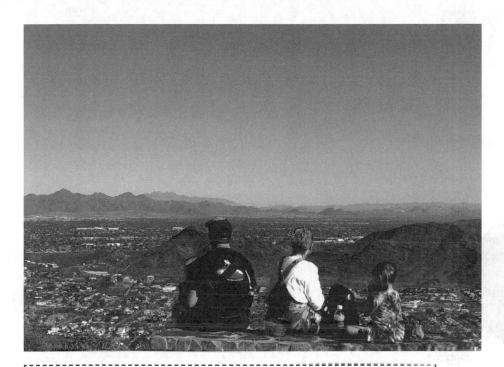

View studded and family-friendly, North Mountain National Trail draws hundreds of visitors to its scenic summit.

eventually emerges at the Quechan picnic area inside North Mountain Park. Complete the 1.6-mile loop by hiking north along the one-way road to return to the Maricopa picnic area. Hikers who crave thigh-pumping steep climbs may choose to do this loop in the opposite direction because the southern trailhead is lower and the trail itself is considerably steeper than the paved service road.

NEARBY ACTIVITIES

The Phoenix Mountains Preserve encompasses many popular hiking trails, including Piestewa Peak (pages 48 and 52), Shaw Butte (page 62), Lookout Mountain (page 36), and Perl Charles. Camelback Mountain (pages 21 and 26), another valley favorite, is southeast of the Phoenix Mountains Perserve.

The newly constructed North Mountain Visitor Center on Seventh Street offers educational classes and interpretive displays explaining the richness of Sonoran Desert landscape.

07 PAPAGO PARK

KEY AT-A-GLANCE INFORMATION

LENGTH: 2.2 miles

ELEVATION GAIN: 140 feet

CONFIGURATION: Loop

DIFFICULTY: Easy

SCENERY: Papago Buttes, unique rock formations, desert, city panoramas

EXPOSURE: Completely exposed

TRAFFIC: Moderate

TRAIL SURFACE: Gravel

HIKING TIME: 1 hour

WATER REQUIREMENT: 1 quart

SEASON: Year-round; hot in summer

ACCESS: 5 a.m. to 11 p.m.; free parking

MAPS: USGS Tempe, trailhead plaque

FACILITIES: Water, ramada, picnic areas

DOGS: Leashed at all times

COMMENTS: This route follows part of the West Park Loop Trail. For more information, visit http://phoenix.gov/parks/hikepapa.html.

GPS Trailhead Coordinates

UTM Zone   12S

Easting   0411380

Northing   3701969

Latitude   N33°27.316'

Longitude W111°57.256'

IN BRIEF

A large oasis amid the sprawling city, Papago Park is to Phoenix what Central Park is to New York. Its distinctive red sandstone buttes and reflective lakes around the zoo are all trademark features of Papago Park. This scenic backdrop provides the setting for a relaxing and view-studded hike.

DESCRIPTION

Few parks in Phoenix offer as many activities as Papago Park. Home of the Phoenix Zoo and Desert Botanical Garden, a golf course, a fire museum, and a sports complex, and studded with many biking, walking, and hiking paths, Papago Park literally has something for everyone.

Papago Park's colorful history dates back to 1879 when it became a reservation for Pima and Maricopa Indians. The park's name was taken from the Papago, a Native American people who inhabited southern Arizona. In the early 1900s the park was designated Papago Saguaro National Monument under Woodrow Wilson's administration, but Congress later rescinded that designation. During World War II a prisoner-of-war camp erected at the base of Papago Buttes housed more than 400 German prisoners. Today, the Army Reserve Motor Park still occupies the area. The City of Phoenix purchased the park in 1959 and has been operating it ever since.

Directions ———————→

From Loop 202, exit onto Priest Drive. Drive north 1.25 miles on Priest Drive, which becomes Galvin Parkway. At the traffic signal for the Phoenix Zoo, turn left into the trailhead parking lot.

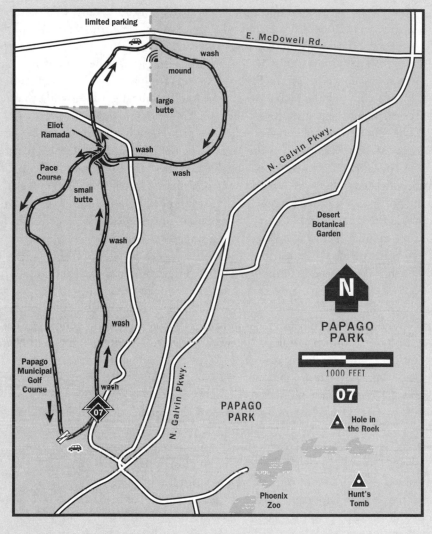

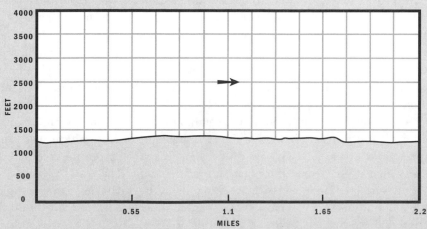

Oddly eroded by wind and rain, several red sandstone buttes lie scattered throughout the 1,200-acre park, providing a scenic backdrop for many of the park's features. These distinctive holey rocks can be seen from nearly anywhere in Phoenix. The largest buttes lie in the northern part of the park, straddling McDowell Road, while Galvin Parkway bisects the park lengthwise. The busy eastern half contains the much-visited zoo and botanical garden, while the quieter western half appeals more to hikers and mountain bikers.

The route suggested here encircles two prominent buttes in the park's western half and comprises part of the West Park Loop Trail. Start from a parking lot west of Galvin Parkway, opposite the main entrance of Phoenix Zoo. The trailhead is located next to a ramada where drinking water is available. Begin by hiking north on a gravel path toward the largest butte. Many confusing use trails crisscross the landscape, but don't worry about getting lost. Just aim straight for the large mound of rock and the elevated ramada at its base.

Approximately 0.6 miles from the trailhead, arrive at Eliot Ramada, where the Phoenix skyline comes into view on the western horizon. Continue across the paved road and pick up a trail that skirts the left side of the butte. Hike toward busy McDowell Road and notice the typical desert flora. Triangle-leaf bursage, brittlebushes, creosotes, palo verdes, and even some fragrant desert lavender line the trail. North of the butte and adjacent to McDowell Road, an old amphitheater lies unused, undoubtedly because of the incessant road noise.

Continue past the amphitheater to a small mound with an excellent northeastern view. All major mountains on the periphery of the East Valley can be seen here. Camelback Mountain dominates the north, while McDowell Mountains, Four Peaks, Red Mountain, and the Superstitions frame the eastern skyline. On a clear day, even needle-like Pinnacle Peak becomes visible. Complete your loop around the largest butte, staying close to the red rock at all forks. As you round the hill's eastern flank, catch a glimpse of the Desert Botanical Garden across Galvin Parkway, Hayden Butte, and Hole-in-the-Rock, an eroded red sandstone butte next to the Phoenix Zoo.

Approximately 1.3 miles from the trailhead, break away from the circumference of the large butte and head downhill toward Eliot Ramada again. From there, aim for the right side of a smaller butte where many wooden signs mark the start of an orienteering course and a pace course. As the trail skirts the small butte, enjoy an open view toward the southwest. Papago Golf Course lies below the trail, while South Mountain, Sierra Estrella, and the White Tank Mountains complete a sweep of the western horizon.

At the southwestern corner of the small butte, head south downhill parallel to the golf course fence. Marvel at the striking contrast between the arid landscape and the greens and fairways inside the golf course, proof positive that the grass is indeed greener on the other side of the fence. The trail passes several junctions and eventually meets the parking lot from which you began, completing a 2.2-mile hike. If you have extra time, consider following the trail all the way around the golf course for an additional 2 miles.

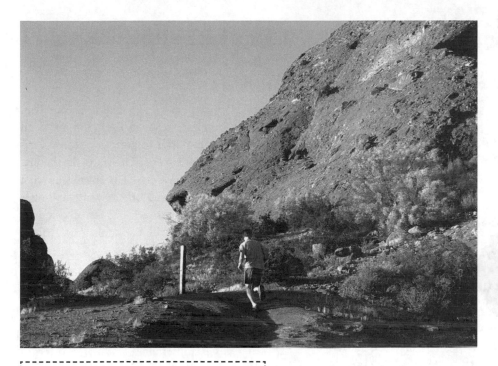

A hiker speeds past sandstone buttes in Papago Park.

Before leaving Papago Park, be sure to visit Hole-in-the-Rock and Hunt's Tomb, two of the park's most popular features. Both of them are located in the eastern half of the park, so you'll need to drive across Galvin Parkway. Make a left after the park gate and follow the signs to Ramada 8. A short but steep trail climbs up to a natural rock window for a splendid sunset vista overlooking the city and the lakes near the zoo. The ancient Hohokam people used the projection of sunlight through Hole-in-the-Rock as a natural sundial.

Farther south in the park and beyond Ramada 16, a white pyramid entombs Arizona's first governor, George W. P. Hunt, and his family. Though the pyramid itself is worth a visit, the view from its western platform is one of the finest in the park. A bench provides the perfect setting for admiring a part of the Phoenix Zoo as well as the desert sky reflected in several lakes around the zoo. With so many attractions, Papago Park is a must-see.

NEARBY ACTIVITIES

The Phoenix Zoo and Desert Botanical Garden are both located within the confines of Papago Park. The park also provides a golf course, a sports complex, picnic areas, and even a fish hatchery. Camelback Mountain (pages 21 and 26), Hayden Butte (page 80), and the Indian Bend Wash Greenbelt (page 85) are all within a short distance of Papago Park.

08 PIESTEWA PEAK: FREEDOM TRAIL

KEY AT-A-GLANCE INFORMATION

LENGTH: 3.8 miles

ELEVATION GAIN: 620 feet

CONFIGURATION: Loop

DIFFICULTY: Moderate

SCENERY: Desert, Piestewa Peak, Phoenix Mountains Preserve

EXPOSURE: Completely exposed, very little shade

TRAFFIC: Moderate

TRAIL SURFACE: Gravel, crushed rock, stone stairs, sharp and uneven rock

HIKING TIME: 2 hours

WATER REQUIREMENT: 2 quarts

SEASON: Year-round; hot in summer

ACCESS: Open 5 a.m.–11 p.m.; free parking

MAPS: USGS Sunnyslope, trailhead plaque

FACILITIES: Water, toilets, ranger station in Phoenix Mountains Park

DOGS: Yes, except on the section shared with Summit Trail 300

COMMENTS: On February 26, 2004, the Phoenix Parks and Recreation department changed the name of this trail to the Freedom Trail. For more information, visit http://phoenix.gov/parks/hikephx.html.

IN BRIEF

There are many reasons to take Freedom Trail over the popular Piestewa Peak Summit Trail (page 52). Some do it to get more scenic variety. Others prefer to get closer to the desert. Some hike it because it is less strenuous than the Summit Trail, and others want a longer hike. Whatever your reason for hiking the Freedom Trail, you will enjoy this loop around Piestewa Peak.

DESCRIPTION

Coiled around the base of Piestewa Peak in the Phoenix Mountains Preserve, Freedom Trail (formerly Circumference Trail) 302 offers a moderate hike and a scenic route through the splendors of Phoenix Mountains Park. In lieu of the towering views from the summit, this trail showcases the best desert flora and fauna in the park and takes you on a wide loop around Piestewa Peak. The Freedom Trail is the second-most popular hike in the Phoenix Mountains Park. Though it shares 0.5 miles with the busy Summit Trail 300, most of the Freedom Trail is relatively devoid of crowds.

The elevation at the trailhead is 1,520 feet. Begin your hike at a well-signed egress from the parking lot located at the northern end of Phoenix Mountains Park. You immediately descend to cross a dry creek and climb

GPS Trailhead Coordinates

UTM Zone   12S

Easting   0405785

Northing   3711738

Latitude   N33°32.574'

Longitude   W112°0.929'

Directions

Exit SR 51 at Lincoln Drive, and drive east 0.5 miles. Turn left onto Squaw Peak Drive, and continue 0.5 miles to the gated entrance to Phoenix Mountains Park (formerly Squaw Peak Park). Go through the gate and follow the road 0.5 miles until it dead-ends at the Apache picnic area.

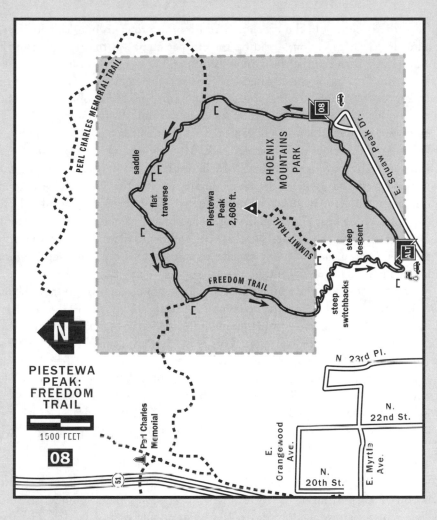

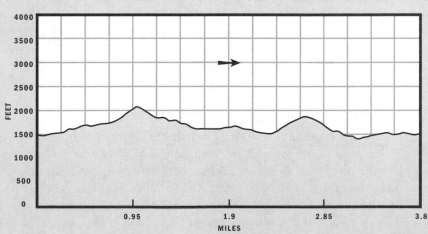

up the other side to join the Freedom Trail loop. I prefer to hike this loop in a counterclockwise direction, avoiding the steeper climb on the first part of the Summit Trail. Turn right at the T intersection and head north along the obvious trail. As you walk along the crushed-rock surface up a gentle incline, admire the abundant desert plants around you. Tall saguaros, prickly cholla, hardy creosotes, and nearly leafless palo verde trees line the trail. In the spring, Mexican poppies and brittlebush blossoms paint the mountainsides gold. This part of the Freedom Trail coincides with Nature Trail 304, complete with many educational plaques detailing various plants and their desert habitat. The basin in which you are hiking hosts the richest variety of desert flora in the Phoenix Mountains Preserve. Try to identify all of the following species of cacti as you hike: buckhorn cholla, teddy bear cholla, giant saguaro, strawberry hedgehog, pincushion, prickly pear, and fishhook barrel cactus. Depending on the time of day and time of year, you can also spot many species of birds here. Look for cactus wrens, mockingbirds, quails, owls, and hawks.

At 0.5 miles from the trailhead, an obvious sign directs you to take the left fork at a trail junction. Stay on the combined Trail 302 and Trail 304. Another tenth of a mile farther, pass a plaque detailing the giant saguaro cactus and a memorial bench dedicated to Janet. This is where Perl Charles Memorial Trail 1A merges into the Freedom Trail. You've already climbed 200 feet from the trailhead, but a steeper climb awaits. Look up to see the peaks and saddles directly in front of you. Keep left and follow the trail as it climbs up steep switchbacks toward the saddle on the right. At 0.75 miles and an elevation of 1,830 feet, follow the combined Trail 302 and Trail 1A to the left at a well-signed junction.

One mile into the hike, top out on a prominent saddle point at an elevation of 2,090 feet, the highest on the Freedom Trail. Two memorial benches provide convenient resting places to reward your efforts. Take a moment to enjoy the view here before heading down the western side of the saddle. The trail descends steeply via a series of tight switchbacks. As you descend, you can see a trail in the basin below heading for a saddle to the northwest. Resist the temptation to take this unmarked trail, which meets the Freedom Trail at 1.15 miles at an elevation of 1,890 feet. Instead, follow the main trail south along a fairly flat and long traverse on Piestewa Peak's northwestern slope. Soon you should see a white triangular sign confirming that you are still traveling on Trail 1A, which coincides with the Freedom Trail here.

Hike along the gentle traverse to a bench dedicated to Mark Hoff at 1.5 miles. A ring of peaks surrounds you, with only a small window of city views opening to the southwest. Continue hiking gently downhill along the trail as it rounds the western side of Piestewa Peak. At 1.75 miles, reach the halfway point on the Freedom Trail and a bench dedicated to Richard Daleiden, where you can rest and catch a view of downtown Phoenix. This spot is also where Trail 1A leaves the Freedom Trail and heads downhill toward the west. In the shadow of

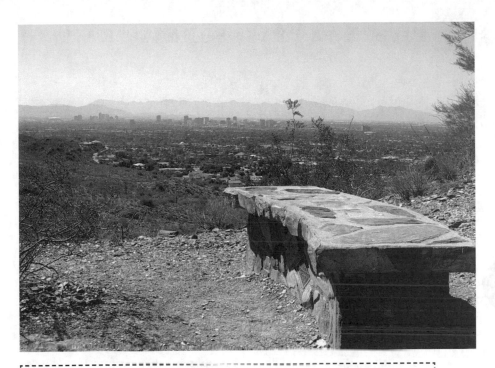

The Richard Daleiden memorial bench along the Freedom Trail overlooks the Phoenix skyline.

towering Piestewa Peak, continue traversing the hill southward until you reach a trail junction at 2.25 miles. From here, take the left fork and follow the Freedom Trail steeply uphill along tight switchbacks.

Half a mile of hard work later, come to a saddle at an elevation of 1,900 feet where the Freedom Trail meets Piestewa Peak Summit Trail 300. A reminder to those who enjoy hiking with four-legged friends: dogs are not allowed on the Summit Trail. If you intend to complete the Freedom Trail loop, remember to leave your pets at home. Descend along the Summit Trail 0.5 miles until just before reaching the parking lot at the base of the mountain. The Freedom Trail breaks away from the Summit Trail and turns north, paralleling the paved road inside Phoenix Mountains Park. Hike another 0.6 miles of mild inclines to complete the 3.8-mile loop and return to the trailhead at the Apache picnic area.

NEARBY ACTIVITIES

The Phoenix Mountains Preserve offers many other trails, including Perl Charles Memorial Trail 1A, Piestewa Peak Summit Trail 300 (page 52), Shaw Butte Trail 306 (page 62), and North Mountain National Trail 44 (page 40). Some trails are accessible to mountain bikes. Historic Murphy Bridle Path lies along Central Avenue, 2 miles to the west. Camelback Mountain, another valley favorite, is only 4 miles to the southeast.

09 PIESTEWA PEAK: SUMMIT TRAIL

KEY AT-A-GLANCE INFORMATION

LENGTH: 2.4 miles

ELEVATION GAIN: 1,190 feet

CONFIGURATION: Out-and-back

DIFFICULTY: Moderate to difficult

SCENERY: City panorama, desert, Phoenix Mountains Preserve

EXPOSURE: Completely exposed, very little shade

TRAFFIC: Very heavy

TRAIL SURFACE: Stone stairs, gravel, sharp and uneven rock

HIKING TIME: 1.5 hours

WATER REQUIREMENT: 1–1.5 quarts

SEASON: Year-round; hot in summer

ACCESS: Open 5 a.m.–11 p.m.; free parking

MAPS: USGS Sunnyslope, trailhead plaque

FACILITIES: Water, toilets, ranger station in Phoenix Mountains Park

DOGS: No

COMMENTS: This is the most popular hiking trail in Phoenix. Formerly known as Squaw Peak, this mountain was recently renamed Piestewa Peak in honor of Lori Piestewa, a Tuba City soldier who lost her life in Operation Iraqi Freedom. For more information, visit http://phoenix.gov/parks/hikephx.html.

GPS Trailhead Coordinates

UTM Zone   12S

Easting   0405067

Northing   3711381

Latitude   N33°32.376'

Longitude   W112°1.391'

IN BRIEF

For decades, Piestewa Peak (formerly Squaw Peak) Summit Trail 300 has carried the title of Phoenix's most popular hiking trail. More people trample this well-trodden path up magnificent Piestewa Peak than any other trail in the Phoenix metropolitan area. This hike has become an institution in Phoenix culture and requires enough oomph to challenge even the fittest athletes. The summit offers a gorgeous panoramic view that justifies its huge popularity.

DESCRIPTION

The 2,608-foot Piestewa Peak towers over the Phoenix Mountains Preserve. Its pointy arête is one of the most prominent features on the Phoenix skyline. During mild weather, literally thousands of people hike Summit Trail 300 every day, making it the second-most popular trail in Arizona. Only the Bright Angel Trail in Grand Canyon National Park attracts more visitors. Piestewa Peak's convenient location makes it a local favorite for aerobic exercise, and the panoramic view from its summit also places this mountain high on the to-do list for Phoenix visitors.

From the moment the sky brightens in the morning until well after nightfall, a seemingly endless line of people dot the Summit

Directions

Exit SR 51 at Lincoln Drive, and drive east 0.5 miles. Turn left onto Squaw Peak Drive and continue 0.5 miles to the gated entrance to Phoenix Mountains Park (formerly Squaw Peak Park). Take the first left inside the gate to reach the Summit Trailhead. If the small parking lot at the trailhead is full, try a picnic area inside the park.

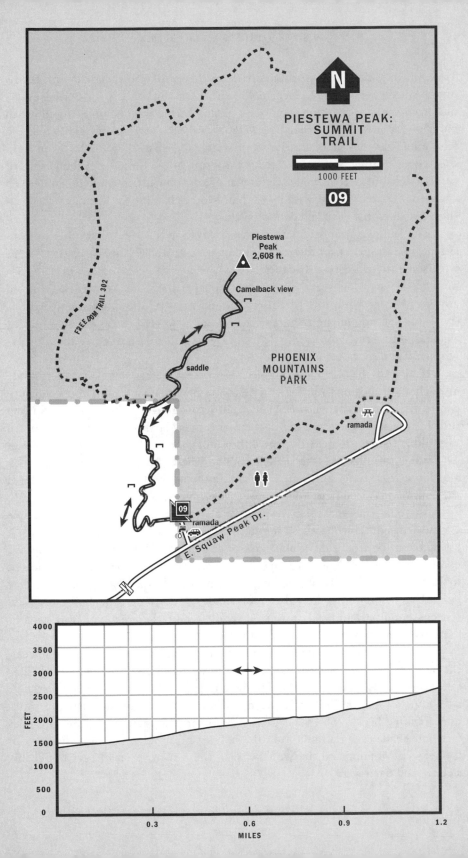

N

PIESTEWA PEAK:
SUMMIT
TRAIL

1000 FEET

09

Piestewa
Peak
2,608 ft.

Camelback view

saddle

PHOENIX
MOUNTAINS
PARK

FREEDOM TRAIL 302

ramada

09

ramada

E. Squaw Peak Dr.

FEET

4000
3500
3000
2500
2000
1500
1000
500
0

0.3   0.6   0.9   1.2
MILES

Trail, making it a people-watching hotspot. If you like to socialize with fellow hikers, there is no better place in Phoenix. On this trail, I have seen everyone from cane-assisted nonagenarians to slumbering infants bouncing along in mom's backpack. You'll meet overweight weekend warriors trying to shave a few pounds as they labor up the steep stairs, and glistening goddesses in tight sportswear jogging past you on their daily run. You'll hear the exclamations of camera-wielding tourists and the chitchat of gossiping office workers. Some even come for a chance to flirt with more than Mother Nature. I'd bet many relationships began with a chance meeting on this trail.

The Summit Trail originated as a pack trail in the 1930s but has seen consistent improvement over the years. Today, it's a veritable staircase of stony steps with some sharp exposed bedrock thrown in to twist your ankles in case of a misstep. Though landscape along the trail appears barren and rocky, rugged Sonoran Desert flora dots the hills around you. Creosote bushes and various species of cacti dominate the area. Occasional palo verde trees provide limited shade. In the spring, golden brittlebush flowers add a dash of color to an otherwise gray and rocky terrain.

Hiking up the 1,190 vertical feet to Piestewa Peak is no small undertaking. Your challenge begins with the search for an open parking spot, if you happen to come on a particularly nice day. The small parking area at the trailhead is often full. Instead, try parking at any of the picnic areas farther up the road. You can hike along the Freedom Trail (page 48) or along the road to get to the trailhead. The Summit Trail starts at a shaded ramada where you can slather on sunblock and fill up your water bottle from a drinking fountain. Once you start climbing, the consistently steep steps pump up your heart rate and adrenaline in a hurry.

As you climb the steep trail, several memorial benches provide ample excuses and convenient places for you to rest and catch your breath. As an interesting diversion from the arduous task of climbing the hill, try to see if you can count the number of benches along the Summit Trail. One such bench dedicated to Robert D. Hill at 0.4 miles from the trailhead has a small palo verde tree behind it, yielding some late-afternoon shade. At 0.5 miles, the trail mercifully flattens out a bit and heads toward a saddle where the Freedom Trail joins it. Stay to the right to continue toward the summit.

At two-thirds of a mile from the trailhead and an elevation of 2,030 feet, the Summit Trail jumps over a saddle to the western side of the mountain. This saddle overlooks an interior basin below and the SR 51 freeway in the distance. At about 0.9 miles, climb up a steep hill and head straight toward the trail's most inviting bench, which has a large palo verde draped over it and provides welcome shade even on the hottest days. Take a rest here and enjoy the view of Camelback Mountain to the west because the rest of the trail gets noticeably steeper and narrower.

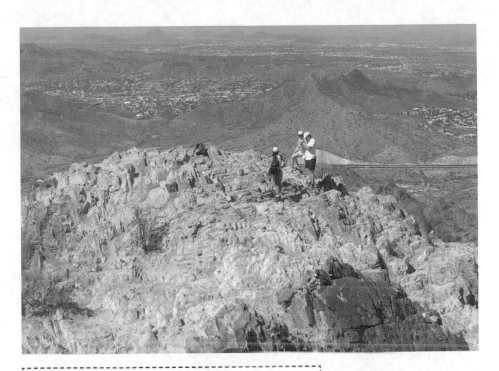

Hikers rejoice upon reaching the rocky summit of Piestewa Peak.

While grinding out the last 0.3 miles, you pass by several old metal hitching posts. While the days of using pack animals on this trail are long gone, these posts are painful reminders that a horse or mule would come in handy right about now. The last few feet of trail near the summit requires a little careful stepping and clambering, especially if you try to get to the absolute tallest point on the mountain where the USGS survey disk lies cemented into the ancient Precambrian granite. Most people settle for a rock outcropping a few feet lower than and just to the west of the true summit. From the 2,608-foot Piestewa Peak, enjoy the sweeping vistas in all directions. Unlike the wide summit of Camelback Mountain, chiseled Piestewa Peak gives you even better open views. You can see the antenna-covered North Mountain and Shaw Butte to the northwest, downtown Phoenix and Chase Field (formerly Bank One Ballpark) to the south, Camelback Mountain to the southeast, and the McDowell Mountains to the northeast. The top of Piestewa Peak is also a great place to catch a beautiful Arizona sunset if you happen to be up here at dusk.

Descend the same route back to the parking lot. For a little variety, and especially during hot summer months, try hiking the Piestewa Peak Summit Trail at night. A line of flashlights can often be seen dancing up the mountain on a clear night. Under a bright full moon or when low clouds reflect the bright

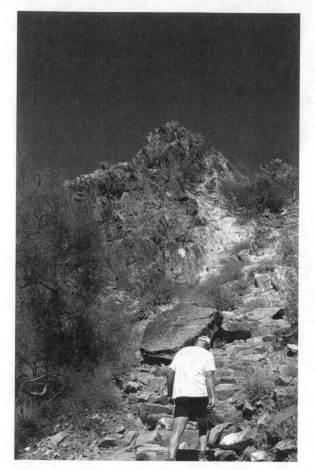

A hiker tackles the final steps just below Piestewa Peak.

city lights, you hardly need artificial lighting at all. Watching the city lights from the top of Piestewa Peak is also a wonderfully romantic way to spend an evening.

NEARBY ACTIVITIES

The Phoenix Mountains Preserve offers many other trails, including Perl Charles Memorial Trail 1A, Freedom Trail 302 (page 48), Shaw Butte Trail 306 (page 62), and North Mountain National Trail 44 (page 40). Some trails are accessible to mountain bikes. Historic Murphy Bridle Path lies along Central Avenue, 2.5 miles to the west. Camelback Mountain, another valley favorite, is only 2 miles to the southeast.

QUARTZ RIDGE TRAIL 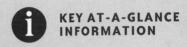 10

IN BRIEF

Dotted with breathtaking views of Piestewa Peak and Camelback Mountain, Quartz Ridge Trail offers yet another scenic jaunt through the Phoenix Mountains Preserve. Though it sits in the middle of the city, this trail traverses many secluded desert basins where you get a real sense of wilderness.

DESCRIPTION

Quartz Ridge Trail 8, along with alternates 8A and 8B, lies in the easternmost part of the Phoenix Mountains Preserve and spans its entire length. Parts of these three trails as well as a small section of Nature Trail 304 form an enjoyable loop. Three trailheads serve this network, offering ample opportunities to pick a balloon, loop, or out-and-back route to suit your hiking tastes. Add a shuttle vehicle, and you have even more options for several one-way hikes.

Directions ————————➤

40th Street Trailhead: Exit SR 51 onto Shea Boulevard and drive east 0.8 miles to 40th Street. Turn south and follow 40th Street 1 mile to the trailhead parking lot.

32nd Street Trailhead: Exit SR 51 onto Lincoln Drive and drive east 2 miles to 32nd Street. The trailhead parking lot is located on the northeastern corner of 32nd Street and Lincoln Drive.

Piestewa Peak Trailhead: Exit SR 51 onto Lincoln Drive and drive east 0.5 miles. Turn left onto Squaw Peak Drive and continue 0.5 miles to the gated entrance to Phoenix Mountains Park (formerly Squaw Peak Park). Go through the gate and follow the road 0.5 miles until it dead-ends at the Apache picnic area. Hike a short distance northeast on Nature Trail 304 to access the loop.

---

i KEY AT-A-GLANCE INFORMATION

LENGTH: 4.4–5.5 miles
ELEVATION GAIN: 400–550 feet
CONFIGURATION: Balloon (optional one-way with vehicle shuttle)
DIFFICULTY: Easy to moderate
SCENERY: Desert, Phoenix Mountains Preserve, city views
EXPOSURE: Mostly exposed
TRAFFIC: Moderate
TRAIL SURFACE: Gravel, rock
HIKING TIME: 2–3 hours
WATER REQUIREMENT: 2 quarts
SEASON: Year-round; hot in summer
ACCESS: Sunrise to sunset; free parking
MAPS: USGS Sunnyslope, trailhead plaque
FACILITIES: None at 32nd Street Trailhead; water, restroom, and ramada at 40th Street Trailhead
DOGS: Yes, leashed at all times
COMMENTS: Many trailheads serve the Quartz Ridge Trail and its alternates, giving you plenty of options to customize the length and difficulty of this hike. For more information, visit http://phoenix.gov/parks/hikephx.html.

GPS Trailhead Coordinates

UTM Zone 12S
Easting 0407614
Northing 3714489
Latitude N33°34.071'
Longitude W111°59.764'

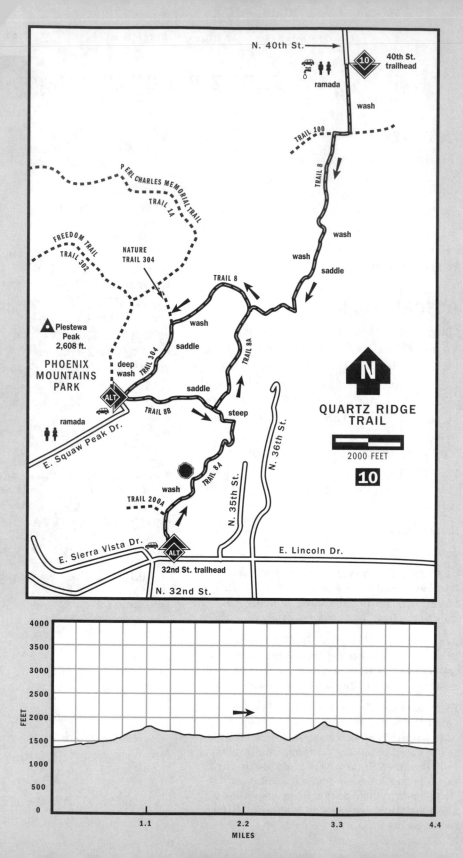

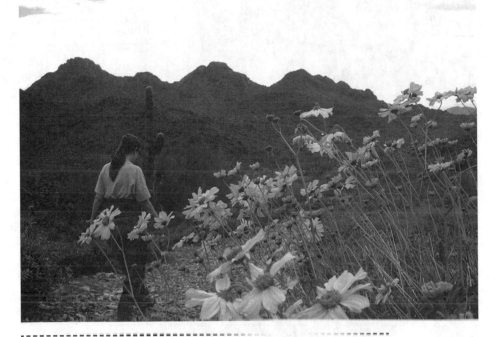

Stacy Herman of Phoenix passes blooming brittlebush along the Quartz Ridge Trail.

The official trailhead for Quartz Ridge Trail is located at the end of 40th Street south of Shea Boulevard. It is also the only trailhead of the three that provides parking for horse trailers. This trailhead takes you on the longest but mildest route through the Quartz Ridge area.

Begin by walking south from the eastern end of the large parking lot on a wide rocky path. Desert plants such as the triangle-leaf bursage and palo verde dominate the landscape. At 0.4 miles, the trail meets Charles M. Christiansen Memorial Trail 100 at a marked intersection. Though it is counterintuitive, you need to turn right onto Trail 100 and hike about 300 feet to find the southbound continuation of Quartz Ridge Trail 8. Trail markings are fairly good here, but it is always a good idea to take along a trail map because many smaller use trails crisscross the mountain preserves and form numerous unmarked intersections. It is easy to get sidetracked. When in doubt, just go straight through any trail junctions.

Hike south on Trail 8 through the open valley with the mountains directly in front of you. Near 0.9 miles, take a slight bend toward the east and head up a basin. As the trail gently climbs, cross some dry washes typical of desert hillsides. Wildflowers are also common sights near north-facing foothills during spring, and you'll likely see some purple lupine and Mexican gold poppies here. At 1.25 miles, reach a wide saddle with an inviting bench. A giant quartz boulder lies on the hill to the left.

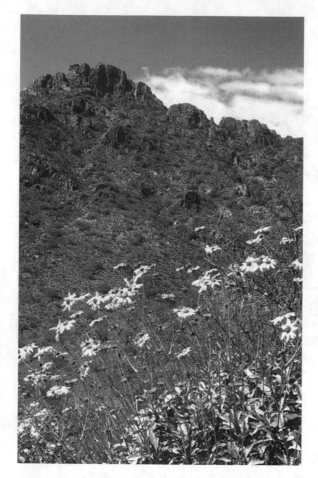

A large basin opens across the saddle, where the only sign of civilization is a conspicuous house on the opposite hill. Follow the trail over the saddle as the slope levels out again. A bit farther into the basin, Trail 8 makes a sharp bend toward the west and heads downhill. A large patch of teddy bear cholla thrives here on warmer south-facing slopes.

At 1.7 miles, you enter a surprisingly deep and wide wash where the intersection with Trail 8A demarks the beginning of a 2.1-mile loop. You can hike this loop in either direction. I describe the circuit in a counterclockwise direction in order to keep trail-hopping to a minimum, but going clockwise is actually easier. Turn right at the trail junction and remain on Trail 8 as it winds through the dry wash. Several trail markers guide you through the twists and turns until you eventually emerge from the wash onto a wide highway-like thoroughfare.

Follow Trail 8 as it bends southeast, staying left at all trail junctions marked and unmarked. The jagged summit of Piestewa Peak dominates the view as you begin a gentle ascent toward the 1,800-foot saddle at the head of this inner basin. Quartz Ridge Trail 8 passes imperceptibly into Phoenix Mountains Park and ends at the prominent saddle where it merges into Nature Trail 304.

Cross the saddle and begin a steep descent along Trail 304. At 2.7 miles, reach the well-marked intersection with Trail 8B, which branches left. Should you have a shuttle vehicle stashed at the Piestewa Peak Trailhead, Trail 304 continues another 500 feet and terminates at the Apache picnic area inside Phoenix Mountains Park. Those hiking the full loop should turn left onto Trail 8B to embark upon the toughest stretch of trail on the entire circuit.

Trail 8B quickly climbs uphill and follows a ridge eastward. The path is steep and rocky and will raise your heart rate in a hurry. If you need a breather, be sure to turn around for an awesome view of Piestewa Peak. A half mile of hard climbing takes you to a 1,925-foot saddle, the highest point of the entire hike. Camelback Mountain pops into view ahead, and the junction of Trails 8A and 8B lies just over the saddle. Take note of this junction because it provides access to the 32nd Street Trailhead.

To complete the loop, turn left at the 8A–8B junction and head north on Trail 8A. This section of trail, though covered in loose rock, descends a hill that is considerably milder than the one on Trail 8B, which is why hiking the loop clockwise would be easier. Continue north 0.7 miles back to the Trail 8 junction inside the deep wash. Turn right and retrace your steps on Trail 8 to finish the hike.

If you prefer a more challenging loop, begin your hike from the 32nd Street Trailhead instead of the one on 40th Street. Trail 8A starts from the eastern end of a small parking lot with a head-on view of Camelback Mountain. Then the trail rounds a hill and turns away from the city and into a quiet mile-long basin. Hike past the Trail 200A junction, a dry wash, some small hills, and then a huge quartz boulder. At the head of the basin, ascend the steep hill via a series of switchbacks and straights, which eventually lead you to the Trail 8A and Trail 8B junction. From there, hike the Quartz Ridge loop in either direction. No matter from which trailhead you begin your hike, the Quartz Ridge trails offer plenty of variety and scenery, an attractive alternative to the hustle and bustle of the crowded Piestewa Peak trails nearby.

NEARBY ACTIVITIES

The Phoenix Mountains Preserve encompasses many popular hiking trails including Piestewa Peak (pages 48 and 52), North Mountain (page 40), Lookout Mountain (page 36), and Perl Charles. Camelback Mountain (pages 21 and 26), another valley favorite, is southeast of the Phoenix Mountains Perserve.

11 SHAW BUTTE TRAIL

KEY AT-A-GLANCE INFORMATION

LENGTH: 4.2 miles

ELEVATION GAIN: 800 feet

CONFIGURATION: Loop

DIFFICULTY: Moderate

SCENERY: Shaw Butte, Phoenix Mountains Preserve, city panorama, desert

EXPOSURE: Completely exposed

TRAFFIC: Moderate

TRAIL SURFACE: Gravel, pavement, packed dirt, rock

HIKING TIME: 2 hours

WATER REQUIREMENT: 2 quarts

SEASON: Year-round; hot in summer

ACCESS: April–September, 5 a.m.– 8:30 p.m.; October–March, 6 a.m.– 7 p.m.; free parking

MAPS: USGS Sunnyslope

FACILITIES: Water, no restrooms

DOGS: Yes, leashed at all times

COMMENTS: This scenic loop visits the top of Shaw Butte and yields impressive panoramas of north-central Phoenix. For more information, visit http://phoenix.gov/ parks/hikenort.html, or call (602) 495-5540.

GPS Trailhead Coordinates

UTM Zone 12S

Easting   0400389

Northing 3718542

Latitude N33°36.225'

Longitude W112°4.461'

IN BRIEF

Shaw Butte Trail 306 may be the best all-around hike in the Phoenix Mountains Preserve. It offers a challenging hike to the summit, a scenic loop through the desert floor, panoramic overlooks around nearly every turn, and fewer crowds than Piestewa Peak.

DESCRIPTION

Located at the northwestern corner of the Phoenix Mountains Preserve, Shaw Butte offers another popular and challenging hike in the heart of Phoenix. Its antenna-studded summit overlooks most of north and central Phoenix. Much like neighboring North Mountain, this well-established trail to the top of Shaw Butte is used by nearby residents for regular exercise. However, the 4-mile Shaw Butte Trail 306 is quite a bit longer than North Mountain National Trail (page 40) and therefore caters to those in search of a longer excursion. It also

---

Directions

From SR 51: Exit onto Cactus Road and follow it west 4 miles to Central Avenue. Note that past the Cave Creek Road intersection, Cactus Road becomes Thunderbird Road. Turn south onto Central Avenue and continue 0.3 miles to the trailhead parking area. If the parking lot is full, wait in line until a spot becomes available. Do not park in the nearby residential area.

From Interstate 17: Exit onto Thunderbird Road and drive east 2.5 miles to Central Avenue. Turn south on Central Avenue and drive 0.3 miles to the trailhead.
   Note: Alternate access points are located at Mountain View Park on 7th Avenue, North Mountain Visitor Center on 7th Street, and at 15th Avenue and Yucca Street. However, they require additional connecting trails.

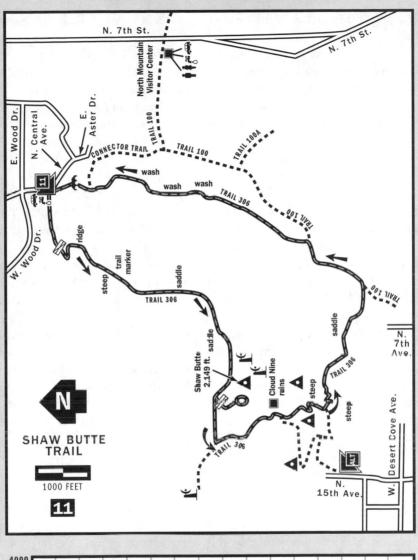

N. 7th St.

N. 7th St.

North Mountain Visitor Center

E. Wood Dr.

N. Central Ave.

E. Aster Dr.

TRAIL 100

TRAIL 100

TRAIL 100A

CONNECTOR TRAIL

TRAIL 100

W. Wood Dr.

wash

wash   wash

TRAIL 306

TRAIL 100

ridge

trail marker

steep

saddle

TRAIL 306

TRAIL 100

saddle

N. 7th Ave.

N

SHAW BUTTE
TRAIL

Shaw Butte
2,149 ft. saddle

Cloud Nine
ruins

steep

TRAIL 306

steep

W. Desert Cove Ave.

1000 FEET

11

TRAIL 306

N.
15th Ave.

W.

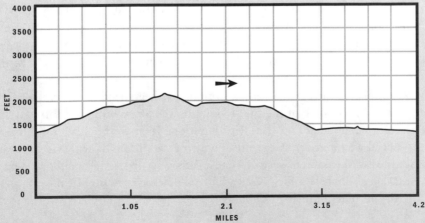

FEET

4000
3500
3000
2500
2000
1500
1000
500
0

1.05   2.1   3.15   4.2
MILES

tends to be less crowded than North Mountain and Piestewa Peak, adding to its appeal.

Panoramic views abound along the Shaw Butte Trail, and a new perspective opens around each bend. This scenic loop hike takes on many personalities. The most popular section climbs a paved road up the northeastern ridge of the mountain. Past the summit, the trail begins a steep and rugged descent. The loop around the base of the mountain provides a gentle stroll through a secluded basin. There's something for everyone here, and the total distance is just right for a morning hike. For these reasons, the Shaw Butte Trail may be the best all-around hike in the Phoenix Mountains Preserve.

On most loop trails, hiking in one direction is easier than the other. For Shaw Butte Trail 306, the easier route is counterclockwise. From the rather small trailhead parking lot, begin by ascending an obvious and wide dirt road on the northeastern side of the mountain. This steep and rocky track passes a gate at 0.25 miles and then bends sharply uphill where sections of broken pavement remind you that this is a service road for the towers atop Shaw Butte. Attain the ridgeline at 0.4 miles with a good view of North Mountain and Piestewa Peak toward the southeast.

Turn southwest on top of the ridge with open views to either side. The towers at the summit still seem quite far. Continue following the wide road as it steadily climbs. The slope levels off as the trail passes a patch of fishhook barrel cacti and reaches a saddle point at 0.8 miles, which overlooks the wide basin between Shaw Butte and North Mountain and the Pointe Tapatio Cliffs Resort. To the east, outlines of the Superstition Mountains and Four Peaks guard the horizon. The trail resumes its climb toward the summit and reaches another saddle at 1 mile from the trailhead. This vista point provides a clear view down Seventh Avenue toward downtown. South Mountain and the Sierra Estrellas can be seen in the distance.

Finish the ascent on gravel, and pass another gate at 1.25 miles. Just beyond this gate, find an obvious trail junction where the service road continues toward the summit and Trail 306 heads downhill toward the west. Take the short detour along the service road to visit the 2,149-foot summit of Shaw Butte. Scenery from the top is impressive, as you might imagine, but numerous antennas strewn about the wide peak obscure your view. The constant buzz from transformers also detracts from the experience. Don't worry; plenty of vistas await you farther along the trail, so return quickly to the trail junction just below the summit.

Many people turn around at the summit and head back to the trailhead, but they then sacrifice some of the finest views on the Shaw Butte Trail. If you have the time, I recommend you complete the loop. Turn west at the trail junction and descend an intensely steep hill down to a saddle point with views toward the southwest. A concrete service road heads west from this saddle to service antennas on a subpeak, which costs a half-mile detour to visit. Turn south at the saddle to continue hiking Trail 306.

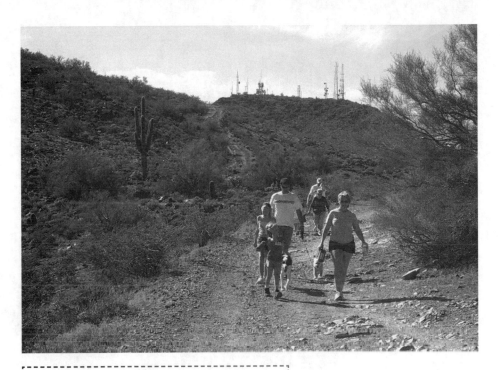

An entire family enjoys the scenery along Shaw Butte Trail.

The next trail section is relatively flat as it hugs the western side of Shaw Butte, with steep drop-offs to the right. At 1.9 miles, you'll reach a trail junction and what appears to be a concrete bunker directly ahead. This is all that remains of Cloud Nine, a fancy restaurant and club that burned to the ground in 1964. Though most of the building is covered in graffiti and concrete rubble, the top of Cloud Nine commands an impressive panoramic view and is definitely worth a visit.

The trail is poorly marked here and can get confusing. Resist the temptation to descend to the west, and take the trail hugging the old foundations of Cloud Nine. Past the ruins, the trail descends to another vista point and then continues downhill on steep and scree-covered switchbacks where every turn offers a scenic perspective on the valley below. A quarter mile below Cloud Nine, you'll reach a lookout where the trail splits again. Turn left down the smaller trail and you'll soon see a trail marker confirming this is the correct route.

Descend the steep switchbacks toward the interior of the basin below. Pass two marked trail junctions in the basin, staying to the left and heading for a narrow gap on the hill flanked by rocky outcrops. Over this small saddle, the trail drops into the main drainage between Shaw Butte and North Mountain. Hikers who seek more of a challenge may choose to go clockwise and climb up these steep sections toward the summit.

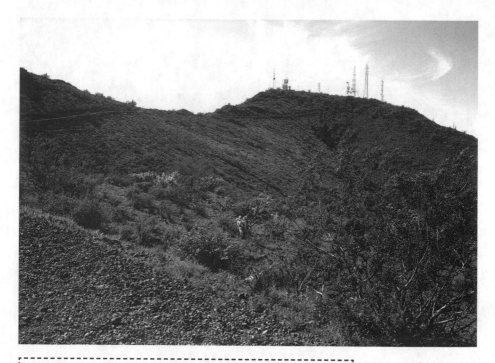

Looking up toward the antenna-studded summit from the Shaw Butte Trail.

The remainder of the hike is a warm-down for those hiking counterclock-wise. Shaw Butte Trail 306 merges with Christiansen Memorial Trail 100 at the bottom of the basin, just past a dry wash. The combined trail turns left and heads northeast. A quarter mile farther the trail forks at an unsigned junction. Take the left fork to remain on the Shaw Butte Trail, which meanders through the scenic basin and crosses several washes. One mile beyond the fork, Trail 306 skirts a dirt berm and returns to the trailhead on Central Avenue.

NEARBY ACTIVITIES

The Phoenix Mountains Preserve encompasses many popular hiking trails includ-ing Piestewa Peak (pages 48 and 52), North Mountain (page 40), Lookout Moun-tain (page 36), and Perl Charles. Camelback Mountain (pages 21 and 26), another valley favorite, is southeast of the Phoenix Mountains Preserve.

SOUTH MOUNTAIN: NATIONAL TRAIL 12

IN BRIEF

National Trail is the longest and grandest of all trails in South Mountain Park. It offers sweeping city vistas, secluded desert valleys, interesting rock formations, ancient Hohokam petroglyphs, historic abandoned mineshafts, and an all-day hike to delight hardy outdoor enthusiasts.

DESCRIPTION

Touted as the largest city park in the country, South Mountain Park spans more than 16,000 acres of desert and mountain preserves at the southern edge of Phoenix. Ironically, the most recognizable feature in South Mountain Park is the man-made forest of television, microwave, and radio antennas atop the 2,690-foot Mount Suppoa. At night the blinking aircraft-obstruction lights on these antennas can be

----

Directions ⟶

Pima Canyon Trailhead: Exit I-10 at Baseline Road. Drive west on Baseline Road 0.6 miles to 48th Street. Turn south on 48th Street, which soon becomes Pointe Parkway. Follow this curvy road 1 mile, skirting the Pointe South Mountain Resort. Just past Guadalupe Road, turn right onto 48th Street and then make an immediate left turn to enter Pima Canyon Park. Drive to the parking lot at the western end of the park.

San Juan Trailhead: Exit I-10 at Baseline Road and drive west 6 miles to Central Avenue. Turn south onto Central Avenue and drive 1.5 miles to the park entrance. Once inside the park, drive 2.2 miles to the junction of Summit Road and San Juan Road. Take San Juan Road west 4 miles until it ends at the San Juan Lookout. Note: San Juan Road is currently open only one weekend per month. Check the Web site for latest road conditions.

KEY AT-A-GLANCE INFORMATION

LENGTH: 15.5 miles
ELEVATION GAIN: 1,350 feet
CONFIGURATION: One-way
DIFFICULTY: Moderate, but long
SCENERY: Desert, city overlooks, mountain vistas, abandoned mineshafts
EXPOSURE: Completely exposed, very little shade
TRAFFIC: Heavy on eastern half, light on western half
TRAIL SURFACE: Packed dirt, gravel, bedrock
HIKING TIME: 7.5 hours
WATER REQUIREMENT: 4 quarts, 5–6 quarts during summer
SEASON: Year-round; hot in summer
ACCESS: Pima Canyon entrance 5 a.m.–7 p.m., Central Avenue entrance 5 a.m.–10 p.m.; free parking
MAPS: USGS Guadalupe, Lone Butte, and Laveen; park map available from visitor center and posted on plaques at trailheads
FACILITIES: Ramadas, picnic areas, visitor center, ranger station, toilets; drinking water available
DOGS: Yes, leashed at all times
COMMENTS: Visit http://phoenix .gov/parks/hikesoth.html, or call (602) 495-0222.

GPS Trailhead Coordinates

UTM Zone 12S
Easting 0408338
Northing 3691757
Latitude N33°21.775'
Longitude W111°59.157'

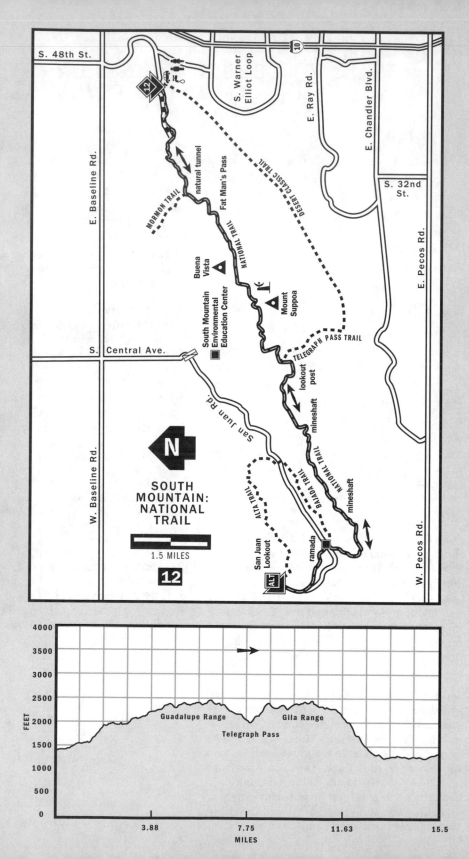

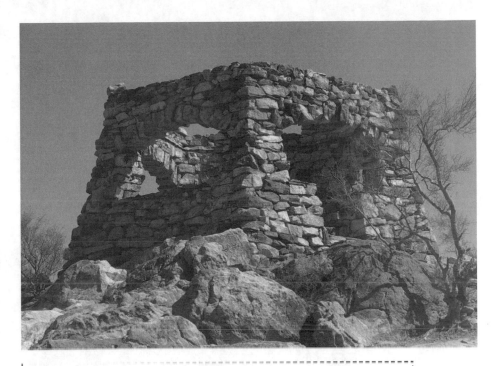

An old lookout tower still guards Telegraph Pass, which roughly bisects South Mountain.

seen from nearly anywhere in the valley and serve as a welcome beacon for the directionally challenged. Visitors to South Mountain, however, don't care for the antennas. They come to enjoy a wide variety of recreational activities, including hiking, mountain biking, horseback riding, picnicking, and sightseeing.

National Trail, the longest in the park, offers day hikers a complete South Mountain experience. In addition to being a superb hike showcasing the best features of the park, National Trail is also one of the premier mountain-biking trails in the country. On weekends, dozens of mountain bikers share the trail with just as many if not more hikers. Running east–west along the top of South Mountain's two longest mountain ranges, National Trail intersects almost every other trail in the park. If you plan to hike the whole 15.5 miles along this trail, prepare to spend an entire day enjoying its many wonders. You also need to arrange a ride to take you from one end of the trail back to the other.

I prefer to hike this trail from east to west, facing the scenic Sierra Estrella mountain range and avoiding an otherwise steep uphill on the western end. Begin your hike from the parking lot at the western end of Pima Canyon Park, located in the shadows of the Pointe South Mountain Resort. The first 1.3 miles is a gentle promenade along a wide and level dirt road. On weekend mornings, prepare to share this road with many speedy mountain bikers and slow baby strollers. The road ends in a wide turnaround. Petroglyphs left by the ancient Hohokams can be found here on the backside of some boulders at the western end of this circular area. At the northwestern end of the turnaround, find the obvious trail markers

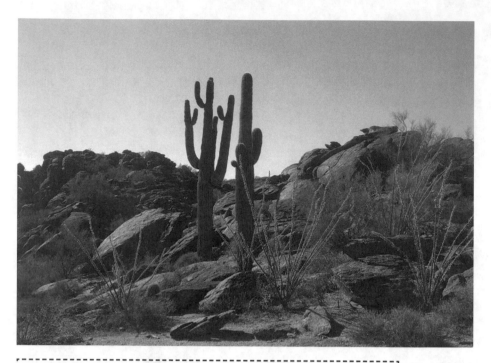

Saguaros and ocotillos thrive in the harsh desert along South Mountain National Trail.

for National Trail, which heads uphill. As you hike, watch out for mountain bikers speeding downhill. Although foot traffic has the right of way, sometimes bikers can't see you or stop in time. After a gentle half-mile climb, walk along the top of a ridge and enjoy the open views of the Phoenix skyline to the north.

At 2.6 miles, National Trail intersects Hidden Valley Trail (page 31), a particularly scenic and secluded bypass that rejoins National Trail 0.5 miles later. Hidden Valley is a popular detour for National Trail hikers, and its length is similar to the circumnavigated section along National Trail. Hidden Valley Trail, however, is harder to follow and requires a little scrambling over rocky obstacles. If you opt for this half-mile jaunt through Hidden Valley, you will be treated to a natural rock tunnel, a quiet valley with scenic rocks, and a nine-inch-wide crack through two large boulders, ironically named Fat Man's Pass. Take off your backpack and squeeze through sideways. Try the natural slide on the smooth rock surface immediately after going through Fat Man's Pass. Claustrophobics and portly hikers need not worry; there is an easy bypass route over the boulders. Just beyond Fat Man's Pass, Hidden Valley Trail merges back into National Trail at 3.2 miles.

If you choose to stay on the smoother and easier-to-follow National Trail, you can still visit the rock tunnel and Fat Man's Pass. They are only a few feet from either end of Hidden Valley Trail. Simply return to National Trail after you check out these formations. An added advantage of staying on National Trail is that Mormon Trail junction at 2.75 miles offers a convenient escape from your commitment in case you are hesitant about finishing this long hike. Mormon Trail leads you to the Mormon Loop Trail, which then loops back to the dirt road and Pima Canyon Park.

Continue hiking west along National Trail after Fat Man's Pass, facing the array of antenna towers on Mount Suppoa, the tallest point in South Mountain Park. At 4.5 miles, look to your left for the Chinese Wall, a dark-colored dike of Tertiary period granite and diorite. The trail reaches Buena Vista Lookout at 5 miles. Cross the paved parking area to find the trail on the other side of the road. After a small hill and at 5.7 miles, the trail joins a paved service road. Walk west along this road for 50 yards to pick up the trail again, which then heads straight for the massive antennas on the summit of Mount Suppoa. The trail skirts the fenced-off antenna complex on its northern side. Roughly 2,500 feet in elevation, this trail section is the highest accessible point in South Mountain Park. Do not dawdle too long though. Rumor has it that the Federal Communications Commission allows its technicians to work only two-hour shifts here because of the high-power transmitters.

At 7.5 miles and with the antennas now safely behind you, continue hiking National Trail, which runs along a rocky ledge above Summit Road. Look for strange-looking elephant trees with smooth red bark and fragrant leaves. The trail drops down to the road and meets the Telegraph Pass Trail (page 109) at 8 miles from the trailhead. From this saddle point, you can see the matchbox-like houses in Ahwatukee to the south and the tall buildings in downtown Phoenix to the north. Congratulations! You are now halfway through the hike.

The western half of National Trail runs atop the Gila Range and sees much less traffic than the eastern Guadalupe range. Expect to encounter fewer crowds and hardly any mountain bikers. From Summit Road climb a steep section of trail to Telegraph Pass Lookout. The Army Signal Corps built this roofless watchtower in 1873 to guard a telegraph line running from Maricopa Wells all the way to the territorial capital of Prescott. This is a great place to rest and enjoy the views.

National Trail then climbs Goat Hill atop the Gila Range at an elevation of 2,300 feet, overlooking a small kart racing course at the base of the mountain and the Phoenix skyline in the distance. Just beyond Goat Hill, pass the Ranger Trail junction at 9.6 miles and continue hiking along a ledge on the southern side of the hill. Clusters of furry teddy bear cholla dot the steep hill below you. Enjoy the scenery here in relative isolation, and notice that the trail is obviously less worn than the first 8 miles. Many abandoned mineshafts lie just off the trail in the next few miles. A particularly large one can be found at 10.8 miles at trail-marker number 39. Most of the mineshafts have been sealed, but avoid the temptation to climb into any dark and potentially unsafe mineshaft openings.

National Trail finally begins its descent from the Gila Range at 12 miles from the trailhead. Hike down the steep hill as the trail winds through a scenic but desolate narrow canyon with colorful rocks. At 13 miles, cross a dry wash and climb toward a notch where the trail bends into the wide valley between the Gila Range and the Ma Ha Tuak Range to the north. Hike along the valley floor toward San Juan Road. National Trail intersects Bajada Trail at 13.9 miles and crosses San Juan Road shortly thereafter. The elevation in the valley is 1,250 feet, the lowest of the entire hike.

The final 1.5 miles of this long hike are relatively flat and uneventful as it parallels the road, skirting the southern tip of the Ma Ha Tuak Range below Maricopa Peak. The 15.5-mile National Trail ends at the San Juan Lookout where you should have a vehicle or a ride waiting.

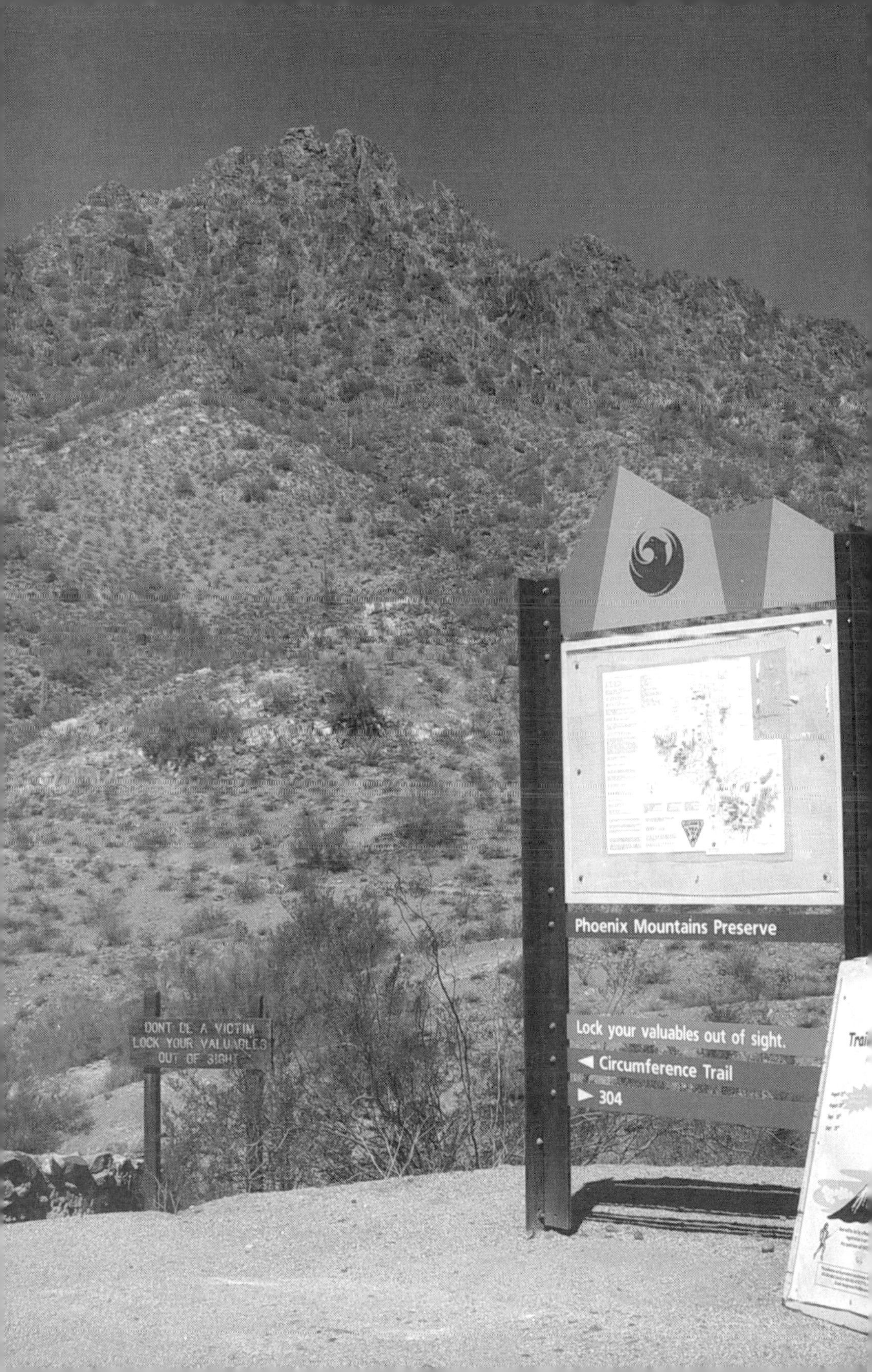

DONT BE A VICTIM
LOCK YOUR VALUABLES
OUT OF SIGHT

Phoenix Mountains Preserve

Lock your valuables out of sight.

◄ Circumference Trail
► 304

Trail

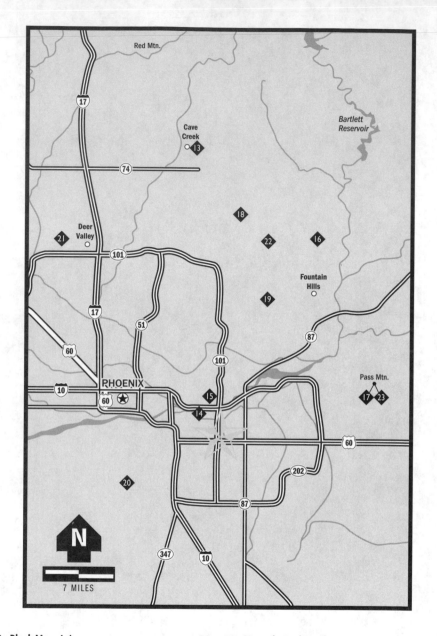

Red Mtn.

Bartlett
Reservoir

Cave
Creek ○ 13

17

74

18

Deer
Valley ○   21

22   16

101

Fountain
Hills ○

19

17

51

87

60

101

Pass Mtn.

PHOENIX   15   17 23

10   60

14

60

202

20

87

N

347   10

7 MILES

PHOENIX SUBURBS:
AHWATUKEE, CAVE CREEK, GLENDALE, MESA, SCOTTSDALE, TEMPE

13 BLACK MOUNTAIN

KEY AT-A-GLANCE INFORMATION

LENGTH: 2.4 miles

ELEVATION GAIN: 1,225 feet

CONFIGURATION: Out-and-back

DIFFICULTY: Difficult

SCENERY: City panorama, desert, unique geology

EXPOSURE: Completely exposed

TRAFFIC: Light to moderate

TRAIL SURFACE: Packed dirt, crushed rock, rocky

HIKING TIME: 1.5 hours

WATER REQUIREMENT: 1.5 quarts

SEASON: Year-round; hot in summer

ACCESS: Open sunrise to sunset; free parking

MAPS: USGS Cave Creek

FACILITIES: None

DOGS: Yes, leashed at all times

COMMENTS: Cave Creek's answer to Camelback and Piestewa Peak

IN BRIEF

Hikers in north Phoenix have several nearby options for regular exercise hikes. Black Mountain ranks at the top of that list for a quick workout and a splendid view from its summit.

DESCRIPTION

Looming over northern outposts Cave Creek and Carefree like a dark fortress, Black Mountain is as forbidding as it is inviting. To unfamiliar hikers, Black Mountain presents some challenges in terms of finding a suitable trailhead, adequate parking, and acceptable access to the summit. However, once you overcome those challenges, the short but challenging hike up Black Mountain rivals the best short hikes in Phoenix.

Named for the black slate and phyllite that comprise much of the mountain, Black Mountain has long been the pride of the twin communities. Cave Creek and Carefree were once separated from urban sprawl and held a distinct mystique to city dwellers. As new development blurred the lines between western outposts and suburbia, these communities have grown to embrace change.

GPS Trailhead Coordinates

UTM Zone   12S

Easting   0412778

Northing   3743494

Latitude   N33°49.792'

Longitude   W111°56.598'

Directions

From East Valley: Take Loop 101 to Scottsdale Road. Drive north 12 miles to Cave Creek Road. Turn west on Cave Creek and follow it 1.25 miles to School House Road. Turn south on School House Road and find small parking area on right side.

From Phoenix: Take Loop 101 to Cave Creek Road. Drive north 10 miles to Carefree Highway (AZ 74). Continue north on Cave Creek Road 3 miles to School House Road.

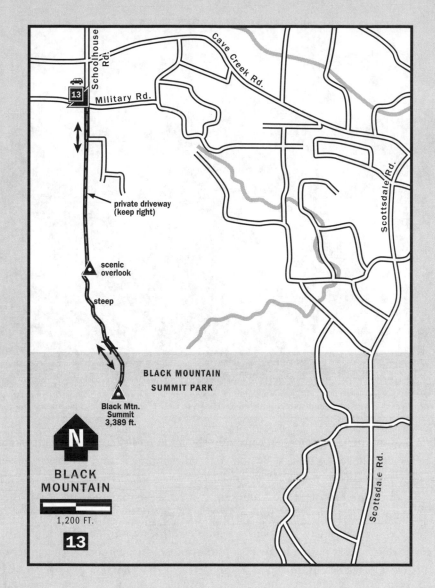

Schoolhouse Rd.

Cave Creek Rd.

Military Rd.

13

private driveway
(keep right)

Scottsdale Rd.

scenic
overlook

steep

BLACK MOUNTAIN

SUMMIT PARK

Black Mtn.
Summit
3,389 ft.

Scottsdale Rd.

N

BLACK
MOUNTAIN

1,200 FT.

13

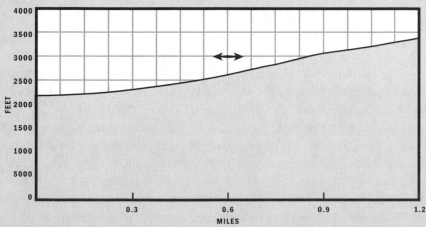

4000

3500

3000

2500

2000

1500

1000

5000

0

FEET

0.3   0.6   0.9   1.2

MILES

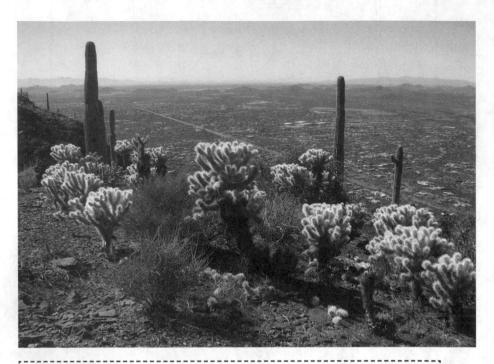

Teddy bear chollas and saguaros accentuate an open view of Cave Creek from Black Mountain.

Black Mountain has often been caught in the middle of that change—a struggle between the old versus new, seclusion versus development, and preservation versus growth.

Though the top of Black Mountain is a preserve managed by BLM, there has been no officially sanctioned way for hikers to reach the summit. Land owners, conservationists, and various municipalities continue to struggle over access, while hikers patiently await a resolution so they can enjoy the sweeping views from Black Mountain's ridges and crest. Over the years, however, a de facto trail and easement have emerged on the north side of Black Mountain, along School House Road, and that's where we begin our hike.

Walk south on School House Road with the mountain directly in sight. Beyond Military Road, begin a gentle ascent past homes in the area. As you approach the foothills, pavement gives way to a packed-dirt road and eventually a jeep trail up the northern flanks of Black Mountain. Don't be discouraged by this bit of road hiking; there's plenty of pristine desert ahead.

A third of a mile past Military Road, veer right at the entrance of a private driveway and find a small trail to the left of the main dirt road (which is off-and-on closed to hikers). Turn away from the road here and hike the narrow trail next to the private driveway. Sonoran Desert flora abounds as jojobas, triangle-leaf bursage, mesquite trees, and saguaros line the trail. You begin to feel your heart rate increase in proportion to the slope.

A half-mile past Military Road, the trail becomes rockier and steeper as it steadily climbs. Smooth gravel and packed dirt degrade into broken rock, and a variety of cacti encroach on the narrow trail. At 0.6 miles, a marker carved into rock declares that you are crossing into a Maricopa County park. Soon after the sign, the narrow trail reaches a wide lookout and meets the extension of the dirt road you left earlier. This is roughly the halfway point of the hike and a good vantage point for a short rest break. Turn around and gaze back down the trail to see how far you have already hiked. On the northern horizon, New River Mountains frame the town of Cave Creek.

Resume your ascent along a wide ridge toward the summit of Black Mountain. Watch your footing on the sharp rocks that line this rugged trail. Jojobas, buckhorn cholla, and flat-top buckwheat thrive here. At 0.75 miles, the trail becomes formidably steep and ascends a rocky staircase made for giants. Take your time laboring up these steep inclines, knowing that a scenic panorama awaits you on the summit.

Nearly 1 mile past the starting point at Military Road, top out on the summit ridge as the trail thankfully levels slightly. Here you have the best opportunity to view up close the black metamorphic rock that gave the mountain its name. Actually, only the western half of Black Mountain exhibits these dark ancient stones. The eastern half consists of much younger granite. The black slate and phyllite are some of the oldest exposed rocks in the state and rival those found at the bottom of the Grand Canyon in age.

Finish the last quarter mile with expansive views of surrounding cityscape and distant mountain ranges. The summit of Black Mountain measures 3,398 feet in elevation, considerably higher than Camelback Mountain (page 26) and Piestewa Peak (page52), and your hard work is rewarded by a panoramic view that will take your breath away. To the east, the horizon presents familiar silhouettes of Four Peaks, McDowell Mountains and Tom's Thumb (page 118), and the Superstition Mountains. To the west lie the Bradshaws and the White Tanks. And to the south, metropolitan Phoenix stretches for as far as the eye can see.

Take plenty of time to soak in the views. Retrace your steps to descend Black Mountain.

NEARBY ACTIVITIES

North of Cave Creek, Spur Cross Ranch Conservation Area offers several hikes through pristine desert in the shadows of Elephant Mountain (page 215). Cave Creek Recreation Area (page 210) lies 3 miles due east of Black Mountain. Bartlett Reservoir and Seven Springs Recreation Area are both accessible via Cave Creek Road.

14 HAYDEN BUTTE PRESERVE AND TEMPE TOWN LAKE

KEY AT-A-GLANCE INFORMATION

LENGTH: 4.3 miles

ELEVATION GAIN: 350 feet

CONFIGURATION: Loop

DIFFICULTY: Easy

SCENERY: City panorama, desert, Tempe Town Lake, urban hiking

EXPOSURE: Completely exposed

TRAFFIC: Moderate to heavy

TRAIL SURFACE: Packed dirt, pavement, sidewalk, rocky trail on top of Hayden Butte

HIKING TIME: 2 hours

WATER REQUIREMENT: 2 quarts

SEASON: Year-round; hot in summer

ACCESS: Open sunrise to sunset; metered parking available near Sun Devil Stadium

MAPS: USGS Tempe

FACILITIES: No facilities at the trailhead, drinking water and restrooms available during the hike

DOGS: Yes, leashed at all times

COMMENTS: Best urban hike in Phoenix. For more information, visit www.tempe.gov/parks, or call (480) 350-5200.

GPS Trailhead Coordinates

UTM Zone 12S

Easting 0413132

Northing 3698702

Latitude N33°25.557'

Longitude W1116.105'

IN BRIEF

This scenic route showcases the best hotspots near downtown Tempe, a city known for its ties to Arizona State University. Though not entirely a hiking trail, this tour visits a mountain preserve, wanders through a lakeside park, and hits a trendy business district.

DESCRIPTION

The recently constructed Tempe Town Lake turned the drab and dry Salt River bed near downtown Tempe into a beautiful park for a multitude of recreational activities. Desert along the banks of the Salt River has been transformed into biking and jogging paths. Boat docks and ramps line the lakeshores. Lush green grassy areas replaced barren dirt lots. Shiny office and residential buildings sprang up on the shore, with more planned. The flurry of development has made the area a prime target for exploration and a perfect setting for urban hiking.

Your lakeside adventure begins at Hayden Butte Preserve Park in the shadows of Sun Devil Stadium, home of Arizona State University's Sun Devils and, for a while, the National Football League's Arizona Cardinals. Near the southwest entrance to the stadium and at the intersection of Veterans Way and College Avenue, find the Hayden Butte

Directions

Exit Loop 202 at Scottsdale Road. Drive south 0.8 miles to Sixth Street. Turn west on Sixth Street and follow it 0.25 miles until it ends at Veterans Way. Turn northwest on Veterans Way and proceed 0.3 miles to the southwest entrance of Sun Devil Stadium. You can also take the Metro light rail to Sun Devil Stadium.

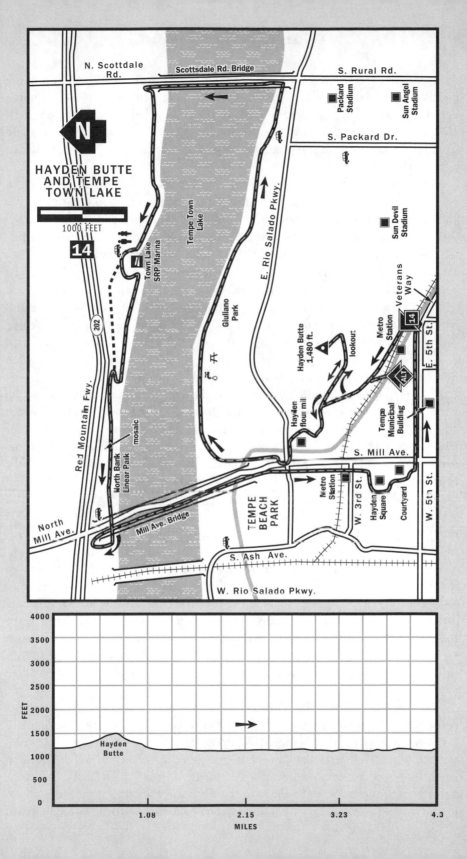

N

HAYDEN BUTTE
AND TEMPE
TOWN LAKE

1000 FEET

14

N. Scottdale Rd.

Scottsdale Rd. Bridge

S. Rural Rd.

Packard Stadium

Sun Angel Stadium

S. Packard Dr.

Tempe Town Lake

E. Rio Salado Pkwy.

Sun Devil Stadium

Town Lake SRP Marina

Giuliano Park

Hayden Butte 1,480 ft.

lookout

Metro Station

Veterans Way

14

E. 5th St.

ALT

202

Red Mountain Fwy.

mosaic

North Bank Linear Park

Hayden flour mill

Tempe Municipal Building

S. Mill Ave.

W. 5th St.

North Mill Ave.

Mill Ave. Bridge

TEMPE BEACH PARK

Metro Station

W. 3rd St.

Hayden Square

Courtyard

S. Ash Ave.

W. Rio Salado Pkwy.

FEET

4000
3500
3000
2500
2000
1500
1000
500
0

Hayden Butte

1.08   2.15   3.23   4.3

MILES

Park sign and the trailhead for the Leonard Monti Trail. Walk west along the packed-dirt trail to start your ascent to the top of Hayden Butte, formerly known as Tempe Butte or "A" Mountain because of the huge letter "A" on its southern face. Interpretive signs posted along the trail explain the history of the area and some of the desert flora and fauna you might encounter. There's even a sign to explain the "A" sign.

Running parallel to the Metro light rail tracks, the trail soon meets an alternate access point behind the police station. Make sure you don't park illegally in the Tempe Police parking lot. Turn uphill here until you reach the paved service road at 0.25 miles. Hike up the steep paved road to a vista point offering spectacular views overlooking the Arizona State University campus. Pass through a gap in the fence behind you to explore the top of Hayden Butte. The handrail-assisted walk up the rocks and cement stairs takes you past the giant "A" and up to the summit for an even better view. From this vantage point 300 feet above the city, you can see into Sun Devil Stadium, look down on Tempe Town Lake, watch the airplanes take off and land at Sky Harbor International Airport, or just relax and listen to the sounds of life in Tempe. At night, Hayden Butte is also a favorite among locals for watching the city lights.

Retrace your steps and head back down the service road. Follow it all the way down to the base of historic Hayden Flour Mill, the large abandoned white building at the bottom of the hill. Many landmarks in Tempe were named after Charles Trumbull Hayden, often considered the father of Tempe, which at one time was called Hayden's Ferry. The Hayden family founded and operated the mill for three generations. The first mill was built at this location in 1874, and the version you see today was erected in 1918. Charles Hayden's son Carl, who was born in the Monti's building across the street, went on to serve in the U.S. House and Senate for more than 57 years. The Hayden Flour Mill ceased operations in 1997, but it remains as a defining landmark in Tempe history.

From one of the oldest buildings in town, head directly north toward one of the newest. The service road ends at a gate near the mill. Walk beyond the gate to Rio Salado Parkway, and cross the street at the crosswalk by the Mill Avenue bridges. The silver and glass buildings ahead of you are part of the Hayden Ferry Lakeside development, a complex of residential, retail, and office buildings built on the site of the original Hayden's ferry service. With Camelback Mountain on the horizon, proceed north between the bridge and the buildings until you come to the edge of the lake.

Tempe Town Lake, like most lakes in Arizona, is artificial. However, its construction is unique because the dams that create the 2.5-mile-long lake are actually inflatable rubber bladders. With Hayden Butte and Sun Devil Stadium on your right, walk east along the southern shore of the lake through Giuliano Park. At 1.2 miles from your starting point, there is a shaded picnic area with a drinking fountain. Straight ahead in the distance, the Superstition Mountains loom on the horizon. The mountain with the yellowish stripe is Pass Mountain

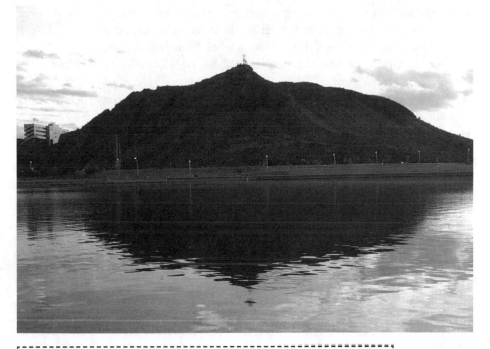

Hayden Butte and Sun Devil Stadium cast their reflections onto Tempe Town Lake.

near Usery Park. The distinctive shape of Four Peaks can be seen to the northeast, and the giant camel of Camelback Mountain slumbers across the lake to the north.

Cement retaining walls line the banks of the lake, and on each seat in the wall, there's an artistic ceramic tile embedded in the concrete. Six hundred such tiles display icons and prose around the lake, composing a book of tiles called "words over water" and providing an interesting diversion during your hike. At 1.8 miles, climb up to the sidewalk on Scottsdale Road and cross over to the northern side of the lake. While on the Scottsdale Road bridge, pause to admire the reflection of Hayden Butte and Sun Devil Stadium in the lake, a scene that's especially beautiful at sunset. Make a 180-degree turn at the northern end of the bridge and descend the ramp to reach the lakeshore once more. Now walk west along the northern shore, past Papago Stables, to the marina at 2.4 miles from your starting point. There are restrooms and drinking water available here as well as a fountain called the Marina Water Muse.

Continue your westward stroll along the North Bank Linear Park. At 3 miles, pass by a tunnel under Loop 202. Notice the 545-foot glittering mosaic called "River Then, River Now, and River Future" snaking along the wall. Interpretive signs explaining various desert plants add an educational dimension to the hike. Proceed through the parking area under both Mill Avenue bridges, and then climb up to the sidewalk on the western side of the western bridge.

Constructed in 1931, the western bridge is the older of the two. Cross over the lake on the western bridge to return to the south shore, completing a loop around the lake. Incidentally, this loop is wheelchair friendly.

At the intersection of Mill Avenue and Rio Salado Parkway, find the main entrance to Tempe Beach Park and Monti's La Casa Vieja Restaurant. Tempe Beach Park received a complete makeover when the lake was constructed and is now a favorite venue for outdoor concerts and events. Built by Charles Trumbull Hayden in 1871, Monti's has the distinction of being the longest continuously occupied building in Tempe.

Continue walking south along the western side of tree-lined Mill Avenue, the liveliest street in town. Home of many bars, restaurants, and shops, Mill Avenue is the cultural center of Tempe. Just past the Metro station and traffic light at Third Street, detour west into the amphitheater at Hayden Square, another popular spot for outdoor concerts. Pass through Hayden Square and emerge on the cul-de-sac next to the gazebo. Look for a large staircase on the western end of the building. Behind this staircase is an entrance to the best-kept secret on Mill Avenue, a charming courtyard with a gazebo and a waterfall hidden from the noisy crowds. Catch your breath here and enjoy the small boutique shops. You can exit from the courtyard to the east and emerge back onto Mill Avenue.

Proceed south again on Mill Avenue until you come to its intersection with Fifth Street. Though not as storied as San Francisco's Haight and Ashbury, this junction is the heart of Tempe culture. Turn east onto Fifth Street to finish your urban adventure. On your way back to Sun Devil Stadium and Hayden Butte Park, note the lavish Tempe Mission Palms Resort and the inverted pyramid shape of the Tempe municipal building.

NEARBY ACTIVITIES

Mill Avenue near the campus of Arizona State University offers many restaurants, bars, shops, and other diversions. Papago Park (page 44), home of the Phoenix Zoo and Desert Botanical Garden, is 2 miles to the northwest. Fans of urban hiking can also take advantage of recreational activities along Indian Bend Wash, which the locals call the "Greenbelt" (page 85).

INDIAN BEND WASH GREENBELT 15

IN BRIEF

The Greenbelt Pathway snakes through a wide swath of greenery in the middle of a thriving desert city, providing a lush oasis for numerous outdoor activities. The Indian Bend Wash Greenbelt not only controls the city's seasonal floods but also creates ample open spaces for recreation and the setting for an outstanding urban hike.

DESCRIPTION

Flooding in a desert may seem improbable, but seasonal storms can easily overcome the often inadequate drainage systems in arid areas. While attempting to solve this problem, Scottsdale planners back in the 1960s had a stroke of genius. They constructed the Indian Bend Wash Greenbelt, an innovative flood-control system and desert oasis rolled into one. Taking advantage of the seasonal nature of flash floods, the city built a row of parks in Indian Bend Wash offering its residents a plethora of outdoor pursuits. The Greenbelt channels occasional floodwater toward the Salt River while accommodating a wide variety of recreational activities.

KEY AT-A-GLANCE INFORMATION

LENGTH: 5 miles
ELEVATION GAIN: 100 feet
CONFIGURATION: One-way
DIFFICULTY: Easy
SCENERY: Parks, golf courses, lakes, Camelback Mountain
EXPOSURE: Mostly exposed, except for occasional tree cover
TRAFFIC: Moderate to heavy
TRAIL SURFACE: Pavement, grass
HIKING TIME: 3 hours
WATER REQUIREMENT: 2 quarts
SEASON: Year-round; hot in summer
ACCESS: Sunrise to 10 p.m.; free parking
MAPS: USGS Tempe, Paradise Valley
FACILITIES: Parking, water, restrooms, picnic areas, various recreational facilities
DOGS: Yes, leashed
COMMENTS: The Greenbelt Pathway runs through a unique system of parks built along Indian Bend Wash. For more information, visit www.scottsdaleaz.gov/parks, or call (480) 312-park.

Directions ——————————➤

Take Loop 101 to any of the following exits: McKellips Road, McDowell Road, Thomas Road, Indian School Road, Chaparral Road, and McDonald Drive. Turn west and drive approximately 1–1.5 miles to the Indian Bend Wash Greenbelt. Parking is available throughout the park system.

To hike the suggested 5-mile one-way route, park one vehicle at McKellips Lake Park, approximately 0.3 miles west of Hayden Road, and another vehicle at the northern end of Chaparral Park, on Hayden Road south of McDonald Drive.

GPS Trailhead Coordinates

UTM Zone 12S
Easting 0415288
Northing 3701539
Latitude N33°27.102'
Longitude W111°54.730'

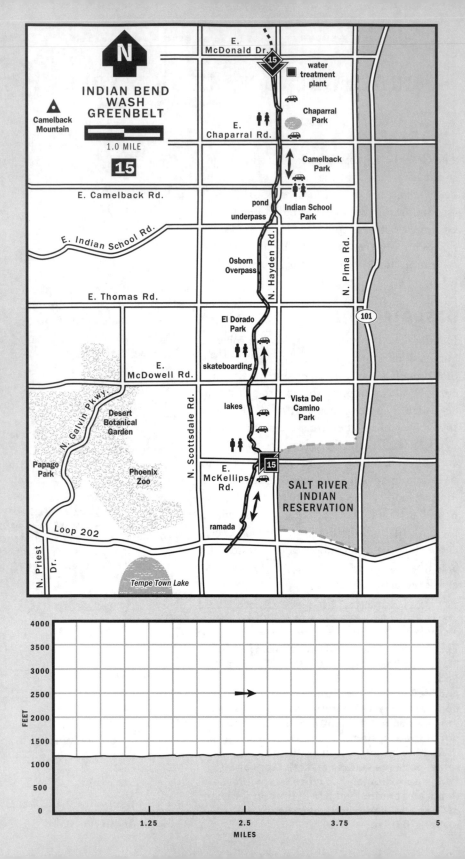

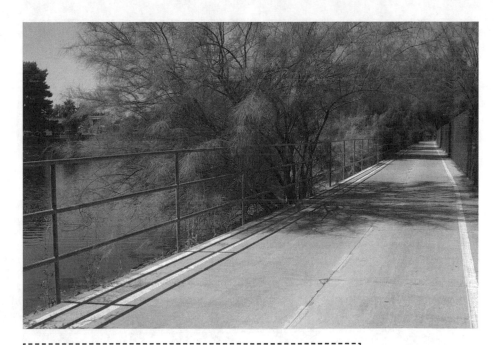

The Greenbelt Pathway runs next to a scenic pond and under shady trees.

The Greenbelt spans nearly 12 miles from Tempe Town Lake north to Cactus Road. While private golf courses consume some of the Greenbelt, its southern half is easily accessible to the general public. Bounded roughly by Hayden and Miller roads, the Greenbelt encompasses miles of parks, lakes, golf courses, picnic areas, and various sporting venues. Tunnels and overpasses protect visitors from traffic, and a multiuse Greenbelt Pathway carries patrons on foot, skates, and wheels through the park system.

Over the years, the Greenbelt has steadily gained popularity and has become one of Scottsdale's prime attractions. It's just one of the many reasons why Scottsdale has been honored as the Most Livable City by the U.S. Conference of Mayors and as a Sports Illustrated Sportstown. The Greenbelt is a haven for health-conscious joggers, bikers, and skaters, active sports teams, stroller-pushing parents, idle picnickers, and even migratory birds. In this tranquil setting, the Greenbelt Pathway offers an excellent urban hike and plenty of people-watching opportunities.

Many parking lots throughout the Indian Bend Wash Greenbelt provide convenient access to its amenities, and you can hike as little or as much as you'd like. A reasonable scenic route is the 5-mile stretch from McKellips Road to McDonald Drive. South of McKellips Road, the Greenbelt runs along Rio Salado Golf Course and then through an undeveloped section before terminating at the northern shore of Tempe Town Lake. North of McDonald Drive, the Greenbelt Pathway passes Saguaro High School and skirts another string of golf courses near the resort-studded McCormick Ranch.

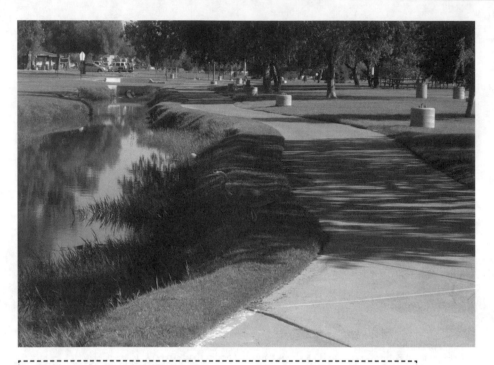

A blue heron rests in the shady banks of Indian Bend Wash along the Greenbelt Pathway.

Begin your hike from McKellips Lake Park, where you will find the Greenbelt Pathway's signature green sign. Many paved walkways cross the park system, and it really doesn't matter which route you take. You can even cut through the grass if you'd like. However, if you wish to stay on the official Greenbelt Pathway, look for its telltale yellow center line, which keeps bikers and skaters heading in opposite directions from colliding with each other.

McKellips Lake Park encircles a large lake where many migrating waterfowl make their homes. It's the southernmost lake in Scottsdale and a pleasant place to relax. As you walk north, the pathway passes imperceptibly into Vista Del Camino Park, which boasts tree-lined walkways next to a quaint canal. Ducks and even herons share the shade with human visitors. The park continues past curvy Roosevelt Street where a playground and spray pad keep kids entertained on a warm summer day. A softball field and a disc-golf course lie on the western side of the waterway.

Cross McDowell Road via the underpass and enter Eldorado Park, the second major park along the Greenbelt Pathway. Embedded within Eldorado Park is a large concrete skating facility called Wedge Skate Park. This relatively new addition to Eldorado Park allows inline skaters to show off their stunt skills. The pathway veers slightly east and comes parallel to 77th Street. Sand volleyball courts, a large playground, and another lake line the trail. Cross the street where 77th Street bends into Murray Lane, and continue hiking north. A large parking lot and a public aquatic center lie at the intersection of Murray Lane and Miller Road, just west of 77th Street.

The Greenbelt Pathway then cuts through Coronado Golf Course via a shaded passage lined with palo verde trees and sandwiched between the golf course and a lake. Continue north through the golf course and cross Thomas Road via another underpass. At 2.5 miles from McKellips Road, follow the Greenbelt Pathway as it passes over Osborn Road with a large driving range to the right and Osborn Park on your left. The path straightens and rides atop a small berm in the shade of pine trees.

Skirt the edge of some housing developments and veer slightly east again until you reach a pond at the intersection of Indian School and Hayden Road. Cross under Indian School Road, and enter the third major park along Indian Bend Wash. Indian School Park caters to a wide variety of sports enthusiasts. There are baseball diamonds, and basketball, tennis, racquetball, and volleyball courts. Even horseshoe and bocce ball fans won't be disappointed. The Greenbelt Pathway runs along the western side of Hayden Road whereas most of the sporting facilities lie across the street. There are several tunnels to keep you safe from speeding traffic should you desire to cross the road. Club SAR at the intersection of Camelback Road and Hayden Road has an indoor training facility for boxing, weights, and aerobic exercise.

The half mile between Camelback Road and Chaparral Road has just become the newest part of the entire Greenbelt. A former eye-sore, Villa Monterey Golf Course along the east side of Hayden Road has been commpletely remodeled into an open-space park. The newly created Camelback Park now covers both sides of Hayden Road just north of Scottsdale Culinary Institute located on Camelback Road.

At Chaparral Road, the Greenbelt Pathway crosses Hayden Road and meets the fourth and final large park on the Greenbelt. Chaparral Park boasts a large lake that caters to fishing buffs and offers a wheelchair-accessible fishing pier. Within the lake, a small island harbors migratory birds and keeps them out of the reach of kids and dogs. The fishing pier is an excellent place to catch the reflection of a desert sunset over Camelback Mountain. North of the lake, pass the public pool and more baseball and soccer fields. Finish the 5-mile hike near the new water-treatment plant and off-leash dog park just south of McDonald Drive.

NEARBY ACTIVITIES

Located west of the Greenbelt on Osborn Road, Scottsdale Stadium hosts the San Francisco Giants' spring training. Tempe Town Lake lies at the southern tip of the Greenbelt and offers additional recreational activities. Camelback Mountain (pages 21 and 26) and Papago Park (page 44) provide other hiking trails and are both within 3 miles of the Greenbelt.

16 MCDOWELL MOUNTAIN REGIONAL PARK: SCENIC TRAIL

KEY AT-A-GLANCE INFORMATION

LENGTH: 4.5 miles

ELEVATION GAIN: 300 feet

CONFIGURATION: Loop

DIFFICULTY: Easy

SCENERY: McDowell Mountains, Four Peaks, desert

EXPOSURE: Completely exposed

TRAFFIC: Light

TRAIL SURFACE: Sand, gravel, packed dirt

HIKING TIME: 2.5 hours

WATER REQUIREMENT: 1.5 quarts

SEASON: Year-round; hot in summer

ACCESS: Open 6 a.m.–8 p.m. (10 p.m. Fri.–Sat.); trail closes at sunset; $6 per vehicle entrance fee

MAPS: USGS Fort McDowell; park map available at the entrance and visitor center

FACILITIES: Toilet, drinking water, picnic areas, visitor center, horse corral, competitive track, youth camp

DOGS: Yes, leashed at all times

COMMENTS: This easy hilltop hike offers excellent views of the McDowell Mountains and Four Peaks. For more information, visit www.maricopa.gov/parks/mcdowell, or call (480) 471-3523.

GPS Trailhead Coordinates

UTM Zone 12S

Easting 0433480

Northing 3727907

Latitude N33°41.448'

Longitude W111°43.105'

IN BRIEF

McDowell Mountain Regional Park covers more than 21,000 acres of desert wilderness at the base of the McDowell Mountains. Take the easy Scenic Trail to a hilltop to enjoy expansive views of surrounding mountains and plains.

DESCRIPTION

Though named for the McDowell Mountains, this large regional park doesn't actually contain much of its namesake mountain range. Instead, the park spans 21,099 acres of mostly low-lying desert plains encircled by Tonto National Forest, the Fort McDowell Indian Reservation, Fountain Hills, and the McDowell Mountains. What the park lacks in altitude, it makes up for in variety. More than 50 miles of multiuse trails offer hikers, equestrians, and bikers plenty of recreational opportunities. A competitive track and youth camps round out the park's diverse offerings.

Scenic Trail is the perfect introductory hike to McDowell Mountain Regional Park. Winding around Lousley Hills at the park's eastern edge, this pleasant loop trail takes visitors through a sandy wash and then atop

Directions

From Loop 101, exit onto Shea Boulevard. Drive east on Shea Boulevard 9 miles, and turn north onto Fountain Hills Boulevard. Follow Fountain Hills Boulevard, which eventually becomes McDowell Mountain Park Drive, 7.5 miles to McDowell Mountain Regional Park. Turn west into the park, and pay the entrance fee at the gate. Continue along the main road inside the park 3 miles, and then turn right onto Schallmo Drive, which terminates at the large trailhead staging area.

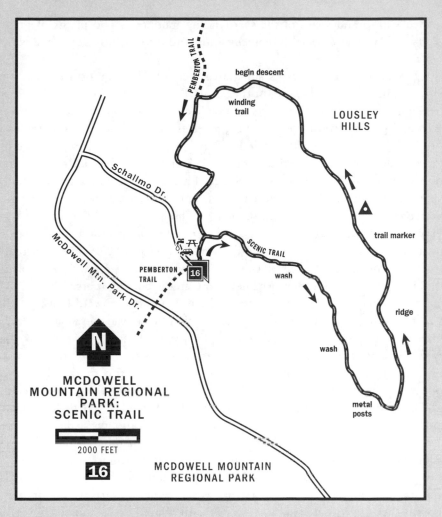

PEMBERTON TRAIL

begin descent

winding trail

LOUSLEY HILLS

Schallmo Dr.

trail marker

McDowell Mtn. Park Dr.

SCENIC TRAIL

PEMBERTON TRAIL

16

wash

ridge

wash

N

MCDOWELL MOUNTAIN REGIONAL PARK: SCENIC TRAIL

2000 FEET

metal posts

16

MCDOWELL MOUNTAIN REGIONAL PARK

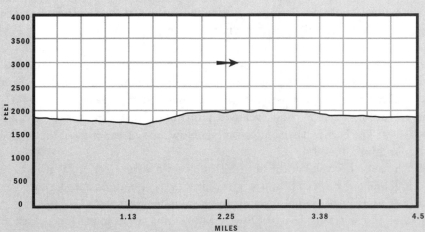

FEET

4000
3500
3000
2500
2000
1500
1000
500
0

1.13   2.25   3.38   4.5

MILES

a ridge with grand views of the surrounding mountains and plains. Beginner hikers and families especially appreciate this trail for its gentle slopes and varied scenery.

From the large trailhead staging area, begin by hiking north on the Pemberton Trail, the park's longest. At the Scenic Trail junction, turn right and leave the Pemberton Trail. The smooth and level Scenic Trail meanders across sparsely vegetated plains toward Lousley Hills, a series of rambling slopes to the east. Stroll along jojoba bushes, triangle-leaf bursage, and mesquite trees, and cross a dry wash at 0.3 miles from the trailhead. Behind you, the McDowell Mountains span the southwestern skyline. Rocky East End Peak and antenna-studded Thompson Peak stand out against the horizon. You can even see the steep service road reaching the saddle to the left of Thompson Peak. This service road served as a challenging hike to the summit of Thompson Peak before development in Fountain Hills overran the trailhead. The city of Scottsdale is currently developing plans to turn the McDowell Mountains into a preserve with plenty of public access. Look for exciting new trails in the coming years.

Continue past the remnants of an old fence, and hike toward Lousley Hills, which are covered in brittlebush and accentuated by occasional saguaros. At 0.5 miles, turn left and enter a wide and sandy wash. The soft sand cushions your every step but can also take the spring out of your stride. Follow the wash 0.2 miles toward the southeast amid some driftwood. There a trail marker directs you to leave the wash and head to the right. Continue hiking into the gap between the hills, toward the Superstition Mountains off in the distance. Triangle-leaf bursage and canyon ragweed shrubs line the trail, and many drooping cadaverous trees and limbs litter the landscape. It's hard to imagine how these plants can perish along the wash while their brethren on the drier slopes seem to thrive.

At a fork in the trail near 0.9 miles, bear left and follow the triangular trail markers mounted on stubby rebar posts. The trail returns to the dry wash shortly thereafter. Watch for the strategically placed tree limbs blocking off errant paths. Continue along the streambed until a sign directs you to break away from it at 1.2 miles. A tenth-mile farther, the trail crosses another dry wash near some metal posts and then climbs up the left bank of the basin.

At 1.5 miles, contour around the tip of the hill and continue the gradual ascent toward the north among fields of brittlebush and with Four Peaks to the east. Taking this loop counterclockwise saves the best scenery for last. As you gain elevation, views expand ever wider until you reach the top of a ridge at 1,975 feet. The earlier basin and wash lie below, and open views of the McDowell Mountains abound.

The next 1.5 miles of the Scenic Trail is my favorite section. Walking along the ridgeline of Lousley Hills, it seems that views get better around every corner and over every little bump. It's amazing how much perspective you gain in just 300 feet of elevation. The McDowell Mountains, especially jagged East End Peak, stand out sharply against the desert plains at their feet. Black Mountain

A lone saguaro in McDowell Mountain Regional Park braves the approaching storm.

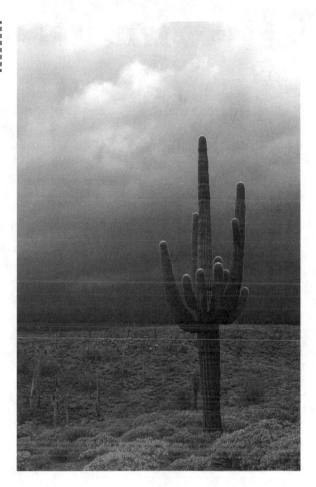

and the New River Mesa can be seen to the northwest, while the massive Mazatzal Range lies to the northeast. Scenic basins flank the trail as you hike along the ridgeline.

Near 3.3 miles, the trail begins to descend a winding path with the wide-open plains in front of you. Cacti are conspicuously absent here. Scenic Trail terminates at a second junction with the Pemberton Trail. Turn left here, and return to the trailhead along the Pemberton Trail for a total hiking distance of 4.5 miles.

NEARBY ACTIVITIES

McDowell Mountain Regional Park offers excellent trails for mountain biking. The Pemberton, Stoneman Wash, Tonto Tank, and Bluff trails form large loops that cover the plains and hills inside the park. The nearby Fountain Hills' main attraction is its 600-foot man-made fountain; it provides another idyllic setting for a casual hike.

17 PASS MOUNTAIN TRAIL

KEY AT-A-GLANCE INFORMATION

LENGTH: 7.4 miles

ELEVATION GAIN: 730 feet

CONFIGURATION: Loop

DIFFICULTY: Easy

SCENERY: Desert, mountain views, city views

EXPOSURE: Mostly exposed, little shade

TRAFFIC: Light

TRAIL SURFACE: Packed dirt, gravel, rock

HIKING TIME: 3.5 hours

WATER REQUIREMENT: 2.5 quarts

SEASON: Year-round; hot in summer

ACCESS: Open 6 a.m.–8 p.m. (10 p.m. Fri.–Sat.); trail closes at sunset; $6 per vehicle, no charge at alternate trailhead

MAPS: USGS Apache Junction

FACILITIES: Restrooms, drinking water, picnic areas, camping, archery range; no services at alternate trailhead

DOGS: Yes, leashed at all times

COMMENTS: For park information, visit www.maricopa.gov/parks/ usery or call (480) 984-0032.

GPS Trailhead Coordinates

UTM Zone 12S

Easting   0443645

Northing   3703814

Latitude   N33°28.444'

Longitude W111°36.441'

IN BRIEF

Pass Mountain Trail forms a large loop around its namesake landmark in the East Valley. This pleasant and easy trail offers grand views of the Goldfield Mountains, Four Peaks, and the Superstition Mountains.

DESCRIPTION

Usery Mountain Regional Park borders Tonto National Forest and encompasses 3,648 acres of mountain preserves at the western end of the Goldfield Mountains. The Wind Cave Trail (page 123) is the main attraction in the park and draws the most visitors. However, those who take the time to explore Pass Mountain Trail, one of the best loop hikes in the area, experience expansive views to the east that easily outshine the Wind Cave's panoramas.

Pass Mountain Trail begins inside Usery Park, but most of it actually runs through Tonto National Forest. Encircling the mountain of the same name, Pass Mountain Trail

----

Directions ——————————————————➤

From US 60, exit onto Ellsworth Road. Drive north 6.5 miles and then turn east into Usery Mountain Regional Park. Pay at the entrance station. Once inside the park, proceed 1 mile and turn left onto Wind Cave Drive. Park at the Wind Cave Trailhead, and access the Pass Mountain Trail here. The official trailhead is located at the horse staging area deeper inside the park.

To reach the alternate trailhead, exit US 60 onto Signal Butte Road. Drive north on Signal Butte Road 0.5 miles, then east on Southern Avenue 1 mile, and finally north on Meridian Road 5 miles. The alternate trailhead is at the end of Meridian Road. You can avoid paying the Usery Park entrance fee here, but there are no services.

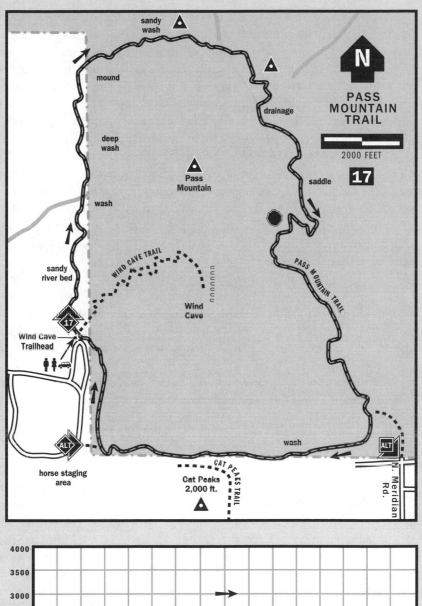

PASS
MOUNTAIN
TRAIL

2000 FEET

17

sandy
wash

mound

deep
wash

wash

sandy
river bed

Wind Cave
Trailhead

horse staging
area

Pass
Mountain

WIND CAVE TRAIL

Wind
Cave

drainage

saddle

PASS MOUNTAIN TRAIL

wash

CAT PEAKS TRAIL

Cat Peaks
2,000 ft.

N. Meridian Rd.

ALT

ALT

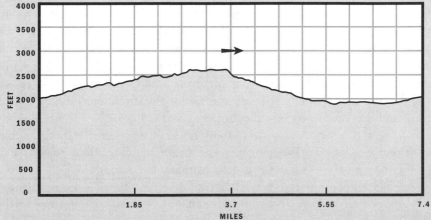

takes visitors from the desert floor, through dry washes, across mountainsides, and up to a saddle with outstanding views. The trail is easy to navigate and gentle on the lungs and legs, making it ideal for a family day hike.

I prefer to start from the Wind Cave Trailhead for this loop, though the official trailhead is located at the horse staging area. Those in the know may also use the alternate trailhead located on national-forest land to avoid paying the park's entrance fee. Note that hiking the loop clockwise avoids a steep climb and renders the 730 feet of elevation gain almost insignificant.

First find Pass Mountain Trail at the signed junction just north of the Wind Cave Trailhead restrooms. Turn left here to begin the clockwise loop. The initial stretch of the loop runs north along the park boundary in the shadows of Pass Mountain. As you hike across dry washes and through typical Sonoran Desert scenery, take note of the huge "Phoenix" arrow on Usery Mountain to the west. The Air Explorers Boy Scout Post built it in the 1950s to guide lost pilots. We can only hope that no pilot ever needed the sign for navigation.

The trail climbs almost imperceptibly as it traverses the valley floor and goes in and out of dry washes. Look for typical desert plants such as the giant saguaro, teddy bear cholla, brittlebush, and jojoba. Red chuparosa flowers display their tubular shapes along sandy wash bottoms and often attract hummingbirds. Literally translated as "rose sucker," the word chuparosa also means hummingbird in Spanish.

At 0.9 miles, the trail draws near the park's boundary fence. Soon after reaching the fence, descend into a deep drainage and climb up the other side to the top of a mound. If you happen to be here on the hour, look northwest into the gap between Usery Mountain and One Mountain for Fountain Hills' famous geyser jetting high into the air. The trail bends to the east and crosses the fence into Tonto National Forest at 1.5 miles from the trailhead. Continue hiking east along the desert floor and cross a wide wash bed into a stand of chain-fruit cholla. Along with the teddy bear cholla, these prickly plants share the common name "jumping cholla," indicating that the slightest wind can cause their sharp needles to jump out at you. Don't worry; the trail leaves plenty of buffer space.

The trail ascends a gentle slope from the valley floor to the top of a mound approximately 2 miles from the trailhead. Suddenly, a stunning vista of the Goldfield Mountains springs into view. A wide and lush valley opens in front of you, and the larger Salt River basin is visible to the northeast. After winter storms, snow-capped Four Peaks complete the scenic panorama. Proceed east along the trail with the yellowish volcanic Goldfield Mountains directly in front of you, and descend slowly into the large basin at 2.4 miles.

The next mile or so along Pass Mountain Trail is the most scenic stretch on the entire circuit, offering sweeping views of the surrounding hills as the trail itself hugs the steep northeastern slopes of Pass Mountain. Winding along the contours of the mountainside, the trail stays relatively level and provides ever-expanding views around each corner. Devoid of tall saguaros, the landscape features smaller

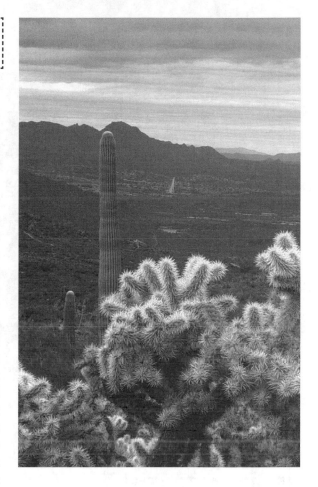

Chain-fruit chollas accent a distant view of the fountain in Fountain Hills along Pass Mountain Trail.

bushes such as palo verde, brittlebush, and jojoba. After a wet winter their flowers paint the slopes a brilliant gold.

The trail eventually bends south and comes to a wide, flat saddle at 3.6 miles and 2,600 feet. A spur trail takes off east along the northern side of the next hill, but stay on the main trail heading south. A wide view of East Mesa and Apache Junction opens straight ahead. Just over the saddle, the trail dives steeply into the next basin near some large rock outcroppings. Hiking the loop clockwise ensures that you descend this 500-foot hill instead of climbing it. Notice the brilliant contrast of colors here among the green plants, chartreuse lichen, yellowish volcanic tuff, and rust-colored rocks.

At 4 miles, pass between two large boulders where the western end of the majestic Superstition Mountains comes into view. The trail slowly curves around the basin and heads southeast toward the sprawling city, exposing more and more of the view toward the Superstitions. At 5.3 miles, an unmarked spur trail forks to the east, crosses a deep wash, and leads to the alternate trailhead at the end of Meridian Road. If you parked at that trailhead, look carefully because there are several small side trails here.

The trail soon bends toward the west and then skirts the southern end of Pass Mountain and the edge of Tonto National Forest. You can almost see into the homes across the street as you hike west on noticeably rockier terrain. Cross a dry wash at 5.8 miles and then continue along a fence marking the Usery Park boundary. Pass the Cats Peak Trail junction a half mile later. After some more wash crossings, come to a sign that points to the Pass Mountain Trailhead at 6.8 miles. Take a left here if you parked at the horse staging area and the official

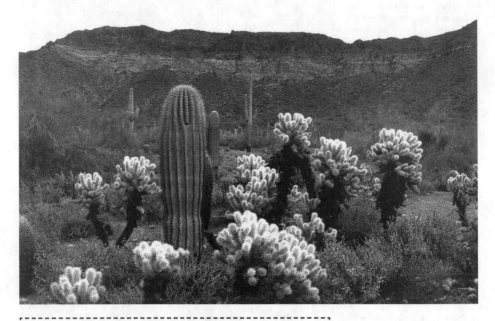

Teddy bear chollas point to the strip of volcanic tuff on Pass Mountain.

trailhead. Otherwise, follow the Pass Mountain Trail north for an additional 0.6 miles, where it re-enters the park to complete the loop near the Wind Cave Trailhead.

NEARBY ACTIVITIES

The popular Wind Cave Trail (page 123) begins at the same trailhead inside Usery Park. The Superstition Mountains to the east present excellent hiking opportunities. Many trails outlined in this book are located in the Superstitions. Salt River Recreation, north of Usery Park, caters to those who wish to relax by floating down the Salt River on an oversized inner tube.

PINNACLE PEAK TRAIL 18

IN BRIEF

Pinnacle Peak Trail offers northeastern valley residents a wonderful place to exercise after work or to spend a weekend afternoon with the family. The trail is scenic and well maintained and has just enough elevation gain to warrant a moderate difficulty rating.

DESCRIPTION

The 3,170-foot Pinnacle Peak rises sharply out of the desert floor like a needle. It is one of the most distinctive landmarks in the Phoenix area, and many resorts have situated themselves in its shadows. Once the rustic fringe of civilization, as evidenced by gritty joints like Greasewood Flat, this area is now a thriving suburbia replete with affluent new homes and golf courses. This interesting juxtaposition of the old west and new development, raw desert and urban sprawl gives the Pinnacle Peak foothills an alluring charm.

Pinnacle Peak is the analogue of Camelback Mountain or Piestewa Peak for those living in the northeastern part of the valley. The recently opened Pinnacle Peak Park and its main trail belong to the City of Scottsdale, which has done a superb job of packing the desert experience into a 3.5-mile out-and-back hike. When you arrive at the park, stop by the visitor center to pick up a trail map and a copy of the native-plant guide, which

KEY AT-A-GLANCE INFORMATION

LENGTH: 3.5 miles
ELEVATION GAIN: 550 feet
CONFIGURATION: Out-and-back
DIFFICULTY: Moderate
SCENERY: Pinnacle Peak, desert, golf courses, city views, desert plants
EXPOSURE: Limited shade, mostly exposed
TRAFFIC: Heavy
TRAIL SURFACE: Packed dirt
HIKING TIME: 1.5 hours
WATER REQUIREMENT: 1.5 quarts
SEASON: Year-round; hot in summer
ACCESS: Open 5:30 a.m.–7:30 p.m.; free parking
MAPS: USGS McDowell Peak, trail map available from visitor center
FACILITIES: Restroom, drinking water, ramada, picnic area, visitor center
DOGS: No
COMMENTS: Pinnacle Peak Trail is a popular hike for northeastern valley residents. For more information, visit www.scottsdaleaz.gov/parks/pinnacle or call (480) 312-0990.

Directions

From Loop 101, exit at Princess Drive. Drive east then north on Pima Road 4.5 miles, then turn east onto Happy Valley Road. Continue 2 miles and turn north on Alma School Road. Drive 1 mile and turn west on Pinnacle Peak Parkway. Drive 0.5 miles to Pinnacle Peak Park.

GPS Trailhead Coordinates

UTM Zone 12S
Easting   0420360
Northing 3732112
Latitude   N33°43.670'
Longitude W111°51.620'

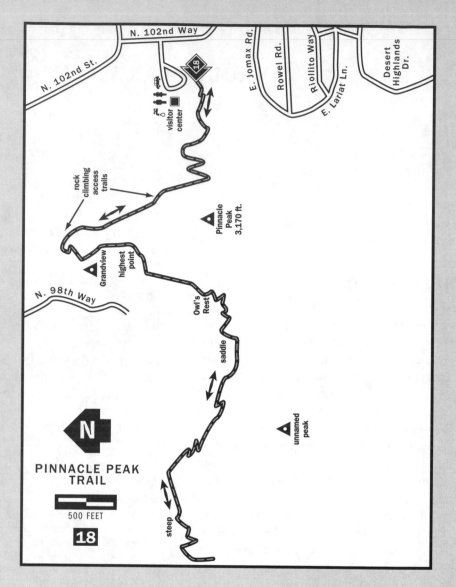

N. 102nd Way

N. 102nd St.

E. Jomax Rd.

Rowel Rd.

Riollito Way

E. Lariat Ln.

Desert Highlands Dr.

18

visitor center

rock climbing access trails

Pinnacle Peak 3,170 ft.

Grandview

highest point

N. 98th Way

Owl's Rest

saddle

unnamed peak

N

PINNACLE PEAK TRAIL

500 FEET

18

steep

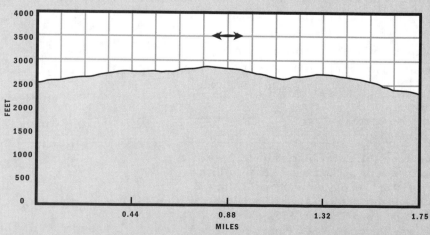

4000
3500
3000
2500
2000
1500
1000
500
0

FEET

0.44   0.88   1.32   1.75

MILES

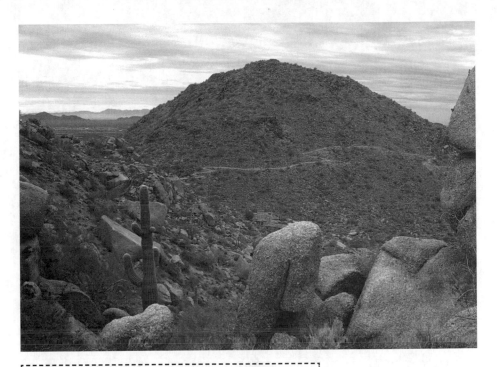

Trailside boulders frame a distant hill along Pinnacle Peak Trail.

explains the desert flora along the way. This interpretive trail tries to be all things to all people, and for the most part succeeds. Hikers share the trail with joggers, rock climbers, tourists, families, and on rare occasions even equestrians.

Begin the hike near the visitor center at a well-marked trailhead in the shadows of Pinnacle Peak. The wide and manicured trail swirls around the base of the mountain among a rich assortment of desert flora that an arboretum would be proud to own. Numbered signs identify various plants such as Christmas cholla and desert mistletoe, two of the most interesting species. The Christmas cholla is a cactus but looks like a shrub, and desert mistletoe is a parasitic plant that lives in leguminous host trees like mesquite, acacia, and palo verde, plants that, along with the giant saguaro cactus, define the Sonoran Desert. Refer to your plant guide for more detailed explanations.

After one-quarter mile, the trail begins to ascend some switchbacks, overlooking the visitor center, parking lot, and northern Scottsdale. The silhouette of Four Peaks graces the eastern horizon. At 0.4 miles, the trail levels out and heads northwest. A small side trail on the left allows rock climbers with ropes and harnesses to access the craggy summit of Pinnacle Peak. If you are not Spiderman, remain on the main trail and head toward the smaller hills directly in front of you. Another rock-climbing access trail splits off to the right near the northernmost part of the trail. The Pinnacle Peak Trail makes a 180-degree bend and climbs south to the Grandview lookout at 0.65 miles. Rest here and

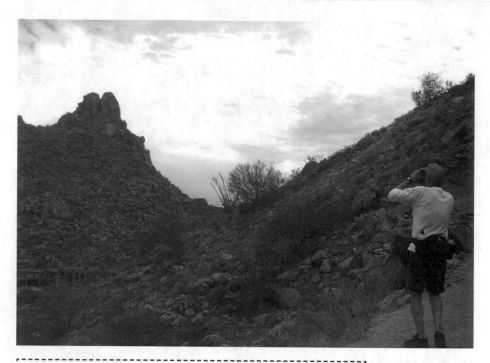

A hiker pauses to admire the 3,170-foot summit along the Pinnacle Peak Trail.

survey the landscape below. Lush green golf courses and blue lakes contrast sharply with the brown desert and sand-colored houses. Embedded in the circular brickwork like tick marks on a clock face, etched wooden logs point to numerous landmarks in the distance, such as Four Peaks and Granite Mountain. Shortly after Grandview, the trail climbs to its highest point at 2,889 feet.

Owl's Rest, at 0.9 miles, is another scenic lookout, this time with nautilus-shaped brickwork. It is perched above a steep hill and provides a convenient rest stop on the return hike. Descend the scenic switchbacks west of Owl's Rest, ducking around large boulders, to a saddle point in the trail at 2,625 feet. The trail climbs once again, up the flank of an unnamed 3,000-foot hill west of Pinnacle Peak. Gauge your progress by the obvious distance markers located at every quarter mile. Near the 1.25-mile marker, the trail reaches its second crest at 2,725 feet and then flattens out.

The final half mile of the Pinnacle Peak Trail is the steepest part of the hike. It drops 400 feet via switchbacks to a shady rest spot at the western boundary of Pinnacle Peak Park. Should you choose to continue hiking in that direction beyond the park boundary another 0.3 miles, you would end up on the Jomax Trail located behind a housing development on Jomax Road. Most people turn around at the park boundary after a good rest because the first half-mile climb on the return trip will surely raise the heart rate. Return to the visitor center along the same trail.

NEARBY ACTIVITIES

Rock climbers with proper equipment can scale Pinnacle Peak via a special climber's access trail at 0.4 miles on the Pinnacle Peak Trail. Tom's Thumb (page 118) in the McDowell Mountains presents a challenging hike to another popular rock-climbing destination. Nearby Pinnacle Peak Patio is a western-themed restaurant once hailed as the largest of its kind in the world and famous for its policy of shearing off the neckties of any patrons who dare to enter wearing one. Reatta Pass and Greasewood Flat offer more old-time western fun another mile north along Alma School Road.

19 SUNRISE TRAIL

KEY AT-A-GLANCE INFORMATION

LENGTH: 5 miles

ELEVATION GAIN: 1,350 feet

CONFIGURATION: One way or out-and-back to summit from either end

DIFFICULTY: Moderate

SCENERY: City panorama, desert, McDowell Sonoran Preserve

EXPOSURE: Completely exposed

TRAFFIC: Moderate–heavy

TRAIL SURFACE: Packed dirt, gravel, rocky

HIKING TIME: 3 hours

WATER REQUIREMENT: 2 quarts

SEASON: Year-round; hot in summer

ACCESS: Open sunrise to sunset; free parking

MAPS: USGS Sawik Mountain, Trailhead plaque, McDowell Sonoran Preserve map

FACILITIES: Lost Dog Wash: Restrooms, water, trail volunteers on weekends; Sunrise Access Area: water

DOGS: Yes, leashed at all times

COMMENTS: Newer trail, but quickly gaining popularity. Visit www.scottsdaleaz.gov/Preserve for more info.

GPS Trailhead Coordinates

UTM Zone   12S

Easting   0424753

Northing   3717956

Latitude   N33°36.028'

Longitude W111°48.704'

IN BRIEF

Fast becoming one of the most popular in-town hikes, Sunrise Trail is a treat for your senses. Enjoy unspoiled desert in scenic McDowell Sonoran Preserve, take in fantastic views of Scottsdale and Fountain Hills, and challenge yourself on a superbly maintained trail to 3,069-foot Sunrise Peak.

DESCRIPTION

Constructed in 2004, Sunrise Trail in the McDowell Mountains hails as one of the newest trails on the Phoenix hiking circuit. Since then, Sunrise has been steadily gaining popularity, first with nearby residents in Scottsdale and Fountain Hills, then as word of mouth spread, with Phoenicians in general. The trail's success comes as no surprise. Its ease of access, proximity to town, multiple trailheads, stunning scenery and views, and perfect balance between challenge and enjoyment appeal to a wide range of hikers. If you can't find something to love about this trail, you might be having a really bad day.

Located on the southeastern tip of McDowell Sonoran Preserve, Sunrise Peak

Directions

Lost Dog Wash Trailhead: Exit Loop 101 at Shea Boulevard and drive east on Shea 4.5 miles to 124th Street. Turn north onto 124th Street and proceed 1.2 miles to the large Lost Dog Wash Trailhead parking area.

Sunrise Access Area: Exit Loop 101 at Shea Boulevard and drive east on Shea 6 miles to 136th Street. Drive north on 136th Street 0.5 miles and turn east onto Via Linda. Follow Via Linda east 1.5 miles to the Sunrise Access Area.

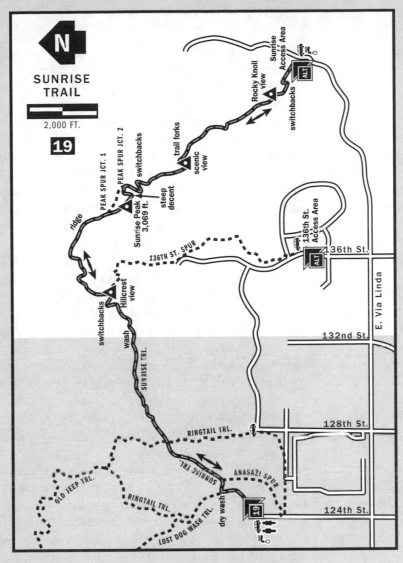

N

SUNRISE
TRAIL

2,000 FT.

19

Rocky Knoll
view

Sunrise
Access Area

switchbacks

trail forks

scenic
view

PEAK SPUR JCT. 1

PEAK SPUR JCT. 2

switchbacks

ridge

Sunrise Peak
3,069 ft.

steep
decent

136th St.
Access Area

136TH ST. SPUR

136th St.

ALT

Hillcrest
view

switchbacks

wash

E. Via Linda

SUNRISE TRL.

132nd St.

128th St.

RINGTAIL TRL.

SUNRISE TRL.

OLD JEEP TRL.

RINGTAIL TRL.

ANASAZI SPUR

dry wash

124th St.

19

LOST DOG WASH TRL.

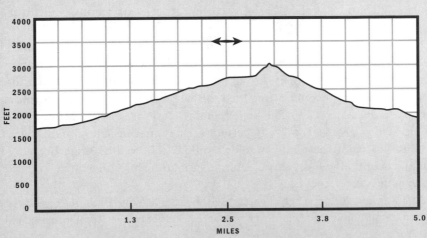

4000
3500
3000
2500
2000
1500
1000
500
0

FEET

1.3   2.5   3.8   5.0

MILES

straddles the mountainous divide between Scottsdale and Fountain Hills. Sunrise Trail skirts this summit and spans a significant portion of the southern McDowells overlooking heavily populated suburbs. Four trailheads service this trail and offer numerous ways to customize your hike. This chapter covers a complete west to east traversal of Sunrise Trail, including a detour to Sunrise Peak. Of course, one drawback to hiking one-way is that it requires a car shuttle.

Stash a car at the Sunrise Access Area, then drive to the well-appointed Lost Dog Wash Access Area located at the end of 124th Street north of Shea Boulevard. Lost Dog Wash was the first major access area built for the preserve and provides access to the southern McDowells. On weekends, volunteers from McDowell Sonoran Conservancy greet visitors there and offer general information, trail maps, helpful advice, safety tips, and even organized hikes. The conservancy is a nonprofit organization that drove the creation of McDowell Sonoran Preserve and partnered closely with Scottsdale city government to fund, acquire, build, and manage the preserve, which when finished will designate 36,000 acres of desert wilderness for conservation. Plans for future trails and access areas are still being finalized, with construction of additional facilities slated to continue for many years.

Begin your hike at the back of the building area and strike out on Lost Dog Wash Trail amid Sonoran desert flora. Brittlebush and palo verde line the wide dirt path. The trail turns north next to a small hill and heads toward antenna-studded Thompson Peak in the distance. At 0.2 miles, cross a dry creek bed and turn right to find the official start of Sunrise Trail. Trail signs in the preserve are easy to find, easy to read, and very informative.

The west half of Sunrise Trail takes a gentle approach to Sunrise Peak, meandering through open desert before climbing toward the summit. Hike along the dry wash for a short distance, but soon you begin a gentle incline. At the next trail junction with Anasazi Spur, stay left to remain on Sunrise Trail, and head northeast toward a saddle between rugged peaks. In front of you, all signs of city life disappear and you are engulfed in the desert hiking experience. Hardy creosote bushes, barrel cacti, and thorny ocotillos dominate the landscape.

Reach Ringtail Trail at 0.7 miles from the trailhead. The second trailhead with access to Sunrise Trail can be found 0.5 miles south of this junction on 128th Street. Continue straight through the trail junction and hike deeper into the preserve, leaving behind a fine view of Scottsdale and distant Camelback Mountain (pages 21 and 26). The slope remains gentle as you hike to and on top of an elevated ridge at 1.3 miles. In certain springs after decent rainfall, brittlebush blossoms paint these hills a golden yellow, followed by brightly colored cactus and ocotillo flowers a month later. A springtime hike on Sunrise Trail can be an exquisite experience.

At 1.8 miles, follow a set of sharp switchbacks as you climb out of the scenic drainage and land on a wide overlook at 2,550 feet in elevation. Sunrise Peak

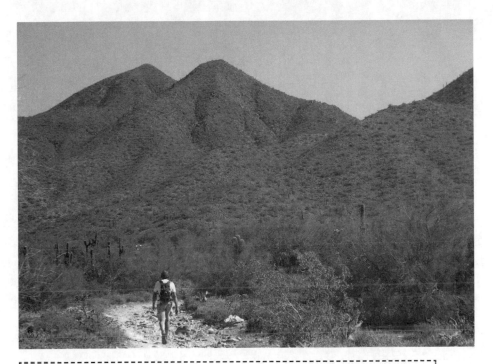

Chris Smith of Phoenix hikes deep into McDowell Sonoran Preserve along the Sunrise Trail.

comes into view in the distance, and you can trace the trail's profile as it cuts across the hill to the north. A narrower trail called 136th Street Spur can take you down to the housing subdivision where you'll find the third trailhead for this hike. But for now, remain on Sunrise Trail as it contours across the hillside. You have an open view toward Camelback, Piestewa Peak (pages 48 and 52), and the downtown Phoenix skyline. After steadily climbing 1,000 vertical feet, the trail finally levels off as it approaches the base of Sunrise Peak.

Find a signed junction with Sunrise Peak Spur at 2.8 miles from the trailhead. This spur trail forms a quarter-mile detour to the summit of Sunrise Peak and then rejoins Sunrise Trail at another junction. Take the spur trail here and head south toward the summit. The spur trail is narrow, rough, and steep, but thankfully short. Upon gaining the summit, a magnificent panoramic view unfolds. To the east, Four Peaks (page 220 Browns Peak) towers over Fountain Hills. If you arrive just past the hour, you'll be treated to a fountain show. Weaver's Needle (page 162 Peralta), Superstition Mountains, and Red Mountain are all visible. To the south and west, metropolitan Phoenix stretches out for many miles. Other rugged McDowell peaks round out the panorama.

The eastern half of Sunrise Trail differs greatly from the western half. It's considerably steeper, more mountainous, and runs through a narrow canyon instead of open desert, yielding a more intimate setting for your descent. For those looking for a more challenging climb, consider starting from the eastern

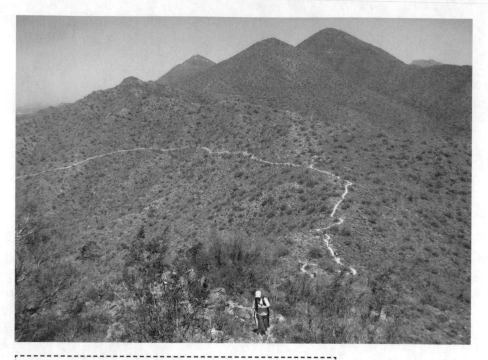

Laurie McGill of Gilbert approaches Sunrise Peak from the Sunrise Trail.

end instead. Be careful though, gravel and steep slopes require you to step judi-
ciously. Follow the spur trail east until it intersects Sunrise Trail once more.
Then, turn right and head down a cactus-laden hill. Tall stands of saguaros and
clusters of fuzzy teddy bear cholla line the trail.

Pass a scenic overlook at 3.8 miles from the trailhead. (This would be a great
place for a rest if you hike up the eastern side.) Teddy bear chollas frame a distant
view of the city below. Below the overlook, Sunrise Trail forks for a short distance
but soon rejoins itself. The steep descent soon gives way to rolling hills, and you
can lift your eyes to admire the scenery again. Reach the smaller Sunrise Access
Area at the end of Via Linda Street, a distance of 5 miles from Lost Dog Wash
Trailhead. Hopefully, your shuttle vehicle is waiting for your arrival.

NEARBY ACTIVITIES

Lost Dog Wash and Ringtail trails in the southern McDowells are also accessible from Lost Dog Wash Trailhead. Frank Lloyd Wright's Taliesin West studio
is located within a short distance of these trails. Other trails in the McDowell
Sonoran Preserve offer longer excursions into the interior of the preserve. Tom's
Thumb (page 118) in the northern part of the preserve is a popular rock-climbing
destination. Nearby McDowell Mountain Regional Park (page 90) contributes
even more options for hiking and biking.

TELEGRAPH PASS TRAIL
AND KIWANIS TRAIL

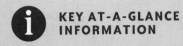
20

IN BRIEF

The only trailhead on the southern side of South Mountain, Telegraph Pass is popular among Ahwatukee residents. It begins as a gentle stroll along the foothills and climbs to the top of Telegraph Pass. Some Hohokam petroglyphs can be seen along this trail.

DESCRIPTION

Some Phoenicians consider the community of Ahwatukee a giant cul-de-sac. In a sense, they are right. Bounded by South Mountain and the Gila River Indian Reservation, the only practical way into and out of trendy Ahwatukee Foothills is via Interstate 10 on its eastern side, which explains the seemingly perpetual traffic jams on said freeway during rush hour. Sometimes it seems quicker hiking to downtown than driving to it. Silly as it may be, I'm sure many frustrated Ahwatukee commuters must have contemplated that option while sitting in traffic. The hypothetical shortcut they would take through South Mountain Park is via Telegraph Pass, which bisects the 11-mile-long mountainous barrier at a point in line with Phoenix's Central Avenue. In fact, during the 1800s, the Army Signal Corps chose this very pass as the optimal route for a telegraph line from Maricopa Wells to Phoenix, and then onto the territorial capital of Prescott. Today, Telegraph Pass is still a prominent and popular saddle in South Mountain Park.

Directions

Exit I-10 onto Chandler Boulevard or Ray Road. Drive west 3.3 miles until these roads intersect. Continue west on Chandler Boulevard 1.75 miles to Desert Foothills Parkway. Turn north onto Desert Foothills Parkway and then follow it 1.2 miles to the trailhead parking lot.

KEY AT-A-GLANCE INFORMATION

LENGTH: 2.4 miles (optional Kiwanis Trail, add 2 miles)

ELEVATION GAIN: 540 feet

CONFIGURATION: Out-and-back

DIFFICULTY: Easy to moderate

SCENERY: South Mountain, city panorama, desert

EXPOSURE: Early-morning and late-afternoon shade; otherwise exposed

TRAFFIC: Heavy on Telegraph Pass, moderate on Kiwanis

TRAIL SURFACE: Pavement, gravel, crushed rock

HIKING TIME: 1.5 hours (optional Kiwanis Trail, add 1 hour)

WATER REQUIREMENT: 1.5 quarts

SEASON: Year-round; hot in summer

ACCESS: 5:30 a.m.–7:30 p.m.; free parking

MAPS: USGS Lone Butte, trailhead plaque

FACILITIES: Water, no toilet

DOGS: Yes, leashed at all times

COMMENTS: Pleasant hike to a scenic pass on South Mountain. For more information, visit http://phoenix.gov/parks/hikesoth.html.

GPS Trailhead Coordinates

UTM Zone 12S

Easting 0400780

Northing 3686826

Latitude N33°19.065'

Longitude W112°3.998'

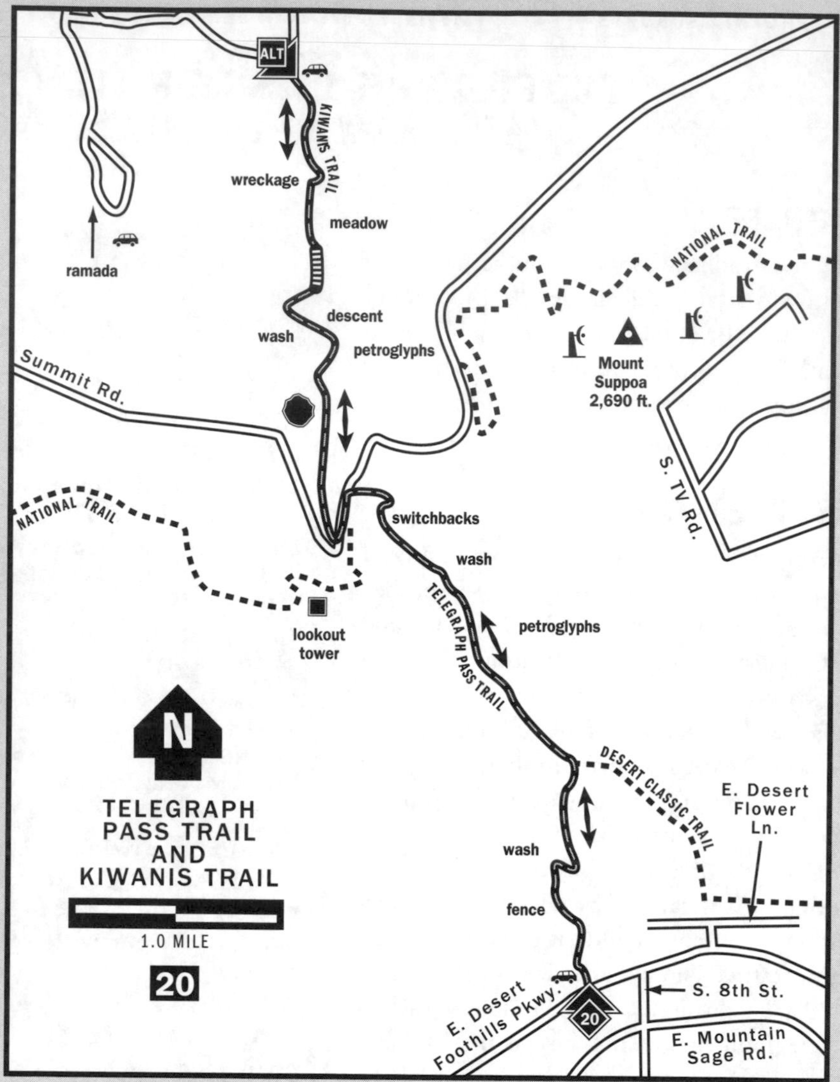

ALT
KIWANIS TRAIL
wreckage
meadow
ramada
descent
wash
petroglyphs
Summit Rd.
NATIONAL TRAIL
Mount Suppoa 2,690 ft.
S. TV Rd.
NATIONAL TRAIL
switchbacks
wash
TELEGRAPH PASS TRAIL
petroglyphs
lookout tower
N
DESERT CLASSIC TRAIL
E. Desert Flower Ln.
TELEGRAPH PASS TRAIL AND KIWANIS TRAIL
wash
fence
1.0 MILE
20
S. 8th St.
E. Desert Foothills Pkwy.
20
E. Mountain Sage Rd.

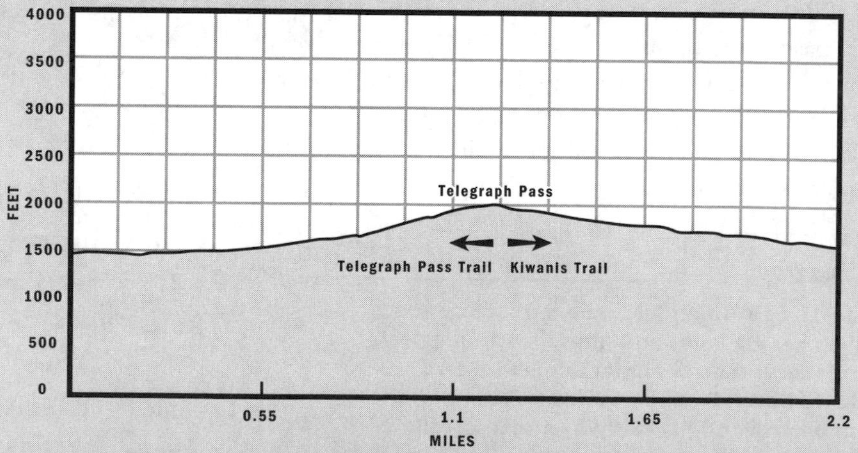

4000
3500
3000
2500
2000
1500
1000
500
0
FEET
Telegraph Pass
Telegraph Pass Trail
Kiwanis Trail
0.55
1.1
1.65
2.2
MILES

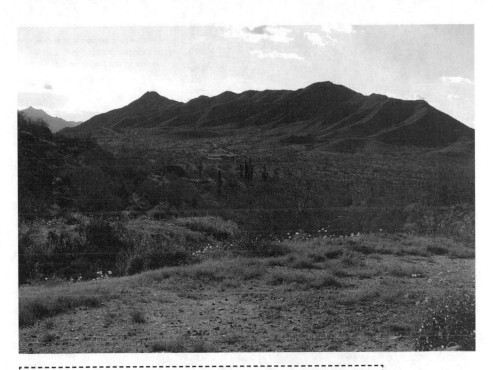

Maricopa Peak and the Ma Ha Tuak Range dominate the view from Kiwanis Trail.

The Telegraph Pass trailhead is the only South Mountain Park entrance on its southern side, making this hike extremely popular among Ahwatukee residents. On weekends, expect to see a steady stream of people, bikes, pets, and strollers on the trail. Don't let the crowds dissuade you; Telegraph Pass Trail is an excellent short hike. The trail leaves the edge of suburbia, runs through desert foothills and up a scenic canyon, and eventually ends at its namesake saddle. Views from Telegraph Pass are worth the 1.2-mile climb, and you also get a dose of history from the Hohokam petroglyphs along the way. If you have extra time, consider hiking over the saddle and down the Kiwanis Trail to visit the interior basin of South Mountain Park. From Telegraph Pass, you can also choose to hike National Trail in either direction for a higher vantage point.

Trailhead parking can be scarce during peak hours, but the trail's short length ensures a high turnover rate so you never have to wait too long for a parking spot. From the parking area, start out north on wide, level pavement that meanders around the fringes of nearby neighborhoods. Mount Suppoa and its forest of antennas loom directly ahead. A low hill, or more appropriately a berm, is on the western side of the sidewalk-like trail. When in season, coulter's lupine and phacelia blanket this hill, adding a dash of blue to the pleasant stroll. Near 0.2 miles, pass a fence that marks the park boundary, and then cross a dry wash a bit farther. The pavement ends at a wide spot 0.4 miles from the trailhead where the Desert Classic Trail begins. A popular mountain-biking trail, Desert Classic runs east 9 miles through the foothills and terminates in Pima Canyon

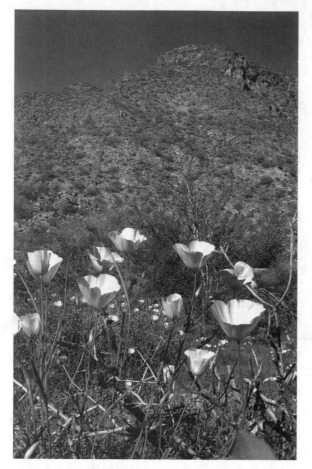

Mexican gold poppies bloom along the Telegraph Pass Trail with Mt. Suppoa in the background.

at the eastern end of South Mountain.

Turn left at the trail junction to continue down Telegraph Pass Trail, which heads northwest into the hills. Now hiking on dirt and gravel and gently climbing, aim for a gap left of the mountaintop. At 0.75 miles, stop to visit petroglyphs left by Hohokams more than 600 years ago. South Mountain Park contains many petroglyph sites, but perhaps none as accessible as this one. A trailside interpretive sign explains the history of the Hohokams and their culture.

Beyond the petroglyph pullout, Telegraph Pass Trail becomes steeper and rockier, especially after trail marker 4. As you hike up the canyon, crossing a dry wash several times, watch out for ambitious trail runners who jog up and down this narrow path daily. At 1.1 miles, begin ascending a few final switchbacks on the right side of the canyon to reach the 2,000-foot-high Telegraph Pass.

A major hub in South Mountain Park, Telegraph Pass bisects two mountain ranges and touches three major trails as well as Summit Road. This prominent saddle commands an impressive view toward Ahwatukee. National Trail runs east–west through the saddle along South Mountain's spine, whereas Telegraph Pass and Kiwanis trails straddle the pass longitudinally.

Though many people turn around at Telegraph Pass, consider spending an extra hour exploring the interior of South Mountain via the Kiwanis Trail. Similar in length and profile to Telegraph Pass Trail, Kiwanis Trail heads north toward the heart of the park. From where Telegraph Pass Trail meets Summit Road at the saddle, turn left and walk next to the road to the apex of a hairpin turn. Cross the road here to access Kiwanis Trail, which dives into a narrow canyon via a series of stony steps.

Kiwanis Trail descends steeply at first but soon levels out considerably. At 0.2 miles beyond Telegraph Pass, buildings in downtown Phoenix come into view in a V-shaped gap between the hills. Directly behind you on the hill, a stone lookout tower built by the Civilian Conservation Corps guards the surrounding landscape. The trail follows the canyon northward past large rock outcroppings that offer some afternoon shade. Though not as prominent as those found on Telegraph Pass Trail, some petroglyphs can be found under a palo verde tree near trail marker 5.

A half mile from the saddle, descend into and cross a dry wash. Then, negotiate some stairs at a steep section a bit farther on the trail, which soon flattens out as it follows the dry wash northward. Look for a rusted wreck in the wash just before the trail enters a small meadow. I always wonder how the wreckage got there amid these rugged hills. About 1 mile from Telegraph Pass, reach the Kiwanis Trailhead in the interior basin of South Mountain where you have a head-on view of the Ma Ha Tuak Range and the massive Sierra Estrella Mountains to the west. Though it would be convenient to shuttle a vehicle to this trailhead via South Mountain Park's Central Avenue entrance, the relatively short hike hardly justifies such a long drive. Return to Ahwatukee the way you came.

NEARBY ACTIVITIES

South Mountain hosts many hiking and biking trails including Alta (page 16), Desert Classic, Mormon (page 31), Ranger, and National (page 40). Many other recreational activities such as picnicking are also available. The Environmental Education Center, near the Central Avenue entrance, has a superb visitor center, complete with a three-dimensional model of the entire park.

21 THUNDERBIRD PARK: H-3 TRAIL

KEY AT-A-GLANCE INFORMATION

LENGTH: 3.6 miles

ELEVATION GAIN: 493 feet

CONFIGURATION: Loop

DIFFICULTY: Easy to moderate

SCENERY: City panoramas, Thunderbird Park, Hedgpeth Hills, desert

EXPOSURE: Completely exposed

TRAFFIC: High

TRAIL SURFACE: Gravel, rock, packed dirt

HIKING TIME: 1.5 hours

WATER REQUIREMENT: 1 quart

SEASON: Year-round; hot in summer

ACCESS: Sunrise to sunset; free parking

MAPS: USGS Hedgpeth Hills, trailhead plaque

FACILITIES: Picnic areas, restrooms, water

DOGS: Yes, leashed at all times

COMMENTS: Pleasant loop hike in Thunderbird Park. For more information, visit www.glendaleaz .com/ParksandRecreation/ parksandfacilities/ thunderbirdpark.cfm

----

GPS Trailhead Coordinates

UTM Zone   12S

Easting   0389885

Northing   3728269

Latitude   N33°41.426'

Longitude   W112°11.326'

IN BRIEF

The H-3 Loop in Thunderbird Park offers a great beginner's hike. This scenic trail takes visitors up the northernmost Hedgpeth Hill and provides ample open views of the city and surrounding mountains. During certain springs, golden brittlebush blossoms completely cover the Hedgpeth Hills.

DESCRIPTION

The City of Glendale acquired the land around Hedgpeth Hills during the 1950s to preserve them and then created Thunderbird Park, which was named after a nearby World War II fighter-training facility. Maricopa County improved the park and managed it until 1984 when the City of Glendale assumed operations. Today, the park is a bustling hotbed of activity for northwestern valley residents.

Thunderbird Park offers 1,185 acres of mountain preserves and approximately 20 miles of hiking trails. The trails and the hills they traverse are all named after Robert Hedgpeth, an early settler in the area. Each trail is designated by "H" and a number. The H-3 Trail and a small section of the H-1 form a convenient loop that is particularly popular among Thunderbird Park patrons. The loop traces a heart-shaped path over and around the northernmost Hedgpeth Hill and presents beautiful panoramic views of the park and the surrounding housing developments.

Directions ⟶

Exit Loop 101 onto 59th Avenue. Drive north on 59th Avenue 1.5 miles to the main entrance of Thunderbird Park, which is just past a hillside amphitheater. Turn west into the park and park at any of the lots near the amphitheater.

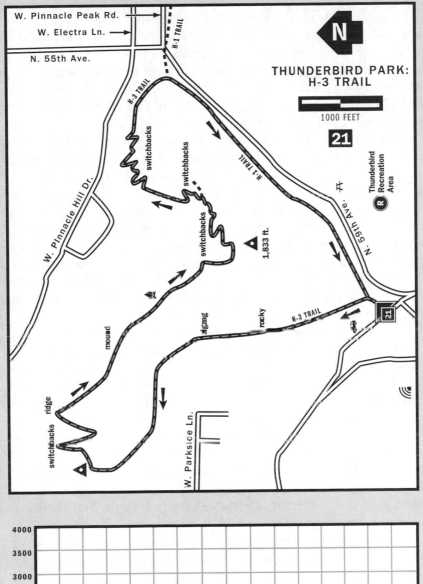

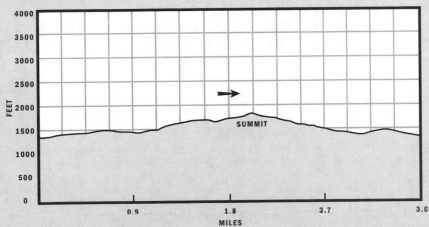

To begin this loop hike, first find the information plaque on the H-1 Trail near the main entrance to Thunderbird Park. Located east of the amphitheater and just south of the first parking area inside the park, this plaque is the ideal place to begin the loop hike. Strike out northeast from the plaque with 59th Avenue on your right, and cross over the paved access road inside the park. About 100 yards from the starting point, find the H-3 junction and turn left to begin hiking the H-3 Trail.

Hike northwest on a wide and gentle packed-dirt trail, which overlooks housing developments in the Arrowhead area. Typical Sonoran Desert vegetation, including palo verde trees, creosote bushes, barrel cacti, and saguaros, surrounds the trail. At 0.3 miles, the trail becomes much rockier. Notice the dark layer of patina, or desert varnish, covering rocks on the trail and giving them a volcanic look. This thin layer of manganese, iron, and clay is only a surface phenomenon. Preferring the hot and dry desert climates, colonies of microscopic bacteria have built the dark coating of desert varnish over thousands of years. The Hohokams, who inhabited central Arizona hundreds of years ago, created petroglyphs on large boulders by etching designs in the desert varnish, exposing the lighter-colored core of the rock.

Generally heading north, the trail makes a short uphill zigzag at 0.5 miles. Numerous brittlebush plants cover the hillside, and new suburbs encroach on the base. Follow the trail as it bends toward the west and then rounds the western end of Hedgpeth Hills, overlooking several horse stables and equestrian training facilities. Pilcher Hill and Ludden Mountain can be seen directly to the north as the trail begins to ascend some switchbacks at 1 mile.

Climb the mild switchbacks 0.2 miles and gain the top of a ridge with an impressive view of neighboring housing developments and distant mountains. Continue climbing a moderate hill to the top of a small mound and piles of boulders at 1.5 miles from the start. Vegetation atop the ridge is somewhat different than on the hillsides. There are noticeably more cacti nestled among lush grasses and not as many brittlebushes.

The gentle ascent resumes after you pass the small mound. Hike up the spine of the hill to a false summit with an old fire ring. Finish the climb along a view-studded ridge to the 1,833-foot summit 1.9 miles from the start. Take a breather here to survey the scenery. The tallest Hedgpeth Hill lies across 59th Avenue to the southeast. Thousands of brittlebush blossoms cover these hills like a golden fleece during the spring. A sea of tile roofs blanket the valley floor. To the southwest, the White Tank Mountains guard the horizon. The Bradshaw Mountains and New River Mesa span the northern skyline, while the McDowell Mountains, Four Peaks, and even Weaver's Needle in the Superstitions can be seen to the east.

From the summit, H-3 Trail descends toward the northeast along a series of switchbacks. At 2.1 miles, pass a spur trail heading straight east to a vista point. Continue down the switchbacks toward a large housing development at the base

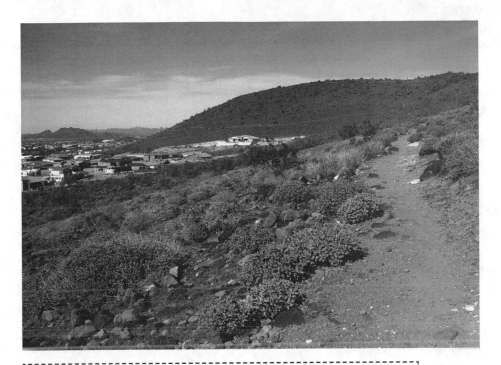

The H-3 Trail winds around brittlebush-covered Hedgpeth Hills and overlooks Glendale.

of the hill. The trail comes so close to the houses at one point that you can see right into their living rooms. Once on the valley floor, the trail circles around the eastern edge of the hill and terminates where it joins the H-1 Trail at 2.8 miles from the start of the loop.

Turn southwest onto H-1 and hike along 59th Avenue between the two Hedgpeth Hills. Noisy traffic whizzes alongside the level trail. Pass a picnic area on the other side of the road at 3.3 miles and the first junction with H-3 0.2 miles farther. Finish this pleasant loop hike just inside the main entrance of Thunderbird Park for a grand total of 3.6 miles.

NEARBY ACTIVITIES

Thunderbird Park contains a bird-watching area and an amphitheater, and its trails also cater to equestrians and mountain bikers. Adobe Dam Recreation Area on the eastern side of the Hedgpeth Hills presents additional opportunities for outdoor activities as it includes a water park, a sports complex, a golf course, kart racing, and even model-airplane flying. White Tank Mountain Regional Park, west of Phoenix, also offers excellent hiking trails.

22 TOM'S THUMB*

KEY AT-A-GLANCE INFORMATION

LENGTH: 4 miles

ELEVATION GAIN: 1,000 feet

CONFIGURATION: Out-and-back

DIFFICULTY: Moderate

SCENERY: City panorama, Tom's Thumb, desert, McDowell Sonoran Preserve

EXPOSURE: Completely exposed

TRAFFIC: Light–moderate

TRAIL SURFACE: Packed dirt, loose gravel, rock and boulders

HIKING TIME: 2.5 hours

WATER REQUIREMENT: 2 quarts, more if you plan to rock-climb

SEASON: Year-round; hot in summer

ACCESS: Open sunrise–sunset; free parking; high-clearance vehicle may be needed after storms

MAPS: USGS McDowell Peak

FACILITIES: None

DOGS: Yes; leashed at all times

COMMENTS: Fun hike to a famous McDowell landmark, and a rock climber's dream. Visit www.scotts daleaz.gov/Preserve for trail maps and information on the McDowell Sonoran Preserve.

GPS Trailhead Coordinates

UTM Zone   12S

Easting   0425762

Northing   3727795

Latitude   N33°41.357'

Longitude   W111°48.100'

Update: In mid-2009, McDowell Sonoran Preserve opened Tom's Thumb Trail, a 5-mile-long trail connecting the proposed North McDowell Access Area to Tom's Thumb and the Windgate Pass Trail. The new trailhead has shifted east by 0.5 miles, bypassing the dreaded boulder-ridden Catacombs gully and making the ascent to Tom's Thumb much easier.

IN BRIEF

Visit a popular landmark in the McDowell Mountains, enjoy commanding views of Fountain Hills and north Scottsdale, and hike through rugged and rocky desert. If you enjoy rock climbing, the Tom's Thumb area also offers challenging climbs.

DESCRIPTION

Look up from most places in Scottsdale and the East Valley, and you'll see the McDowell Mountains and their undulating peaks against the horizon. Look closer and you might find a thimblelike protrusion, known as Tom's Thumb, perched high on the ridgeline. That tiny thimble is actually a 140-foot-tall granite spire popular with local rock climbers. It's even named after climber Tom Kreuser's

Directions

Exit Loop 101 at Princess Drive and turn northeast onto Pima Road. Follow Pima 4.5 miles to Happy Valley Road. Turn east and drive 3.5 miles on Happy Valley, ignoring any NO OUTLET signs. Turn right onto Alameda Road, and then make another right at 119th Way. Turn left at Casitas Del Rio Drive, then left again at Paraiso Drive, which becomes a graded dirt road. Drive 1 mile to an unsigned road (130th Street). Turn right and follow it to the end to the trailhead parking area.

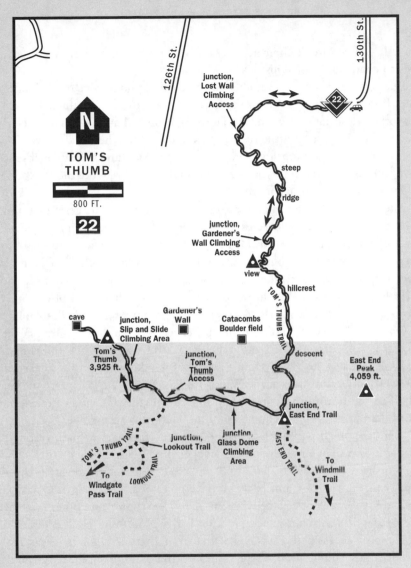

N

TOM'S
THUMB

800 FT.

22

126th St.

130th St.

22

junction,
Lost Wall
Climbing
Access

steep

ridge

junction,
Gardener's
Wall Climbing
Access

view

hillcrest

TOM'S THUMB TRAIL

cave

junction,
Slip and Slide
Climbing Area

Gardener's
Wall

Catacombs
Boulder field

Tom's
Thumb
3,925 ft.

junction,
Tom's
Thumb
Access

descent

East End
Peak
4,059 ft.

junction,
East End Trail

TOM'S THUMB TRAIL

junction,
Lookout Trail

junction,
Glass Dome
Climbing
Area

EAST END TRAIL

LOOKOUT TRAIL

To
Windgate
Pass Trail

To
Windmill
Trail

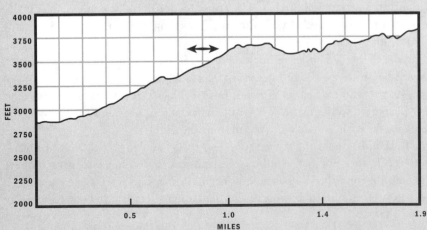

FEET

4000
3750
3500
3250
3000
2750
2500
2250
2000

0.5   1.0   1.4   1.9

MILES

thumb. If you're a rock climber, the Tom's Thumb area boasts many technical routes to challenge your skills.

But you need not be a climber to seek this famous McDowell landmark. Hikers find plenty of reasons to make the short trek to visit this rock. Unlike many other destinations in the McDowells, Tom's Thumb remains relatively unknown because it sits in the rugged and secluded northern part of McDowell Sonoran Preserve. Add a primitive dirt-road approach and a relative absence of housing developments, and you have the makings of a wilderness experience literally within minutes of suburbia.

The McDowell Sonoran Preserve currently covers 16,000 acres of mountain wilderness. Another 20,000 acres of state trust land have been designated for inclusion, but the City of Scottsdale has yet to purchase the land. Funded by taxpayers, this project, once completed, will have set aside one-third of Scottsdale's total landmass for conservation. Construction of gateway access areas, parking, and trails continues throughout the preserve. The southern half of the preserve receives most visitors, while the northern part remains relatively desolate.

One of the newest trails in the preserve, the 5-mile-long Tom's Thumb Trail, takes you through the remote northern McDowells. This trail runs from the parking area to the base of Tom's Thumb, then descends into the heart of the McDowells and terminates at the Windgate Pass Trail. We'll explore the northern half of the trail in this trip description, although you can also take a much longer hike to reach Tom's Thumb from the Gateway Access Area.

From the small parking lot, hike westward on a narrow path through the foothills. The trail begins on relatively level ground, with the tip of Tom's Thumb visible to the west. It may be hard to believe, but you are already at an elevation higher than the top of Camelback Mountain. Jojoba bushes dot the arid landscape, and you may notice a peculiar absence of saguaros and other large cacti.

At 0.3 miles, reach a signed junction for the Half and Half Wall and Lost Wall climbing access path. This is the first of many rock-climbing areas accessible from Tom's Thumb Trail. Stay left and begin climbing uphill. Large boulders flank the trail as you climb higher. The trail steepens, and the gravel may prove slippery if you're not careful with footing. Trekking poles may help, especially on the descent down.

For the next 0.25 miles, climb steep switchbacks and cross several ridges, where you begin to see the full height of Tom's Thumb to the west. If you need a break, stop to admire distant views of Four Peaks, Bartlett Lake, and the Cave Creek Mountains to the north. The trail then contours around the hillside and crosses a wash, with Pinnacle Peak visible to the right.

At 0.75 miles, pass the signed junction to Gardener's Wall, one of several ways to reach this popular climbing destination. Gardener's Wall, a massive granite slab on the hilltop where many rock climbers go to test their mettle, is visible below Tom's Thumb. You might see some distant climbers clinging to cracks on that wall.

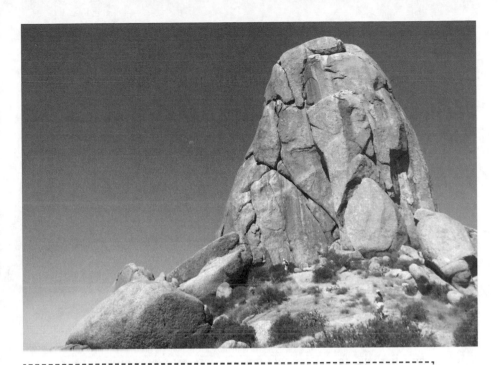

Hikers approach 140-foot-tall Tom's Thumb atop a scenic ridge in the McDowell Mountains.

The steep ascent resumes until you top out on a hillcrest about 1 mile from the trailhead and 3,680 feet in elevation. Take a well-deserved rest here as the trail levels off. Some teddy bear cholla can be seen as you have passed the cold northern face of the mountain onto a warmer hilltop. At 1.2 miles, drop down 100 feet into a wide grassy basin, with the Catacombs boulder field off to your right. Before this new trail was constructed, the only way to access Tom's Thumb was through that treacherous gully. You'll find a variety of wildflowers in this basin during spring and early summer. Some species, such as the Arizona caltrop and black-foot daisy, bloom well into September. Reach the signed junction with the East End Trail atop a prominent view-studded saddle at 1.4 miles. East End Peak towers above your left shoulder and Fountain Hills lies below. If you happen to arrive at this point on the hour, you'll see the fountain's signature plume in the distance. Red Mountain, Pass Mountain (page 94), and Superstition Mountain (page 187, Siphon Draw Trail) line the southeastern horizon. The East End Trail continues south and eventually meets the Windmill Trail, but stay on Tom's Thumb Trail and head west.

From the saddle, pass a small dip and then climb a moderate hill covered in gravel. Pass the Glass Dome climbing access path, and then go through a gap between two large boulders on top of the hill. Odd rock formations abound on top of the McDowells. If you use your imagination, you might see the rocky profile of an old man facing left, with droopy eyes and nose. Pass to the left of this rock to reach another saddle at 1.7 miles from the trailhead overlooking north Scottsdale.

From this saddle, leave Tom's Thumb Trail and turn right, following the climbing access path toward Tom's Thumb and Gardener's Wall. You can see Tom's Thumb from here, but the trail first skirts the left side of a large rock outcropping in front of you. You'll pass one more junction to access a climbing area called Slip and Slide—and wonder why anyone would climb that!

Snaking around huge boulders atop the McDowell ridgeline, you finally come to a stunning view of Tom's Thumb 2 miles from the trailhead. It's hard to imagine this 140-foot monolith is actually the little thimble viewed from town. Approach the base of this spire at 3,830 feet in elevation to get an appreciation for its true height. From this vantage point, you can also view Camelback Mountain (pages 21 and 26) and Piestewa Peak (pages 48 and 52) to the southwest, and Carefree and Bartlett Dam to the northeast.

For an even more spectacular view, you might try climbing to the top of Tom's Thumb. However, doing so requires proper climbing equipment and an expert lead climber. There are routes ranging in difficulty from 5.7 to 5.12a. Consult a rock-climbing guidebook for further details. Needless to say, you shouldn't attempt climbing Tom's Thumb without safety gear and rock-climbing experience.

For nonclimbers, there's another point of interest worth visiting near Tom's Thumb. Work your way around the massive rock tower by ducking through a crevice at the left side of Tom's Thumb. Bushwhack down past some dense shrubs; then turn right and climb back up to the ridge behind Tom's Thumb. You'll be at the opposite side of Tom's Thumb from your approach. Find and follow a faint trail approximately 200 feet northwest, and then veer left off the trail to find a cave that some locals call the Ogre's Den. Visitors past have left some trinkets, a makeshift memorial, a notebook, and even some artwork on the walls. Once satisfied with the cave and Tom's Thumb, return to the trailhead by retracing your steps.

If you would like a slightly longer hike, consider turning right when returning to Tom's Thumb Trail at the second saddle. You'll soon come to a junction with the Lookout Trail. Hiking that trail adds about 1 mile to the trip but takes you to another excellent vantage point called the Lookout. If you set up a car shuttle in advance, you can optionally descend the Tom's Thumb Trail to its terminus, then follow the Windgate Pass Trail west toward the Gateway Access Area, an 8.5-mile, one-way hike.

NEARBY ACTIVITIES

Nearby Pinnacle Peak Trail (page 99) offers a hike equivalent in distance to Tom's Thumb. Many popular McDowell trails are accessible from the southern side of the mountain range; see Sunrise Trail (page 104) for details. Additional access points to McDowell Sonoran Preserve trails are still being planned and constructed. Windgate Pass Trail is the nearest developed trail to Tom's Thumb.

WIND CAVE TRAIL   23

IN BRIEF

The Wind Cave Trail is the most popular attraction in Usery Mountain Regional Park. This moderate hike takes visitors across the desert valley floor, through a dry wash, up the slopes of Pass Mountain, and across a strip of volcanic tuff, and ends at a wind-eroded overhang called the Wind Cave.

DESCRIPTION

Two obvious features stand out in the Usery Mountain range east of Mesa: a huge "Phoenix" sign on the side of Usery Mountain pointing toward town, and a distinctive yellow stripe of volcanic tuff across Pass Mountain. The latter can be seen from most places in Phoenix. Though Pass Mountain isn't as tall as the Superstition Mountains behind it, the yellowish horizontal stripe halfway up its western slopes makes the otherwise ordinary mountain one of the most recognizable landmarks in the East Valley. The Wind Cave, really only an eroded overhang, sits at the southern tip of the volcanic tuff and draws many visitors to Usery Mountain Regional Park. In addition to the cave and the superb views from its lofty setting, the Wind Cave Trail offers a desert experience the entire family can enjoy. My five-year-old nephew relished the opportunity to learn about various kinds of cacti and to climb up and down the rocks. He even spotted a tarantula next to the trail!

Directions

From US 60, exit onto Ellsworth Road. Drive north 6.5 miles and turn east into Usery Mountain Regional Park. Pay at the entrance station. Once inside the park, proceed 1 mile and turn left onto Wind Cave Drive. Parking and restrooms are located at the picnic area.

KEY AT-A-GLANCE INFORMATION

LENGTH: 3.2 miles

ELEVATION GAIN: 820 feet

CONFIGURATION: Out-and-back

DIFFICULTY: Moderate

SCENERY: Wind Cave, Usery Mountains, desert, city panorama

EXPOSURE: Mostly exposed, little shade

TRAFFIC: Moderate

TRAIL SURFACE: Gravel, rock, boulders

HIKING TIME: 1.5 hours

WATER REQUIREMENT: 1 quart

SEASON: Year-round; hot in summer

ACCESS: 5 a.m.–8 p.m. (10 p.m. Fri.–Sat.); trail closes at sunset; $6 per vehicle

MAPS: USGS Apache Junction; map available at park entrance

FACILITIES: Restrooms, drinking water, picnic areas, camping, archery range

DOGS: Yes, leashed at all times

COMMENTS: For park information, visit www.maricopa.gov/parks/usery or call (480) 984-0032.

GPS Trailhead
Coordinates
UTM Zone 12S
Easting   0443645
Northing   3703814
Latitude   N33°28.444'
Longitude   W111°36.441'

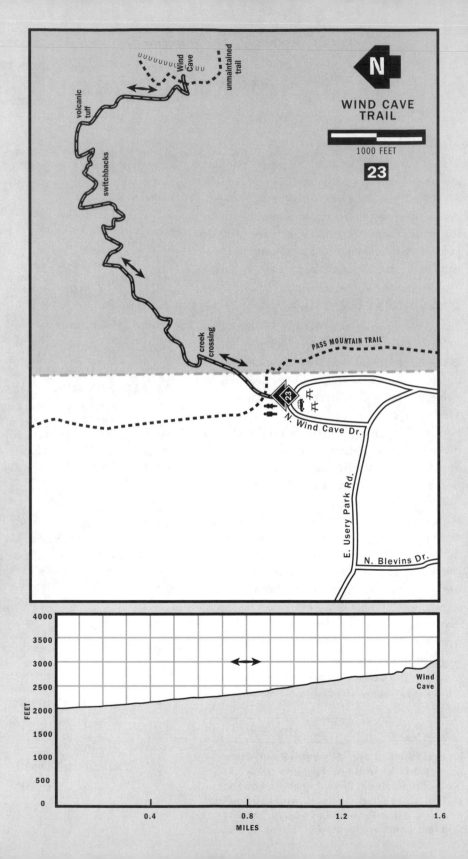

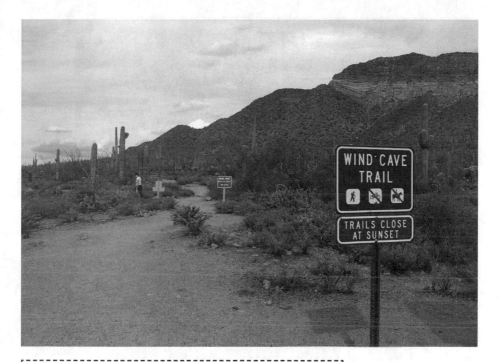

A hiker explores the Wind Cave Trail in Usery Mountain Regional Park.

The Wind Cave Trail begins at a picnic area on Wind Cave Drive, a paved loop 1 mile inside Usery Mountain Regional Park. The guard at the park entrance provides everyone with a detailed map of the park, but this trail is easy to follow and obvious signs make navigation a cinch. Almost immediately, the Wind Cave Trail crosses the Pass Mountain Trail and shoots northeast into the desert. About 450 feet into the hike, cross an equestrian barrier and enter Tonto National Forest. The trail continues to meander along the desert floor. The first half of the trail runs along the gentle base of the mountain, giving you ample time to study the scenery. Typical Sonoran Desert inhabitants such as saguaros, chollas, palo verdes, and creosotes dominate the region, but the variety of cacti is especially rich here. See if you can identify all the following: giant saguaro, buckhorn cholla, teddy bear cholla, chain-fruit cholla, strawberry hedgehog, prickly pear, beaver tail, and fishhook barrel.

At 0.2 miles, the trail crosses a dry creek and continues gently uphill along a wide and nicely graded gravel path. As you get closer to the base of Pass Mountain, the going gets steeper and slightly rougher. Look toward the mountain to find the Wind Cave at the right edge of the band of volcanic tuff. On weekends, many hikers dot the distant trail like ants on a tree trunk. Stands of saguaros cover the hillside, and palo verde trees add a splash of color to the scene. (Many of these palo verde trees contain dark clumps of desert mistletoe, which are parasitic plants that sap nutrients from their gracious hosts, eventually killing

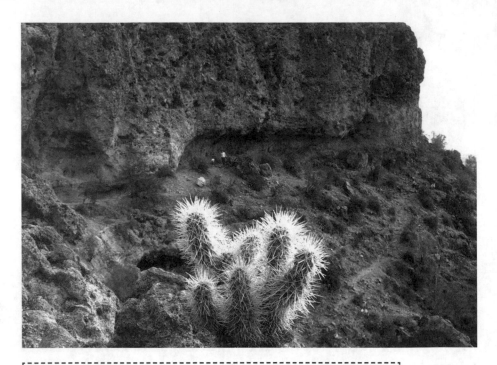

A teddy bear stands in front of the shallow Wind Cave in Usery Mountain Regional Park

them.) While enjoying the serene scenery, you might be surprised to hear barrages of automatic gunfire breaking the silence. Do not be alarmed. The gunshots emanate from the Usery Mountain Shooting Range across the main road and pose no threat, although they may annoy.

Near 0.8 miles the trail begins to climb via a series of switchbacks. The neatly graded gravel degenerates into crushed rock and occasional tall steps that a small child would have to scale on all fours. However, the trail is by no means difficult or unmanageable. If you require a break during the steep ascent to catch your breath, turn and look west toward Usery Mountain. Notice the huge arrow painted on its side where the tail of the arrow spells out and points to Phoenix. You might wonder why this seemingly needless sign exists, and why the Federal Aviation Administration would grant any directionally challenged pilot who needs this sign a license to operate an aircraft. The sign was built as a community-service project by the Air Explorers Boy Scout Post under the direction of an eccentric pilot named Charles Merritt. They constructed the sign during the 1950s from large rocks and several coats of whitewash in order to guide wayward pilots. Whether anyone ever needed its help or cared to admit it is still a mystery. However, the "Phoenix" sign is nevertheless an interesting conversation piece.

Climbing higher, the trail eventually draws level with the base of a wide layer of volcanic tuff. This 25-million-year-old formation consists of compacted volcanic ash and debris, quite different in composition from the rocky granite and basalt found elsewhere on the mountain. High quartz content gives this layer a shimmering glow in the afternoon sun. A coating of chartreuse lichen finishes the tuff, giving it the distinctive color visible for dozens of miles. Continue by traversing the base of the tuff and make your way south toward the hike's destination.

The Wind Cave is at 2,840 feet in elevation, and it really is windy. The shape of Pass Mountain forces moving air masses to slide along its western face toward the south and carved the C-shaped alcove out of the rock over millions of years. Moisture seeping through the smooth but porous walls feeds clusters of rock daisy, which seem to grow downward from the ceiling like chandeliers. On a hot summer day, the shade and breeze in the eroded alcove feel absolutely heavenly. The Wind Cave is a wonderful place to picnic while enjoying the surroundings and the awesome view, but prepare to defend your lunch from resident chipmunks. They are cute and quite friendly.

Though the trail ends at the Wind Cave, adventure seekers can climb to the top of Pass Mountain summit ridge via an unmaintained path at the southern end of the cave or bushwhack up a slope on its northern end. The ridge is only 200 feet higher than the Wind Cave but offers superb views toward the east where you can see the Superstition Mountains in all their glory. The tallest point on Pass Mountain is two-thirds of a mile to the north along the ridge, but reaching it requires significant bushwhacking and is not recommended. It's only another 100 feet higher anyway. Return to the trailhead the same way you came. Be careful going downhill on slippery loose gravel along the trail.

NEARBY ACTIVITIES

Usery Mountain Regional Park offers many other popular trails such as the Blevins Trail and the Pass Mountain Trail (page 94). Other recreational activities available at the park include archery, camping, and picnicking. Fans of firearms can discharge their weapons at the Usery Mountain Shooting Range located at the base of Usery Mountain. The Superstitions Wilderness to the east is a hiker's dream. Many hikes in this book are based in the Superstitions. River rats can visit the Salt River north of the Usery Mountains to swim or to float downstream in an inner tube, a favorite pastime among Phoenix residents.

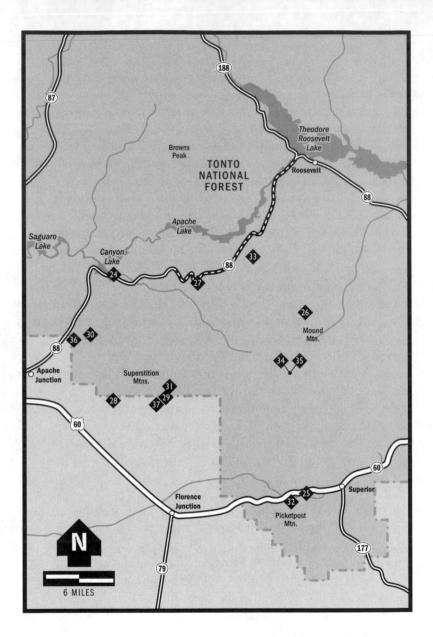

6 MILES

EAST
INCLUDING SUPERSTITION WILDERNESS

24 BOULDER CANYON TRAIL TO LABARGE CANYON

KEY AT-A-GLANCE INFORMATION

LENGTH: 10.5 miles

ELEVATION GAIN: 600 feet (1,500 feet accumulated gain)

CONFIGURATION: Balloon

DIFFICULTY: Moderate to difficult

SCENERY: Canyon Lake, Battleship Mountain, Weaver's Needle, LaBarge Canyon

EXPOSURE: Mostly exposed; some shade inside LaBarge Canyon's mouth

TRAFFIC: Light to Moderate

TRAIL SURFACE: Rock, gravel, sand, some streambed boulder-hopping and scrambling

HIKING TIME: 6 hours

WATER REQUIREMENT: 4 quarts

SEASON: Year-round; hot in summer

ACCESS: Open sunrise to sunset; free parking

MAPS: USGS Mormon Flat Dam and Goldfield

FACILITIES: Restroom, water, restaurant at Canyon Lake Marina

DOGS: Yes

COMMENTS: Some route-finding skills are required for the trek to LaBarge Canyon. For more information, visit www.fs.fed.us/r3/tonto/wilderness/wilderness-superstition-index.shtml.

IN BRIEF

This superb route through Superstition Wilderness packs plenty of scenery into a 10-mile hike. If close-up views of Canyon Lake, Battleship Mountain, Weaver's Needle, and the Superstition Ridgeline aren't enough to motivate you, then tranquil pools and an enticing swimming hole in LaBarge Canyon ought to do the trick.

DESCRIPTION

In addition to legendary lost gold, the Superstition Wilderness harbors treasures of a different kind. Rugged and surreal mountains, tranquil valleys, and trickling springs entertain outdoor enthusiasts seemingly to no end. Dozens of trails and even more unnamed routes cover the 160,200-acre wilderness area. The striking juxtaposition of a harsh desert environment and hidden streams and emerald pools intrigues all who venture into the depths of the wilderness.

Boulder Canyon Trail 103 exemplifies the exceptional beauty of this unique landscape. Offering stunning hills, rocky streams, panoramic views, and even an abandoned mine, this trail has something for everyone. Easy access from the Canyon Lake Marina also makes this trail one of the most popular

GPS Trailhead Coordinates

UTM Zone 12S

Easting 0460800

Northing 3710369

Latitude N33°32.038'

Longitude W111°25.373'

Directions

Drive east on US 60 and exit onto Idaho Road. Drive 2.25 miles north on Idaho Road to SR 88, the Apache Trail. Turn northeast onto SR 88, and follow it 14 miles to the Canyon Lake Marina, which is just past the second one-lane bridge. Turn left into the marina and park in specially marked trailhead parking spots along the fence closest to SR 88.

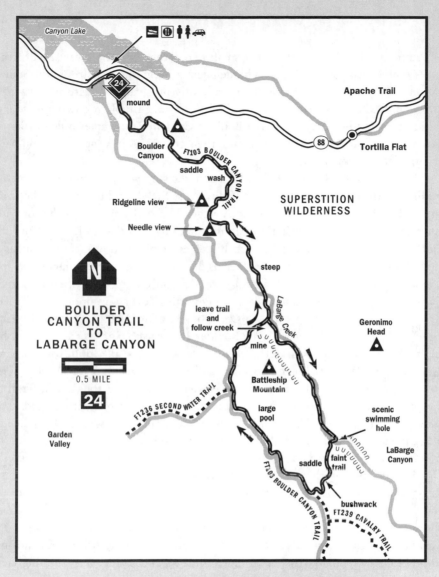

Canyon Lake

Apache Trail

24

mound

Boulder
Canyon

FT103 BOULDER CANYON TRAIL

88

Tortilla Flat

saddle

wash

Ridgeline view

Needle view

SUPERSTITION
WILDERNESS

steep

N

BOULDER
CANYON TRAIL
TO
LABARGE CANYON

0.5 MILE

24

Garden
Valley

leave trail
and
follow creek

LaBarge Creek

Geronimo
Head

mine

Battleship
Mountain

scenic
swimming
hole

FT236 SECOND WATER TRAIL

large
pool

LaBarge
Canyon

FT103 BOULDER CANYON TRAIL

saddle

faint
trail

bushwack

FT239 CAVALRY TRAIL

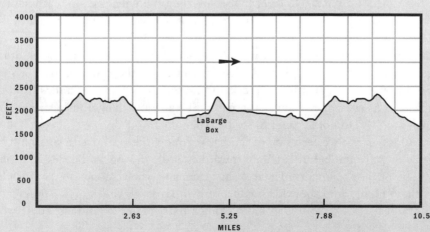

FEET

4000
3500
3000
2500
2000
1500
1000
500
0

LaBarge
Box

2.63   5.25   7.88   10.5

MILES

hikes around. However, only a very small percentage of people venture off trail to visit the "LaBarge Box," truly a hidden gem among the treasures of the Superstitions. Only minutes off the main trail, this box canyon features a narrow rocky gorge framed by sheer cliffs and a large pool suitable for swimming. The route described here begins on the Boulder Canyon Trail, takes a detour along LaBarge Creek to LaBarge Canyon, and then crosses over a saddle to loop back on Boulder Canyon Trail.

Upon arrival at Canyon Lake Marina, make sure you park in the designated trailhead parking against the fence. Walk across SR 88 and begin the hike from a signed trailhead east of the one-lane bridge. The rocky trail hugs the roadside fence and heads east. Keep right at an unsigned fork in the trail, and then turn south heading up a moderately steep hill. Desert plants dominate the hillside, but in spring, colorful wildflowers such as desert mariposa lilies, blue dicks, and Mexican gold poppies can be found here. As you climb, turn often to survey Canyon Lake behind you and expect to enjoy this view again upon your return.

A series of vista points line this part of the trail. At 0.4 miles you'll reach a mound with a bird's-eye view of Boulder Recreation Site to the right. A bit farther, a wooden sign marks the wilderness boundary at a point overlooking Boulder Canyon. The trail turns left uphill where it reaches yet another vista point, this time affording views of the Salt River basin and the Apache Trail to the east. At 1.2 miles you'll reach the top of a 2,360-foot hill with a panoramic view of the entire area. This is the highest point of the hike. Weaver's Needle lies straight ahead, and the entire Superstition Ridgeline can be seen to its right. To its left, a boxy formation called Battleship Mountain flaunts its sheer cliffs.

Past the hilltop the trail descends slightly and follows a ridge to the east. Cross a flat saddle point at 1.7 miles and then skirt the hills. The trail bobs up and down, never finding a comfortable path across the slopes. Jagged rocks loom above you on the left, and a deep valley stretches out to the right. Cross a dry wash at 1.9 miles where a seasonal waterfall flows after significant rainstorms. Another quarter mile farther, the trail rounds a bend to reveal a stunning view of the Superstition Ridgeline. Then ascend some switchbacks and reach another high point at 2,300 feet with closer views of Weaver's Needle and Battleship Mountain.

Turn left over a small rocky saddle to see the entire LaBarge Creek drainage directly below. Dropping 500 feet in elevation, the trail descends a steep and slippery slope down to the creek and then crosses it at 3.25 miles from the trailhead. A word of caution: LaBarge Creek can flow dangerously strong after major storms. Do not attempt to ford it when it's flooded.

Once on the western side of the creek, follow the trail over a small hill but break away from it before it climbs toward a saddle in front of Battleship Mountain. If you pass remnants of a makeshift campsite, you've gone too far. Turn left off the trail and into the wide boulder-strewn LaBarge Creek at 3.5 miles from the trailhead. Make your way south along LaBarge Creek, sandwiched between

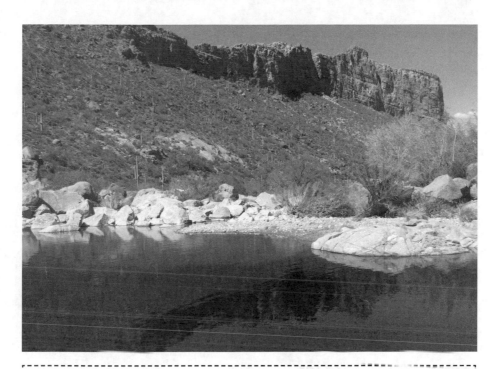

A large swimming hole at the mouth of LaBarge Canyon reflects Battleship Mountain and the desert sky.

massive Battleship Mountain on your right and towering Geronimo Head on your left. There is no trail, but negotiating the rocky creek bottom should present no major problems. A quarter mile after leaving the trail, you should begin to see a sharp mountain ahead and a flat hill to its left. LaBarge Box lies between these landmarks.

Boulder-hopping up LaBarge Creek requires some light scrambling. If you encounter a troublesome area, there's often an easy bypass nearby. Approximately 4.5 miles from the trailhead, you'll hardly believe your eyes: LaBarge Box features an emerald-colored pool at its mouth, a narrow passage carved from stone and guarded by towering vertical cliffs. Welcome to one of the most beautiful places in the Superstitions!

A slick-rock area next to the pool is the ideal setting for a picnic. Spend some time lounging around the rocks and playing in the water. It's worth exploring deeper into the scenic canyon, which first curves left and then right. LaBarge Canyon features massive boulders and large pools and can be quite challenging to negotiate. If you aren't used to scrambling, you won't get very far. Nevertheless, it's worth a visit for the magnificent cliffs that form this narrow passage. Return to the mouth of LaBarge Canyon after your detour. When you are ready to leave, you can either backtrack along LaBarge Creek or opt to circle around Battleship Mountain. Should you choose the latter option, you'll need some route-finding skills. First, find a faint trail beginning at the western end of the pool. Marked by occasional cairns, this narrow use trail zigzags up a steep hill to the saddle at Battleship Mountain's southern tip, where an unobstructed view of Weaver's Needle presents itself.

Over the saddle, the faint trail becomes nearly impossible to follow, but you can see Boulder Creek below. The goal is to head downhill toward the creek. Resist the temptation to turn uphill to the right. Instead, bushwhack down the overgrown slope and then veer right toward Boulder Creek. Once there, look for cairns in the creek bed marking the Boulder Canyon Trail. Only then should you start heading back toward the north.

Boulder Canyon Trail crosses the creek many times and runs along some flat valleys lined by tall chain-fruit cholla. Pass a large pool at 1.4 miles from LaBarge Box, and then find the signed junction with Second Water Trail 236 a half mile farther on the left side of Boulder Creek. Continue north on Boulder Canyon Trail and cross Boulder Creek a final time at 2.2 miles from LaBarge Box. Then climb a hill to the abandoned Indian Paint Mine nestled in red rocks. The mine lies at the saddle just north of Battleship Mountain. Cross this saddle to find the point where you left the trail earlier. From there, retrace your steps 3.5 miles to complete the loop.

NEARBY ACTIVITIES

Canyon Lake is third in a chain of reservoirs in the Salt River valley and provides many opportunities for water sports. There is even a steamboat cruise available from the marina. Lost Dutchman State Park, on SR 88, offers many excellent hikes including the Siphon Draw Trail to the Flatiron (page 134). Tortilla Flat, a small but charming tourist trap, is 2 miles east of the Canyon Lake Marina on SR 88.

BOYCE THOMPSON ARBORETUM: MAIN TRAIL
25

IN BRIEF

Situated in the shadow of Picketpost Mountain, Boyce Thompson Arboretum showcases a unique collection of native desert flora as well as arid land plants from around the world. The park's trail system routes visitors through impressive plant displays set in a naturally scenic landscape.

DESCRIPTION

Boyce Thompson Arboretum State Park has long been a favorite of valley residents and visitors. This unique sanctuary houses a wide assortment of plants, specializing in those typically found in deserts and other arid regions of the world. The arboretum was named for Colonel William Boyce Thompson, an incredibly wealthy and powerful magnate who lived at the turn of the 20th century. Nestled at the base of Picketpost Mountain and next to Queen Creek, the arboretum arranges its displays within a natural desert setting. Nothing seems particularly out of place here, yet some specimens on display come from thousands of miles away.

Blandly named and 1.5 miles in length, the Main Trail connects Boyce Thompson Arboretum's major features while many side paths and loops compete for your attention. A typical traversal of the Main Trail ends up being somewhere between 2 and 3 miles in length with all the inviting detours. As you stroll through the plant displays, look for

KEY AT-A-GLANCE INFORMATION

LENGTH: 1.5–3 miles

ELEVATION GAIN: 100 feet

CONFIGURATION: Balloon with many side trails

DIFFICULTY: Easy

SCENERY: Variety of desert plants, Queen Creek, Picketpost Mountain

EXPOSURE: Partly shaded

TRAFFIC: High

TRAIL SURFACE: Packed dirt, gravel, pavement

HIKING TIME: 2.5 hours

WATER REQUIREMENT: 1 quart

SEASON: Year-round; hot in summer

ACCESS: 8 a.m.–4 p.m.; May–August, 6 a.m.–3 p.m.; last entry at 2 p.m.; $7.50 for adults, $3 for children

MAPS: USGS Picketpost Mountain, park map provided at entrance

FACILITIES: Visitor center, gift shop, restrooms, water, wheelchair accessible

DOGS: Yes, leashed at all times

COMMENTS: An educational and scenic outdoor experience for the entire family. For more information, visit http://arboretum.ag.arizona.edu, or call (520) 689-2723.

GPS Trailhead Coordinates

UTM Zone 12S

Easting   0485254

Northing 3682144

Latitude N33°16.801'

Longitude W111°9.543'

Directions

Leave Phoenix on US 60 and drive east past Florence Junction and Gonzales Pass. Boyce Thompson Arboretum State Park is on the south side of US 60, near mile marker 223.

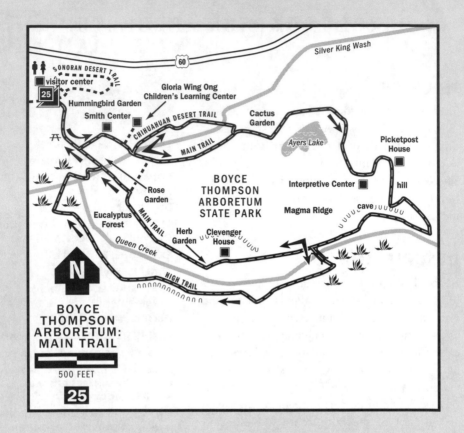

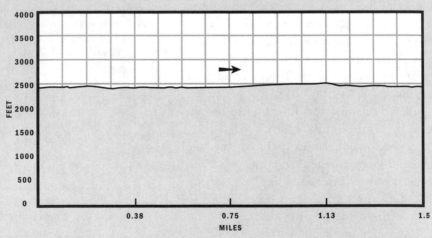

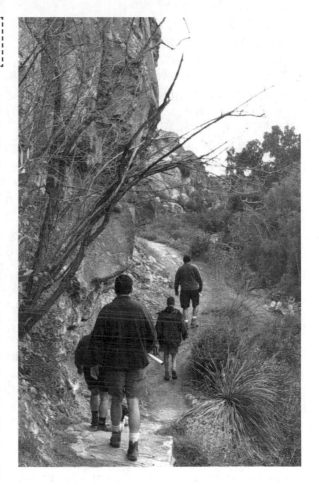

green numbered signs that identify correspondingly numbered plants on the park map. It's a fascinating way to learn about the rich biodiversity of the desert around us.

Inside the main entrance, pass the gift shop and restrooms to begin your self-guided tour. Notice the view of towering Picketpost Mountain to the south. Be sure to visit the quarter-mile–long Sonoran Desert Trail to your left because this loop showcases plants typically encountered on hikes near Phoenix. Curandero is a Spanish word meaning medicine man, and the Curandero Trail, also on this loop, provides interpretive signs that explain medicinal uses for plants native to the Sonoran Desert.

Return to the Main Trail and walk down next to the aloes. You'll soon cross a service road and enter a shaded garden with displays designed to attract hummingbirds. Beyond the Hummingbird Garden, follow signs for the Main Trail and head toward the rose garden and the Smith Interpretive Center. This historic building contains two greenhouses dedicated to cacti and succulents from around the world. The next building on your left is the Gloria Wing Ong Children's Learning Center, where you will likely find interactive displays and educational programs.

The Main Trail forks beyond the Children's Learning Center; I recommend continuing eastward, saving the scenic river walk for last. Near the Cactus Garden, you'll find a strange boojum tree—it looks like someone uprooted a giant carrot and then planted it upside-down. After the Cactus Garden, walk east toward Ayers Lake, a man-made reservoir that holds water for all the gardens in the park and provides a sanctuary for migrating waterfowl.

East of Ayers Lake, the Main Trail becomes rougher as it winds through some rocky hills known as the Magma Ridge, the only segment not recommended for wheelchairs. No gardens grace these scenic rocks, but they are naturally beautiful. Enjoy several interpretive stations with superb views of the rocky terrain and the surrounding area. Near Boyce Thompson Arboretum's eastern edge, the Main Trail passes below the hilltop perch of historic Picketpost House, where Colonel Thompson lived in the early 1900s.

A few steep turns farther, the Main Trail enters a densely wooded riparian zone on the banks of Queen Creek. This is my favorite part of the entire park. Sandwiched between sheer cliffs on the right and tall trees on the left, the trail heads back west under a canopy of shady branches and leaves. A newly constructed suspension bridge provides access to the High Trail, an unimpressive name for an otherwise fine natural trail. There are no plant displays on this trail, and it eventually connects to the picnic area downstream.

Unless you have extra time, I would skip the High Trail and head straight for the Herb Garden where an assortment of fragrant spices delights your olfactory senses. Rub some leaves gently between your fingers and then try to identify their scent without reading the labels. Also inside the Herb Garden, notice the charming Clevenger House built right into the rocky cliff.

Beyond the Herb Garden, pass through a forest of palms and giant eucalyptus trees. If any section of the Main Trail looks unnatural in Arizona, this would be it. The arboretum did an excellent job, however, of putting the tall trees next to Queen Creek where they would be less conspicuous. Finally, finish your exploration of the park by crossing the whitewashed Outback Bridge and returning via the Australian Walkabout. Along the way, browse the old-fashioned wool-shearing shed, which looks like it might belong to an unkempt groundskeeper whose rusted heap of a pickup truck lies nearby.

Boyce Thompson Arboretum is dedicated to "educational, recreational, research, and preservation opportunities associated with arid land plants." It offers enough diversity of flora, seasonal variations, and special events to keep visitors coming back. Before you leave, browse the Demonstration Garden near the entrance for landscaping ideas and perhaps even buy some desert plants or wildflower seeds for your next home-improvement project.

NEARBY ACTIVITIES

Picketpost Mountain looms directly above Boyce Thompson Arboretum. The Picketpost Trail (page 167) is a challenging route to its summit. US 60 also provides access to many hikes in the Superstition Wilderness including Peralta Trail (page 162), Rogers Canyon Trail (page 182), and Lost Goldmine Trail (page 153).

CIRCLESTONE FROM REAVIS RANCH 26

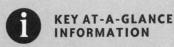

IN BRIEF

Within the depths of Superstition Wilderness, an ancient people built a large ring of stone atop a hill. Circlestone is as remote as it is mysterious. Visitors can ponder its origins in complete solitude while enjoying panoramic views of the surrounding mountains and forests.

DESCRIPTION

Legends of lost gold aside, the Superstition Mountains contain real treasures of an entirely different kind. Cultural gems like the Rogers Canyon cliff dwellings and Hieroglyphic Canyon petroglyphs lie hidden throughout the wilderness area. These remnants of ancient cultures add to the amazing natural landscape and make the Superstitions one of the best places in Arizona to explore.

Of all archaeological sites in the Superstition Wilderness, perhaps none is as grand or as mysterious as Circlestone. Its easiest access route requires an hour's drive on primitive roads from the nearest highway, plus a 10-mile hike through mountainous terrain. Likely receiving only a few dozen groups annually, Circlestone's remoteness serves as its own preservation mechanism.

As its name suggests, Circlestone is a nearly circular ring of primitive walls made of stone. Circlestone lay undisturbed in the middle of nowhere for centuries, and its origin and purpose remain a mystery. For these

----

Directions

This hike begins from Reavis Ranch, which requires a 7.5-mile hike from Rogers Trough Trailhead. Refer to the Reavis Ranch hike for driving directions to Rogers Trough and hiking directions to Reavis Ranch.

KEY AT-A-GLANCE INFORMATION

LENGTH: 6.7 miles (18.7 miles from Rogers Trough Trailhead)

ELEVATION GAIN: 1,150 feet

CONFIGURATION: Out-and-back

DIFFICULTY: Moderate to difficult

SCENERY: Pine forest, high desert, Superstition Wilderness, Circlestone ruins, Mound Mountain

EXPOSURE: Mostly exposed, some shade available near Reavis Creek

TRAFFIC: Very light

TRAIL SURFACE: Gravel, rock, packed dirt

HIKING TIME: 3.5 hours (10 hours from Rogers Trough Trailhead)

WATER REQUIREMENT: 3 quarts (5 quarts from Rogers Trough Trailhead)

SEASON: Year-round; hot in summer

ACCESS: Sunrise to sunset; free parking at Rogers Trough Trailhead

MAPS: USGS Iron Mountain

FACILITIES: None, but perennial Reavis Creek provides an emergency water source

DOGS: Yes

COMMENTS: Best done as a detour from a Reavis Ranch backpacking home base

----

GPS Trailhead Coordinates

UTM Zone 12S

Easting 0485575

Northing 3705575

Latitude N33°29.481'

Longitude W111°9.359'

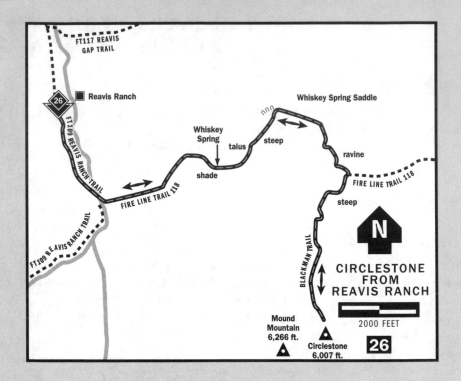

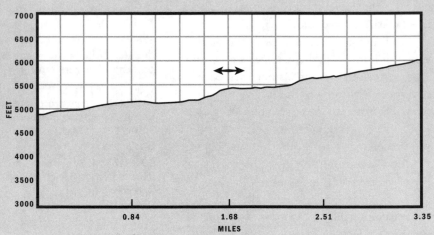

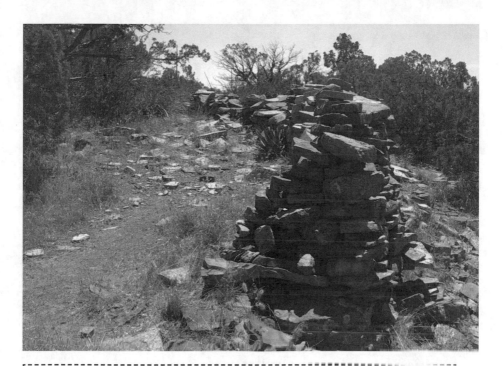

Nameless ancients built a giant circular stone structure in the middle of Superstition Wilderness.

reasons, some have drawn the obvious parallels between Circlestone and Stonehenge. The Circlestone walls consist of large rocks of varying sizes, carefully stacked to five feet high in places. No mortar was used in the walls' construction. Instead, the ancient architects relied on the natural fit of the rock surface. The stone circle measures 133 feet in diameter in most places. Within the confines of the outer wall are some smaller structures that resemble rooms and radial spokes.

Scholars and historians have speculated for years on Circlestone's purpose. Some say it was a stock corral, a trading center, or a defensive stronghold. However, the fact that the nearest water source is miles away makes all these hypotheses unlikely. The prevailing theory is that it was a place for religious gatherings. No one knows for sure who built Circlestone. Its construction techniques seem to predate the Hohokam and Salado people. It is possible that the Anasazi or Hopi built the structure well over 1,000 years ago.

Situated atop a 6,010-foot hill, Circlestone overlooks nearly everything in sight. Only the adjacent 6,266-foot Mound Mountain offers a better view, but there are no trails to its summit. When you arrive at Circlestone, which is nearly 1,000 feet higher than Superstition Peak, you are practically standing on the roof of the Superstitions. To reach this archaeological marvel, it is best to start from a backpacking base camp at Reavis Ranch. While you can certainly hike to Circlestone in a day, you will likely regret it the next morning: it's a 20-mile death march.

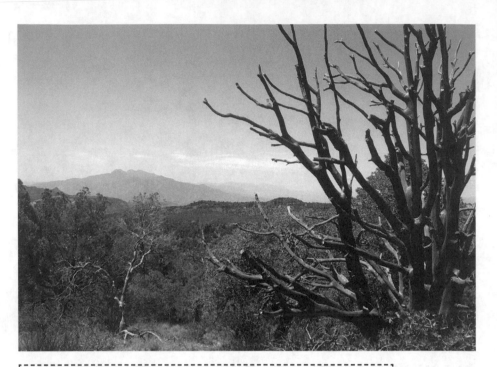

A view toward Four Peaks from the Blackman Trail near Circlestone's hilltop perch.

From Reavis Ranch, head south on Reavis Ranch Trail for about half a mile until you reach the signed Fire Line Trail junction. Turn uphill onto Fire Line Trail 118, which begins a moderate climb out of the shady pine forest and onto exposed slopes. Sharp rocks cover this rugged trail, an indication that very few people have ventured this way. Scrub live oaks and manzanita bushes are the dominant plant species along the trail.

The slope eases near 0.4 miles into the Fire Line Trail, where you reach an open plain. Look to your left for the distant outline of Four Peaks. Continue traversing the open terrain until you cross the usually dry Whisky Spring at 0.75 miles and re-enter a patch of shade. A short distance farther, cross Whisky Spring again and pass a large talus on the side of a hill.

The trail then follows a crumbly creek bed up a steep slope near dark-colored volcanic rock. After a fairly consistent climb, you'll reach Whisky Spring Saddle at 1.3 miles from the beginning of the Fire Line Trail. Pine trees surround this wide and flat saddle, and if you turn back, you can see a wall of large boulders above the treetops. The trail swings toward the southeast and descends slightly.

At 1.7 miles and 5,460 feet in elevation, the trail runs along the side of a hill with a deep ravine to its left. Look for two large cairns on the right side of the trail before it heads downhill. Leave the Fire Line Trail here and turn right onto the unmarked Blackman Trail, which immediately climbs a steep and rocky slope. Thankfully, the slope levels off after 0.2 miles. Veer left at a saddle point and keep aiming for the top of a large nondescript mound to the south.

The Blackman Trail is actually in great condition for the small amount of foot traffic it receives. As it climbs higher along a gentle ridge, your view steadily improves. Circlestone sits atop the 6,010-foot mound, which is 0.9 miles from the beginning of Blackman Trail. From this high perch, you can clearly see Four Peaks, Mound Mountain, and most of the Superstition Wilderness. From the east side of Circlestone, the copper mines in Miami are also visible.

Leave plenty of time to explore the ruins and to soak up the panoramic views. However, remember that the Circlestone walls are very fragile. Take extra care not to topple any of the stones, and make sure you leave the site undisturbed. To get the most out of your visit to Circlestone, consider reading *Circlestone: A Superstition Mountain Mystery* by James A. Swanson before you go. Better yet, take it along as a reference while you are there.

NEARBY ACTIVITIES

Reavis Ranch, the home base for this hike, is itself a popular destination for hikers and backpackers. Rogers Canyon Trail (page 182), which shares a trailhead with Reavis Ranch Trail, leads to a Salado cliff dwelling near Angel Basin. North of Reavis Ranch, a spur trail leads to Reavis Falls (page 172), a scenic waterfall nestled in the wilderness. Many other nearby trails crisscross the Superstition Wilderness.

27 FISH CREEK

KEY AT-A-GLANCE INFORMATION

LENGTH: 3 miles

ELEVATION GAIN: 250 feet

CONFIGURATION: Out-and-back

DIFFICULTY: Moderate in effort, but requires advanced route-finding and scrambling skills

SCENERY: Fish Creek Canyon, rain-forest-like vegetation, cliffs, pools

EXPOSURE: Considerable shade with some clearings

TRAFFIC: Light

TRAIL SURFACE: Heavy scrambling over boulders and along creek bed

HIKING TIME: 4 hours

WATER REQUIREMENT: 2.5 quarts

SEASON: Year-round; hot in summer

ACCESS: Sunrise to sunset; free but very limited parking

MAPS: USGS Horse Mesa Dam

FACILITIES: None

DOGS: Yes, but not recommended because of scrambling

COMMENTS: Very scenic but can be overgrown

GPS Trailhead Coordinates

UTM Zone   12S

Easting   0471547

Northing   3709312

Latitude   N33°31.488'

Longitude   W111°18.425'

IN BRIEF

With spectacular cliffs framing a narrow slot canyon, Fish Creek sports some of the most eye-popping scenery in the Superstitions. However, the price you pay to explore this wonderful landscape is tough scrambling along a tricky creek bed with no trails or route markers.

DESCRIPTION

Fish Creek, or more appropriately upper Fish Creek, is not really a hike. There are no established trails or even route markers such as cairns, flags, or signs. However, Fish Creek does have plenty to offer hikers in terms of beautiful slot canyons bounded by sheer cliffs, intriguing rock formations, and a lush riparian habitat reminiscent of a rain forest. You would never expect to find scenery like this in the middle of a desert wilderness, but that's precisely what makes the Superstitions unique.

Before you get started, be aware that Fish Creek flows through a narrow slot canyon. There is no place to escape should you be caught in a flash flood. Therefore, do not attempt this hike during or after heavy

----

Directions ⟶

Drive east from Phoenix on US 60 and exit onto Idaho Road. Drive north on Idaho Road 2.25 miles and then turn northeast onto SR 88, the Apache Trail. Follow scenic and winding SR 88 25 miles to the Fish Creek Bridge, about 0.5 miles past mile marker 223. Cross the bridge and park in a relatively wide spot along the road, but be careful not to impede traffic. Many trucks towing boats routinely pass this narrow roadway. Part of SR 88 is a graded dirt road, but it should be navigable by most passenger cars.

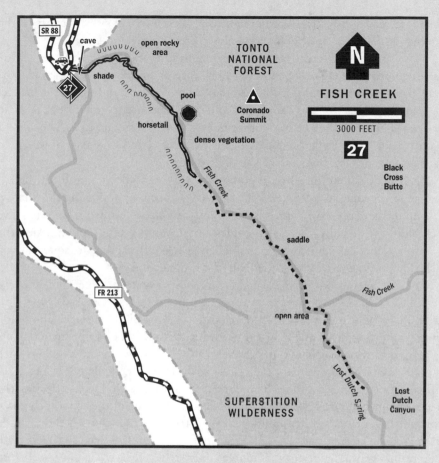

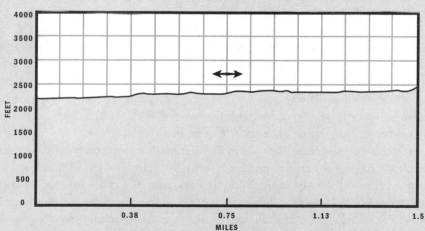

storms. Entering Fish Creek during monsoon season is also risky because of the likelihood of sudden downpours that can trigger a flash flood.

The first obstacle you face when attempting to explore Fish Creek is the task of entering the creek. The Fish Creek Bridge on SR 88 hangs high above the creek bed, with precipitous drop-offs on all sides. When standing on the bridge, you can see the narrow slot canyon and tall cliffs that rise to either side. You can see the pebbly creek bed below, but it's not obvious how to get to it. The trick is to cross back over the bridge from your parking area and find a small trail that leads up to a cave on the western side of the canyon.

It may be counterintuitive to go up when trying to descend into the creek, but the safest route into the creek is at the cave. Begin by following the narrow trail up to the large cave, which is really only an alcove eroded from a massive rock bluff. Incidentally, the cave provides a high vantage point for watching the sometimes comical shuffling of boat-laden trucks attempting to squeeze past each other on the narrow dirt road and the bridge below.

Follow an obvious trail from the cave, down a steep slope, and into the creek bed. Turn right upstream and forge deeper into Fish Creek Canyon. Initially, the pebbly streambed isn't too cluttered and seems quite navigable. Hop around large boulders, and enter a dense forest of lush trees. Water-loving plants such as cottonwoods and willows thrive in Fish Creek, while desert plants such as giant saguaros sprout from shelves on the cliff walls. Pools of various sizes that remain from the last flood lie scattered among large boulders, reflecting the green canopy and an occasional patch of clear sky. Some of these pools stagnate from the lack of fresh water and develop a putrid film of algae and slime, while others remain surprisingly clear and transparent. Each pool seems to teem with life until it eventually dries up. Tadpoles, butterflies, insects, spiders, and frogs all make their homes near the pools.

The going gets considerably tougher about 0.2 miles from the cave. Large boulders and thick bushes seem to block the path no matter which way you turn. Here's where the landscape challenges your scrambling skills and your imagination. Finding a route through the myriad of boulders, pools, and shrubbery isn't easy, but there's usually a way to get through that doesn't require any dangerous moves. Sometimes you have to climb over rocks, while other times you might crawl through an opening under overlapping boulders.

It's difficult to judge distance in Fish Creek because you will likely make very slow progress upstream, and high-tech gadgets like GPS units don't work because of the tall canyon walls. Nevertheless, near 0.4 miles into the hike the canyon opens up, yielding a better view of the imposing cliffs surrounding the canyon. The reddish hue of the rocks contrasts with abundant green leaves and blue sky. Hoodoos are often found on top of the canyon walls, and if you are lucky, a mountain goat or two will also peek down from the cliff's edge.

As you venture deeper into Fish Creek Canyon, the large boulders give way to more water and dense vegetation. Instead of scrambling over rocks, you are now bushwhacking through thick undergrowth. It helps to stay near the canyon

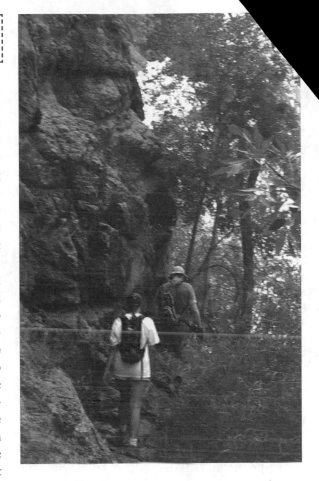

Ample cliff-side scrambling awaits those who venture into Fish Creek's verdant box canyon.

walls on the sides, but you will have to cross the creek often in order to find the optimal route through the brush. The canyon walls exhibit many interesting formations such as recumbent folds where sedimentary layers of rock are folded under intense heat and pressure.

You can explore Fish Creek for as long as you'd like. It eventually leads to Lost Dutch Canyon approximately 3.3 miles from the bridge. It is also possible to make a long one-way hike out of Fish Creek by stashing a shuttle vehicle at the Tortilla Trailhead, which requires a four-wheel-drive to reach. However, most people simply go upstream from the bridge as far as they'd like and then return the same way. A fairly reasonable turnaround point is after about 1.5 miles, which takes a first-time visitor roughly 2.5–3 hours to reach. When choosing your turnaround point, remember that the egress takes roughly half the time of the ingress because you'll have solved many of the tricky scrambling problems on your way in.

NEARBY ACTIVITIES

Canyon Lake, Apache Lake, and Roosevelt Lake are a series of reservoirs on the Salt River with marinas that lie on or near SR 88. The Superstition Wilderness contains hundreds of miles of trails, many of which are accessible via this road. The Reavis Trailhead near Apache Lake leads to Reavis Falls (page 172) and Castle Dome. Boulder Canyon Trail (page 130) starts from the Canyon Lake Marina and offers scenic views toward Weaver's Needle and Superstition Mountain. Other hikes, such as Siphon Draw (page 187) and Massacre Grounds, are located near Lost Dutchman State Park.

LYPHIC TRAIL

147

IN BRIEF

Nestled at the base of Superstition Mountain, Hieroglyphic Canyon boasts one of the best collections of Hohokam petroglyphs in the state. Venture beyond the petroglyphs and follow Hieroglyphic Canyon up to the Superstition Ridgeline for astounding views of Weaver's Needle and the city.

DESCRIPTION

Anchored by a 5,000-foot peak at each end and a long connecting ridge in the middle, Superstition Mountain dominates the East Valley skyline and has some of the best hikes near Phoenix. Hieroglyphic Trail 101 offers an excellent introductory hike for beginners, families, and first-time visitors to the Superstitions. The easily accessible trailhead, relatively short route, and gentle slopes welcome hikers of all levels. Superb views of the majestic Superstitions and a trove of prehistoric Hohokam petroglyphs provide additional incentives for a visit. Advanced hikers and adventure seekers can continue beyond the petroglyphs and follow Hieroglyphic Spring

...H: 3 miles (optional hike to Superstition Ridgeline adds 3.3 miles)

ELEVATION GAIN: 570 feet (optional hike adds 1,700 feet)

CONFIGURATION: Out-and-back

DIFFICULTY: Easy (optional hike is difficult)

SCENERY: Superstition Mountains, Hohokam petroglyphs, pools, desert,

EXPOSURE: Mostly exposed; limited shade available in riparian areas

TRAFFIC: Moderate–heavy to petroglyphs, light beyond

TRAIL SURFACE: Gravel and rock to petroglyphs; boulders and some scrambling beyond

HIKING TIME: 1.5 hours (optional hike adds 3 hours)

WATER REQUIREMENT: 1 quart to petroglyphs (optional hike adds 1.5 quarts)

SEASON: Year-round; hot in summer

ACCESS: Sunrise to sunset; free parking

MAPS: USGS Goldfield

FACILITIES: None

DOGS: Yes, leashed at all times

COMMENTS: For more information, visit www.fs.fed.us/r3/tonto/wilderness/wilderness-superstition-index.shtml.

GPS Trailhead Coordinates

UTM Zone 12S

Easting 0460575

Northing 3694382

Latitude N33°23.386'

Longitude W111°25.477'

Directions

Drive east on US 60 to Kings Ranch Road between mile markers 202 and 203. Turn northeast onto Kings Ranch Road and follow it 2.8 miles. Immediately after crossing a cattle guard, turn right onto Baseline Road and drive east 0.3 miles. Turn left onto Mohican and continue north 0.3 miles. Turn left onto Valley View Drive and follow it as it curves into Whitetail Road. Then turn right onto Cloudview Avenue and proceed 0.5 miles to the large trailhead parking lot. This route may sound complicated, but nearly all other turns are marked with "Dead End" signs.

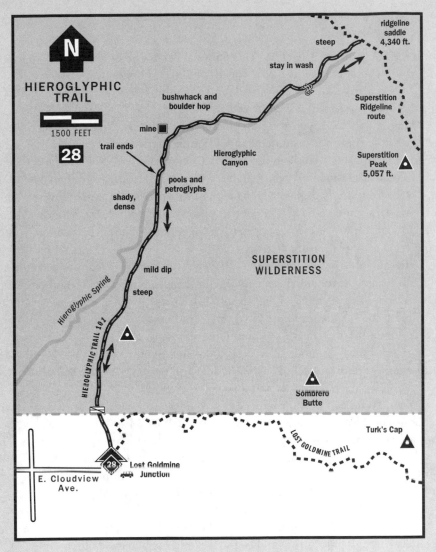

N

HIEROGLYPHIC TRAIL

1500 FEET

28

ridgeline saddle 4,340 ft.

steep

stay in wash

Superstition Ridgeline route

bushwhack and boulder hop

mine

Superstition Peak 5,057 ft.

trail ends

Hieroglyphic Canyon

pools and petroglyphs

shady, dense

SUPERSTITION WILDERNESS

Hieroglyphic Spring

mild dip

steep

HIEROGLYPHIC TRAIL 101

Sombrero Butte

Turk's Cap

LOST GOLDMINE TRAIL

28 Lost Goldmine Junction

E. Cloudview Ave.

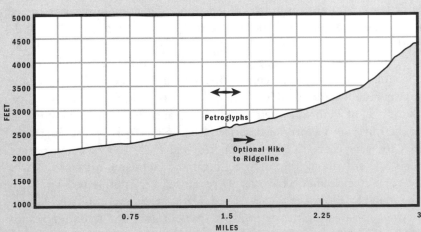

Petroglyphs

Optional Hike to Ridgeline

FEET

MILES

up to the Superstition Ridgeline. This optional excursion doubles the hike length and requires scrambling up an additional 1,700 feet. However, the just reward for your toils is an awesome view of the sprawling city below, the interior of Superstition Wilderness, and Weaver's Needle.

Hieroglyphic Canyon roughly bisects Superstition Mountain from east to west, culminating in a prominent saddle point high on its ridgeline. Near the canyon's mouth lies a cradle of granite bedrock accentuated by a series of small pools. Ancient Hohokams, who inhabited Central Arizona more than 800 years ago, etched hundreds of petroglyphs here onto a canvas of patina-covered boulders. Modern miners and settlers in the region came upon these primitive drawings and mistook them for Egyptian hieroglyphics. Thus, the canyon's name arose from a simple misunderstanding.

Hieroglyphic Trail and Lost Goldmine Trail share a common trailhead, which is located at the northern end of a large parking area at the end of Cloudview Avenue. Begin by climbing a short hill up to a ridge where two wooden signs mark the spot where Lost Goldmine Trail forks to the east. Stay left here, and continue hiking toward the mountain, enjoying clear views of Superstition Peak. To the west, mounds of hoodoos cap sedimentary plateaus like birthday candles atop a double-layered cake. The Flatiron lies on the higher plateau at the extreme western tip of this mountain range.

Near 0.3 miles, cross the Superstition Wilderness boundary fence where typical Sonoran Desert vegetation surrounds you. Triangle-leaf bursage, jojobas, and chollas line the trail, while saguaros and palo verde trees blanket the foothills. The trail becomes rocky as it begins a gentle ascent toward the mouth of Hieroglyphic Canyon. When the slope levels out at 0.6 miles, catch an open view of the city. Pass Mountain, Camelback Mountain, and South Mountain all come into view to the west, while Sombrero Butte, a hat-shaped hill, lies to the east.

Continue your gentle approach to Hieroglyphic Canyon. Soon, the trail parallels Hieroglyphic Spring and begins a moderate but short climb uphill. Skirt a rocky knoll 1.1 miles from the trailhead to enter the mouth of Hieroglyphic Canyon. Mesquite and ironwood trees provide some shade here on a hot day.

At 1.5 miles from the trailhead, reach a large rocky area where eons of water erosion have polished the granite streambed into natural tubs for several small pools. Not quite large enough for a swim but there's likely some water here year-round. Large boulders frame the pools and provide a natural canvas for hundreds of Hohokam petroglyphs. The ancient Hohokam etched scenes from their lives into a layer of desert varnish on the rocks, preserving a slice of history for generations to come. The petroglyphs here show a complex range of subjects and are among the finest collection of Hohokam artwork in Arizona. Sadly, some recent vandals have also left their marks. Another set of petroglyphs can be found by following the creek bed downstream approximately 0.1 mile.

After investigating the petroglyphs, turn around and look out toward the city. The slick rock and pools frame a scenic vista to the south. Hieroglyphic

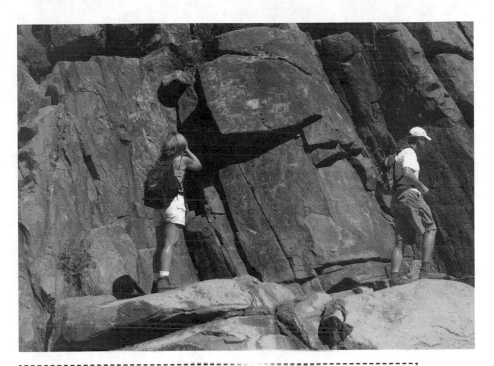

Angie Crownover and Chris Nicholas investigate petroglyphs along the Hieroglyphic Trail.

Trail ends here; casual hikers should return along the same route. Remember that the trail is located on the eastern side of the canyon just above the slick rocks and pools.

For adventurous advanced hikers, an optional trek into the upper reaches of Hieroglyphic Canyon yields some breathtaking views on the Superstition Ridgeline. However, you will need some scrambling and route-finding skills to complete the ascent. This optional segment doubles the total distance and more than triples the elevation gain.

Follow Hieroglyphic Spring upstream from the petroglyph site and stay near the left side of the canyon; you'll pass an old mine shaft at 1.8 miles from the trailhead. Turn east and scramble over large boulders in the dry creek. Vegetation can get dense and overgrown here so pick your way carefully. People rarely venture this far into Hieroglyphic Canyon, so you will likely enjoy complete solitude.

At 2.3 miles from the trailhead, arrive at the apparent confluence of two drainages. Take the left fork even though the faint path looks less traveled than the right fork. A few hundred feet farther, reach the top of a wall where a dark streak of color on the rock indicates there's a waterfall here after significant rainfall. The dense vegetation gives way to open rock faces and porous volcanic tuff as you follow the streambed past a few small pools farther up Hieroglyphic Canyon.

At 2.7 miles, arrive at another slick rock area and then a fork in the stream-bed. Route-finding is tricky here, but occasional cairns mark the way. You want to keep left, but there's another waterfall and some thick brush in the way. Work your way around the steep climb, but return to the slick rock of the streambed when possible. If you find yourself on a steep slope covered in scree and loose rock, you've gone too far to the right. There is actually a faint trail on these scree slopes marked by sparsely spaced cairns. You can try your hand at this route if you are confident; otherwise, stay in the drainage for easier route-finding. The price you pay in the drainage is dense undergrowth and more scrambling, but at least you won't get lost. The high trail is easier to find on your way down.

The final ascent involves steep but manageable scrambling along the wash. A few final switchbacks take you up to a prominent saddle point on the Super-stition Ridgeline at 4,340 feet in elevation, fully 1,700 feet higher than the petroglyph site. The Superstition Ridgeline hike (page 192) passes through this saddle, and you can see the well-worn use trail. Needless to say, the views here are stunning. To the north, a foreshortened Four Peaks towers over the rug-ged interior of Superstition Wilderness. Behind you, the city seems very far away. Turn right and walk up the hill for a spectacular profile view of Weaver's Needle, revealing that it really consists of two rock spires.

Truly masochistic hikers can continue southeast for another 0.7 miles to reach the base of Superstition Peak, which is yet another 700 feet higher. Enjoy the gorgeous views and return via the same route. On the way down, stay left of Hieroglyphic Spring and look for cairns marking your descent. Remember to veer left around the steep waterfalls.

LOST GOLDMINE TF

IN BRIEF

To those who wish to enjoy the Superstition Mountains without scaling steep grades, the Lost Goldmine Trail offers a nearly level jaunt through scenic foothills. Roughly tracing the Superstition Wilderness boundary, this trail skirts rugged cliffs and tall peaks on the southern flank of the Superstitions.

DESCRIPTION

Constructed by volunteers in 2001, Lost Goldmine Trail is one of the newest trails near the Superstition Mountains. This 6-mile trail runs along Superstition Wilderness's southern edge and links Peralta Canyon on the prominent mountain range's eastern end with

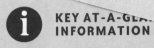

KEY AT-A-GLANCE INFORMATION

LENGTH: 6 miles
ELEVATION GAIN: -330 feet
CONFIGURATION: One-way
DIFFICULTY: Easy
SCENERY: Desert, Superstition Mountains
EXPOSURE: Completely exposed
TRAFFIC: Light
TRAIL SURFACE: Gravel, rock
HIKING TIME: 2.5 hours
WATER REQUIREMENT: 2 quarts
SEASON: Year-round; hot in summer
ACCESS: Sunrise to sunset; free parking
MAPS: USGS Goldfield and Weavers Needle
FACILITIES: None
DOGS: Yes, leashed at all times
COMMENTS: Lost Goldmine Trail actually extends 4 more miles eastward to the Broadway Trailhead, but portions of that route have been under construction recently.

Directions

Hieroglyphic Canyon Trailhead: Drive east on US 60 to Kings Ranch Road. Turn northeast onto Kings Ranch Road and follow it 2.8 miles. Immediately after crossing a cattle guard, turn right onto Baseline Road and drive east 0.3 miles. Turn left onto Mohican and continue north 0.3 miles. Turn left onto Valley View Drive and follow it as it curves into Whitetail Road. Then turn right onto Cloudview Avenue and proceed 0.5 miles to the large trailhead parking lot. This route may sound complicated, but nearly all other turns are marked with "Dead End" signs.

Lost Goldmine Trailhead: Return to US 60 and continue east. Past mile marker 204, turn northeast onto Peralta Road. Reset your trip odometer at this turn. Peralta Road becomes a dirt road after 1 mile, but most cars can safely pass, except after heavy storms. Keep left when the road forks at 5.5 miles from the turnoff. Turn into the signed parking lot for Lost Goldmine Trailhead when the trip odometer reads 7.1 miles. If you reach the Peralta Trailhead, you have gone too far.

GPS Trailhead Coordinates

UTM Zone 12S
Easting   0467138
Northing 3694638
Latitude   N33°23.589'
Longitude W111°21.242'

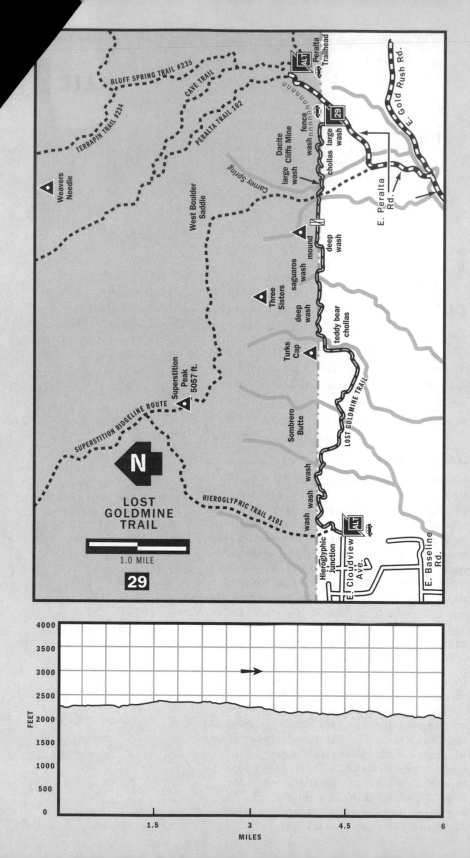

PERALTA TRAILHEAD

BLUFF SPRING TRAIL #235

CAVE TRAIL

TERRAPIN TRAIL #234

PERALTA TRAIL 102

Weavers Needle

West Boulder Saddle

Carney Spring

Dacite Cliffs Mine

fence

large wash

large wash

chollas

29

E. Gold Rush Rd.

E. Peralta Rd.

deep wash

saguaros

mound

deep wash

Three Sisters

deep wash

teddy bear chollas

Turks Cap

Superstition Peak 5057 ft.

SUPERSTITION RIDGELINE ROUTE

N

Sombrero Butte

LOST GOLDMINE TRAIL

LOST GOLDMINE TRAIL

HIEROGLYPHIC TRAIL #101

wash wash wash

Hieroglyphic Junction

E. Cloudview Ave.

E. Baseline Rd.

1.0 MILE

29

FEET

4000
3500
3000
2500
2000
1500
1000
500
0

1.5   3   4.5   6

MILES

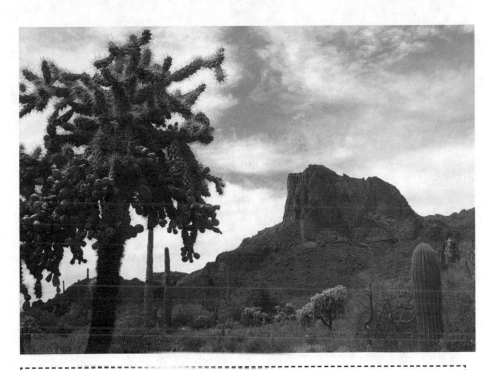

A chain-fruit cholla enlivens the Three Sisters, a prominent rock formation along Lost Goldmine Trail.

Hieroglyphic Canyon in the middle. A disjointed section of this trail extends to Jacob's Crosscut Trail near the Broadway Trailhead at the mountain range's western end. Lying in the shadows of massive cliffs and hoodoo-lined ridges, Lost Goldmine Trail showcases the rugged beauty of the venerable Superstitions and its desert foothills. This trail's relatively level elevation profile and proximity to the city also attract a wide range of hikers, bikers, and equestrians.

Lost Goldmine Trail takes its name from the legend of the Lost Dutchman's Mine, an enduring fable that has captured prospectors' imaginations for more than 100 years. Folks with dreams of finding lost treasure have come from all over the world to comb this region for signs of gold. No gold has ever been found. As recently as 2004, the U.S. Forest Service granted a rare Treasure Trove permit to a group of explorers and archaeologists attempting to locate the Lost Dutchman's Mine. They are not the first and certainly won't be the last to try.

With a shuttle vehicle, you can hike Lost Goldmine Trail in either direction. I chose to go from east to west. Begin the one-way trip from Lost Goldmine Trailhead, which is located at the end of a large parking area just shy of Peralta Trailhead (page 162) on Peralta Road. Hike west into the dense desert vegetation of triangle-leaf bursage, mesquite, palo verde, and various cacti. Superstition Mountain's eastern end features sheer cliffs and jagged peaks. The vertical face of Dacite Cliffs lies to the north. Turning to the northwest, you soon reach the wilderness boundary fence at 0.25 miles. A majority of this trail traces the fence, but don't worry, you are still surrounded by wilderness.

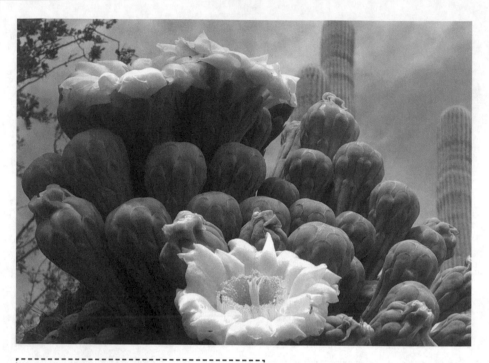

A saguaro in bloom alongside the Lost Goldmine Trail.

Following the fence westward, the trail crosses many dry washes and arroyos that drain seasonal rainfall away from the mountain. Near these dry washes, larger bushes thrive in dense clusters. A particularly deep wash lies 0.6 miles from the trailhead. Somewhere north of this spot at the base of the cliffs, Dacite Cliffs Mine lies hidden from view. Its long, dark mineshaft remains intact and hosts many bats and other nocturnal creatures. Finding the mine and exploring it will be left as an exercise for the adventurous reader. Continuing west along the fence, the trail intersects a dirt road at 0.8 miles, crosses another major wash, and then meets unmarked Carney Springs at 1.1 miles. For ambitious hikers seeking the ultimate challenge, a torturous traversal of the Superstition ridgeline (page 192) begins here and ends inside Lost Dutchman State Park on the opposite side of the mountain range.

Pass the remains of an old stock tank and then cross Carney Spring. At 1.5 miles, go through a gated fence and reach a flat mound where expansive views abound. The jagged rock formations on top of the mountain to your right are the Three Sisters, and the hoodoo-covered 5,057-foot Superstition Peak lurks behind them. Directly west lies Turks Cap and Sombrero Butte. Majestic saguaros dot the landscape while clusters of bristly cholla glow in the sunlight. During spring, a variety of wildflowers add a splash of color to the harsh Sonoran Desert landscape. Not bad for a place only minutes from the city.

Continue hiking west amid forests of saguaros and fields of cholla, through scenic valleys and across gentle slopes. The trail remains fairly level, but there are enough ups and downs to keep you on your toes. At 3 miles from the trail-head, turn south to circumnavigate a craggy hill called Turks Cap. Vegetation thins out on the southern side of Turks Cap, giving a sense of airiness to the hike. Once past Turks Cap, cross a surprisingly wide, smooth dirt road that heads straight into the hills. Superstition Peak is clearly visible now. The trail then rounds Sombrero Butte, a hill in the shape of an inverted hat.

A series of dry washes cut across the trail, which returns to the wilderness boundary at 4.8 miles from the Lost Goldmine Trailhead. Look for a seasonal waterfall and a cave high up on the mountainside. By now the western end of Superstition Mountain can be seen in the distance. The Siphon Draw Trail (page 187) inside Lost Dutchman State Park takes hikers to a prominent feature called the Flatiron, which sits on the western tip of Superstition Mountain.

Descend into a small valley at 5 miles from the trailhead. Housing developments begin to come into view, a sign that the trail's end is near. The Superstitions' dramatic western end seems to get closer and closer. Cross a few more washes as the trail approaches a tall berm. Curve south parallel to the berm for a short distance, and then climb a few switchbacks to the top of the berm, where you'll find the well-marked intersection with Hieroglyphic Trail (page 148). The Hieroglyphic Canyon Trailhead lies on the western side of the berm, a total of 6 miles from the Lost Goldmine Trailhead.

NEARBY ACTIVITIES

Hieroglyphic Trail takes hikers into Hieroglyphic Canyon where they can view some of the finest Hohokam petroglyphs in the state. Popular Peralta Trailhead provides access to Peralta Trail (page 162), Dutchman's Trail, and Bluff Spring Trail. The grueling Superstition Ridgeline hike (page 192) begins at Carney Springs Trailhead, which lies near Lost Goldmine Trail.

30 MASSACRE GROUNDS TRAIL*

KEY AT-A-GLANCE INFORMATION

LENGTH: 5.7 miles

ELEVATION GAIN: 925 feet

CONFIGURATION: Out-and-back

DIFFICULTY: Moderate

SCENERY: Massacre Falls, Superstition Mountains, Four Peaks, desert

EXPOSURE: Mostly exposed, limited shade near Massacre Falls

TRAFFIC: Light

TRAIL SURFACE: Crushed rock, gravel

HIKING TIME: 3 hours

WATER REQUIREMENT: 2.5 quarts

SEASON: Year-round; hot in summer

ACCESS: Sunrise to sunset; free parking

MAPS: USGS Goldfield

FACILITIES: None

DOGS: Yes

COMMENTS: Massacre Falls flows only after storms.

Update: As of 2009, the access road to Massacre Grounds has been blocked off for reforestation. To reach this hike, park at the Crosscut Trailhead on First Water Road. Continue along First Water Road another 0.3 miles to find the old access road. Then, turn right and hike the road for 0.7 miles to reach the original trailhead.

IN BRIEF

Take a relatively short hike into the northern flanks of Superstition Mountain for stunning views of surrounding hills, the distant city, and a seasonal waterfall. The trail also passes near the site where Apaches allegedly slaughtered a Mexican mining crew in the 1800s.

DESCRIPTION

Shrouded in legend and mystery, Massacre Grounds Trail evokes horror and wonder with its gruesome name. The imagination can run wild with phantasms of the Old Wild West if you let it. Fortunately, this relatively short jaunt into the Superstitions delivers nothing but pleasant views of rolling hills, unique rock formations, and the rugged beauty of Superstition Mountain. When in season, wildflowers dominate the foothills at the trail's beginning, and near its terminus, intermittent cascades tumble over a wide cliff face after heavy rains.

GPS Trailhead Coordinates

UTM Zone 12S

Easting   0456995

Northing 3703437

Latitude   N33°28.279'

Longitude W111°27.811'

Directions ⟶

Drive east on US 60 to the Idaho Road exit. Take Idaho Road north 2.25 miles and then turn northeast onto SR 88, the Apache Trail. Follow SR 88 to FR 78, First Water Road, which is a wide dirt road just past the entrance to Lost Dutchman State Park. Turn right onto First Water Road and drive 0.5 miles to the Crosscut Trailhead.

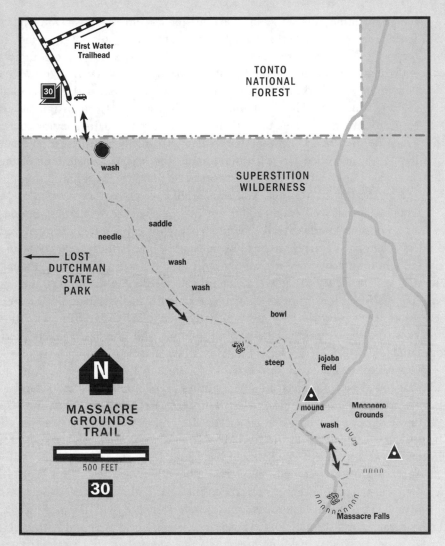

First Water
Trailhead

30

TONTO
NATIONAL
FOREST

wash

SUPERSTITION
WILDERNESS

saddle

needle

← LOST
DUTCHMAN
STATE
PARK

wash

wash

bowl

N

steep

jojoba
field

MASSACRE
GROUNDS
TRAIL

mound

Massacre
Grounds

wash

500 FEET

30

Massacre Falls

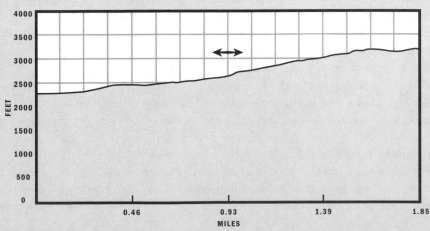

The lore behind this trail's lurid name stems from the Lost Dutchman's Mine legend, an oft-told tale that has contributed to the mystery of these mountains for more than a hundred years. In the 1800s a crew of Mexican miners supposedly met a grisly fate at the hands of Apaches in the vicinity of today's Lost Dutchman State Park. Massacre Grounds Trail passes near the location of this purported ambush. The "Dutchman" Jacob Waltz, a German immigrant and prospector, allegedly came upon their gold mine but took its location to the grave when he died in 1891. Many have since tried to locate the lost gold but none have ever succeeded. To learn more about the legend, consult one of the many available books on the subject or stop by Superstition Mountain Museum on SR 88 on the way to Massacre Grounds Trailhead.

From the unmarked trailhead, begin by crossing the wilderness boundary fence. Follow the gravel trail around a rocky hill capped by lichen-covered boulders. Then cross a dry wash lined by mesquites, hop bushes, and jojobas and head straight for a prominent needle-like spire atop a conical hill. Ignore a small spur trail that branches to the west. Behind the needle, Superstition Mountain is an impressive backdrop for this hike. Vegetation is fairly sparse, but because these foothills face north, they are especially hospitable to wildflowers. After winters with decent rainfall, a field of wild lupine and poppies blankets these slopes and adds vibrant colors to an already scenic setting.

The trail passes the rock spire to its left, climbing a gentle slope to a saddle with gracious views of Superstition Mountain's precipitous cliffs and ridgeline. Then the trail crosses the saddle and begins to turn east into a narrow basin. Hike next to the dry creek, where dense clusters of mesquites and hop bushes thrive. The trail confusingly crosses the creek a few times, passes a small dry waterfall, and then turns left up a steep chalky hill at 1 mile from the trailhead.

At the top of the steep hill, cut across a bowl-like area with Four Peaks to the north and the tip of Weaver's Needle to the east. Follow the trail as it curves around a wide basin and then turns south through a dense field of jojoba bushes. The moderate climb through jojoba bushes takes you up to a mound with excellent views of the Goldfield Mountains, the Salt River valley, and a distant Four Peaks, which appears to have a single flat summit from this vantage point. To the west, the Praying Hands rock formation lies at the cliff's edge, while Pass Mountain frames the distant city.

The trail turns east again, circumnavigating a prominent north-facing cliff and gently climbing to the flat plateau above it. At 1.5 miles from the trailhead, enter and cross a deep wash on the plateau. Avoid the temptation to scramble up this wash—look for a semi-hidden egress on the other side. After crossing the wash, encounter an open rocky plateau dotted with prickly pear cacti where the trail can be somewhat difficult to follow. Look for cairns that mark the way. To the south, you should also be able to see the cliffs over which Massacre Falls flow.

Cross this rocky plateau, heading south. Look for a spur trail going east up a gentle slope, and follow it to a vista point at the tip of a dizzying drop-

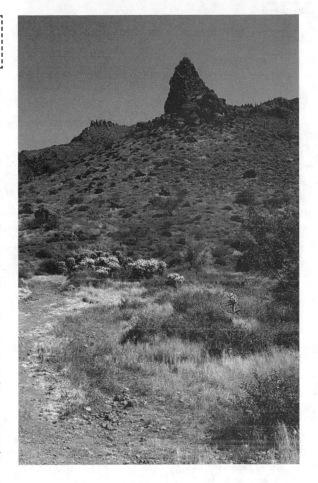

The Massacre Grounds Trail passes a prominent rock spire against a Superstition Mountain backdrop.

off. This is the end of the Massacre Grounds Trail. Now look north across the rolling hills toward Four Peaks. Massacre Grounds lies somewhere in the valley below. Backtrack along the trail that parallels the south-facing cliff to a notch at its western end. Then turn left toward Superstition Mountain and Massacre Falls.

Follow a faint trail south across a gentle slope. Soon you'll cut through some dense bushes and arrive at the eastern tip of the cliff that forms Massacre Falls. The elevation here is 3,200 feet, and with nearly 2,000 feet of mountain still above you, there's plenty of drainage water flowing down the cliff face if you happened to be here after a heavy storm. Even when the cliff is dry, an up-close view is worth the detour. Dark streaks in the reddish rock show the waterfall's path, while lush plants grow at its base. Some atypical wildflowers, such as Texas betony, can be seen here in spring and early summer.

NEARBY ACTIVITIES

Nearby Lost Dutchman State Park provides many hiking opportunities including the popular Treasure Loop and Siphon Draw (page 187) trails. The touristy ghost town of Goldfield and the Superstition Mountain Museum lie on SR 88 on your way back to town. First Water Trailhead, which is located farther east on First Water Road, offers another popular launching pad for hikes into the Superstitions. Trails accessible from there include Second Water Trail, Black Mesa Trail, and Dutchman's Trail. If you continue driving east on SR 88, you'll reach Canyon Lake, Tortilla Flat, Apache Lake, and eventually Roosevelt Lake. Many other trailheads serving the Superstition Wilderness are accessible from SR 88.

31 PERALTA TRAIL

KEY AT-A-GLANCE INFORMATION

LENGTH: 4.6 miles

ELEVATION GAIN: 1,360 feet

CONFIGURATION: Out-and-back (optional return via Cave Trail, add 0.6 miles)

DIFFICULTY: Moderate (difficult if returning via Cave Trail)

SCENERY: Desert, riparian plants, unique rock formations, Weaver's Needle

EXPOSURE: Partial shade during early morning and late afternoon, otherwise exposed

TRAFFIC: Moderate–high on Peralta Trail; sparse on Cave Trail

TRAIL SURFACE: Gravel, crushed rock, smooth rock, boulders

HIKING TIME: 3 hours (4 if returning via Cave Trail)

WATER REQUIREMENT: 2.5 quarts

SEASON: Year-round; hot in summer

ACCESS: Sunrise to sunsetMAPS: USGS Weaver's Needle, Tonto National Forest map, trailhead plaque

FACILITIES: Toilet, no water

DOGS: Yes

COMMENTS: For more information, visit www.fs.fed.us/r3/tonto/wilderness/wilderness-superstition-index.shtml.

GPS Trailhead Coordinates

UTM Zone 12S

Easting   0467714

Northing 3695225

Latitude N33°23.858'

Longitude W111°20.872'

IN BRIEF

The Superstition Wilderness offers arguably the best hiking trails near Phoenix, and the Peralta Trail is one of the most popular hikes in the Superstitions. This moderate hike introduces you to the rugged beauty of the Superstition Mountains without taxing your abilities to their limits. Fremont Saddle, the destination of this hike, rewards visitors with an awesome view of Weaver's Needle, the most famous landmark in the Superstition Mountains.

DESCRIPTION

The mysterious Superstition Mountains hold the legend of the Lost Dutchman's Mine, one of the most enduring tales of lost gold. This world-famous tale of hidden treasure still inspires the occasional prospector to comb the area in hopes of striking it rich. Legend has it that the Peralta family from Mexico owned mining operations in the Superstition Mountains in the 1850s but fled the area after the Apaches massacred their miners near the present-day Lost Dutchman State Park. The Dutchman, in actuality a German immigrant named Jacob Waltz, supposedly came upon a map to a Peralta mine and found hidden

----

Directions

Drive east from Phoenix on US 60. Approximately 23 miles past the Loop 101 junction, the freeway ends and US 60 turns into a divided highway. Just east of mile marker 204, turn north onto Peralta Road, which turns into a graded dirt road after 1 mile. Passenger cars should be fine, but watch out for stream crossings after heavy rains. At 5.5 miles from US 60, follow an obvious sign and take the left fork uphill. Continue until you reach the Peralta Trailhead parking area at 7.5 miles from US 60.

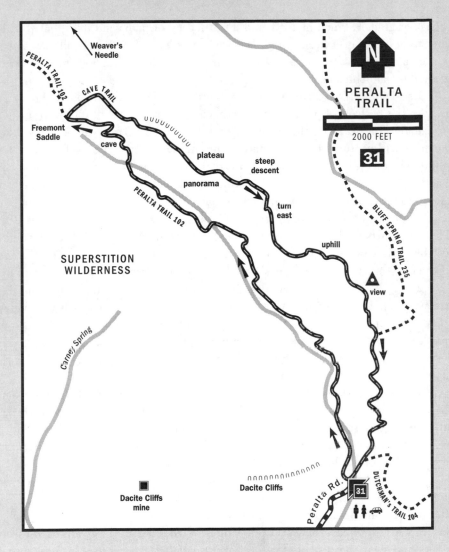

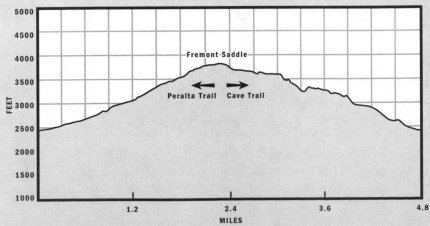

caches of gold. He died in 1891 and left a legacy of maps and tales, but to this day, no gold has ever been found. Weaver's Needle, a 1,220-foot-tall rock spire in the Superstitions, figures prominently in most stories and various maps related to the Lost Dutchman's Mine.

The Peralta Trail takes visitors 2.3 miles up Peralta Canyon to Fremont Saddle, the best overlook from which to view Weaver's Needle. If you haven't yet caught gold fever on the scenic drive to the Peralta Trailhead, the mysterious hills will capture your imagination the moment you step out of the car. As you make your way to the trailhead at the end of the parking area, the imposing Dacite Cliffs tower ominously above you on the left. What spirits lie hidden in these mountains and watch your every move?

Begin by taking a left at the trailhead, and follow signs for Peralta Trail 102. The trail starts fairly level through a desert riparian landscape full of triangle-leaf bursage, canyon ragweed, jojoba, and cactus. Mountains rise on both sides of the canyon and provide some shade during early morning and late afternoon. At 0.25 miles, cross the dry Peralta Creek and begin a gradual climb along the eastern bank of the canyon. A grove of sugar sumacs and other brush provides some shade at 0.5 miles from the trailhead. Continue climbing along the obvious trail to 0.8 miles where the trail seemingly splits. Keep to the right and you'll soon loop back to rejoin the creek bed. At 0.9 miles, another shady thicket with many smooth boulders beckons you to stop and rest.

The well-worn Peralta Trail ascends some cactus-lined switchbacks toward the east at 1 mile from the trailhead. Turn around to catch a glimpse of the ridge atop the western side of the canyon. Perhaps the ghost of the Lost Dutchman lurks among the hoodoos there? Even if your imagination fails to conjure the mysterious prospector, look for his horse in the form of a rearing steed–shaped rock.

At 1.3 miles and an elevation of 3,050 feet, the trail crosses the dry creek again and climbs up some switchbacks on the western side of the canyon. As the trail straightens into a gentle ascent around 1.5 miles, notice nearby jojoba bushes with their teardrop leaves pointing upward. Native Americans used these plants and their sweet fruits for food and medicine. Peer across the canyon to see a layer of pale green volcanic tuff and Geronimo's Cave just above it. There are also some grotesquely eroded rock formations on the eastern side. Look for a ghostly facial impression with two hollow eye sockets and a gaping mouth. The Peralta Trail crosses the creek bed again and climbs up switchbacks on top of multicolored volcanic bedrock. At 2 miles the trail passes next to the entrance of a deep cave. Unfortunately, the ceiling is extremely low, making it difficult to explore, but you can turn around and enjoy a great view of Peralta Canyon below and Picketpost Mountain in the distance. From the cave, continue up the trail another 0.3 miles to reach the obvious Fremont Saddle, where a jaw-dropping view of Weaver's Needle suddenly appears. Peralta Trail continues 4 more miles, but most day hikers turn around here. Take a well-deserved break at the

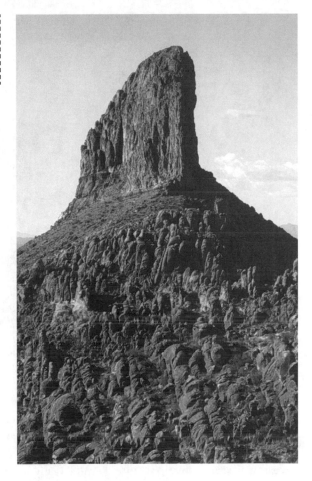

Fremont Saddle along Peralta Trail commands a splendid view of Weaver's Needle deep within Superstition Wilderness.

3,760-foot Fremont Saddle and ogle Weaver's Needle some more before returning the way you came.

If you are feeling adventurous, return via the slightly longer and much less traveled Cave Trail, which requires some scrambling and route-finding skills. Make sure you have a map and compass or map and GPS unit and that you know how to use them if necessary. To take the Cave Trail, depart Fremont Saddle to the east and follow a faint trail marked by cairns. The Cave Trail first goes northeast and then loops around to head south along the pale green volcanic ridge you saw earlier from below. The trail can disappear on the smooth rock surface, so follow cairns carefully and do not drop down into Peralta Canyon. Geronimo's Cave requires some scrambling to visit and is mostly unimpressive, so I recommend you skip it.

At 1.1 miles from Fremont Saddle, the Cave Trail descends steeply off the end of the volcanic ridge. This class-3 descent follows a steep drainage some call the Devil's Slide, which runs down a slick rock face. This route should not be attempted when wet. At the end of the slide is an even scarier drop-off. Be extra careful while shimmying down here, and don't be shy about using your hands and butt for extra traction. After the descent, the trail unexpectedly climbs back up and goes east in several spots. Keep looking for cairns marking the trail. If you don't see one for a while, backtrack and try again. The middle mile of this 3-mile return route is the most confusing, so allow extra time for route-finding.

At 2 miles from Fremont Saddle and on top of a crest, you finally get a warm and fuzzy feeling because you can now look down and see a wide and

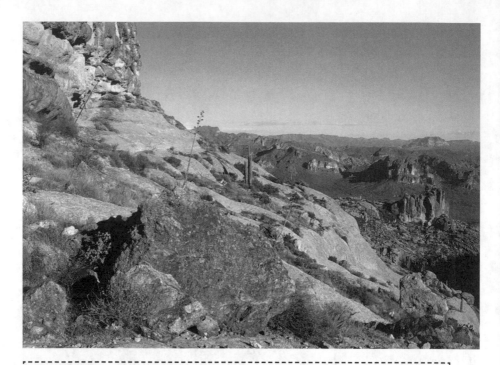

Open views abound from the lichen-covered volcanic tuff that comprises much of the Cave Trail.

obvious trail below. As you heave a sigh of relief while hiking down the hill, check out the view of Miner's Needle to the northeast and the forest of saguaros around you. The Cave Trail joins Bluff Springs Trail at an unsigned junction 2.1 miles from Fremont Saddle. Bear right here and continue south. Take a quick break at a scenic overlook into Peralta Canyon at 2.3 miles, before the trail makes another bend to the east. At 2.6 miles from Fremont Saddle, be sure to make a sharp hairpin turn, marked by a huge cairn atop a ridge. The trail drops down toward the southwest from here and merges with the Dutchman's Trail just before reaching the parking lot.

NEARBY ACTIVITIES

The Superstition Wilderness boasts an excellent network of hiking trails. The Lost Goldmine Trail is located on Peralta Road, just shy of the Peralta Trailhead. The Carney Springs Trailhead, with access to the Superstition Ridgeline (page 192), is only 1.5 miles from the Peralta Trailhead. Lost Dutchman State Park on the northwestern side of the Superstitions offers camping, ranger-led hikes, and access to the Siphon Draw Trail (page 187) where the Ridgeline hike ends. In February and March the annual Renaissance Festival, just east of the Peralta Road turnoff on US 60, comes alive with medieval fun for the whole family.

PICKETPOST MOUNTAIN*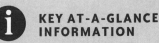

IN BRIEF

The daunting angular shape of Picketpost Mountain intrigues all who drive along US 60 between Phoenix and Superior. A short but challenging trail on the northwestern side of the mountain takes visitors 2,000 feet above the valley floor to a wide summit where, of all things, there is a mailbox.

DESCRIPTION

Drivers heading east on US 60 toward Superior must cross the 2,651-foot Gonzales Pass. When they reach its apex, an amazing view of Picketpost Mountain suddenly appears and almost assaults the field of vision. Rugged, daunting, and fortress-like, Picketpost Mountain rises sharply from the desert floor. Its angular features and steep cliffs pique the imaginations of passersby. Many wonder if it is possible to hike to its summit, and the answer, of course, is a resounding yes.

Despite its imposing appearance, Picketpost Mountain has a well-established and fairly popular trail to its summit. The Picketpost Trail approaches from the northwest and runs up a steep chute cut from sheer cliffs by millennia of erosion. Sweeping panoramic views abound on the summit. The top of Picketpost Mountain is actually quite wide

KEY AT-A-GLANCE INFORMATION

LENGTH: 4.3 miles
ELEVATION GAIN: 1,990 feet
CONFIGURATION: Out-and-back
DIFFICULTY: Difficult
SCENERY: Picketpost Mountain, panoramic views, desert
EXPOSURE: Mostly exposed; limited shade in chute
TRAFFIC: Light
TRAIL SURFACE: Gravel, rock, some scrambling
HIKING TIME: 3.5 hours
WATER REQUIREMENT: 2.5 quarts
SEASON: Year-round; hot in summer
ACCESS: Open sunrise to sunset; free parking
MAPS: USGS Picketpost Mountain
FACILITIES: Restroom, no water
DOGS: Yes
COMMENTS: Spectacular scenery and a challenging climb await those who tackle Picketpost Mountain.

Directions

Drive east from Phoenix on US 60 toward Superior. Past the Florence Junction and beyond mile marker 221, turn south onto unmarked FR 231, the Uno Trail. Follow this dirt road 0.3 miles and then make a sharp left onto paved Saddleridge Trail. Take this paved road 0.75 miles until it ends at the large parking area for Picketpost Trailhead.

GPS Trailhead Coordinates

UTM Zone 12S
Easting 0483630
Northing 3681241
Latitude N33°16.310'
Longitude W111°10.588'

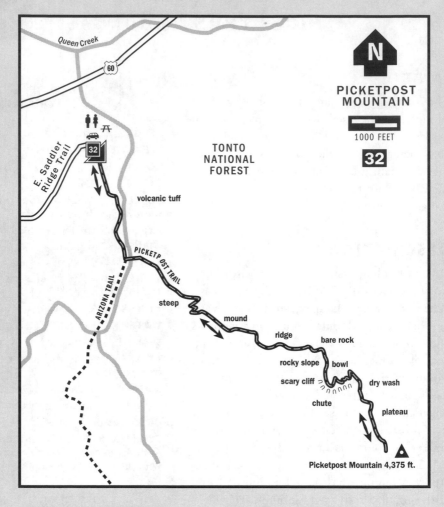

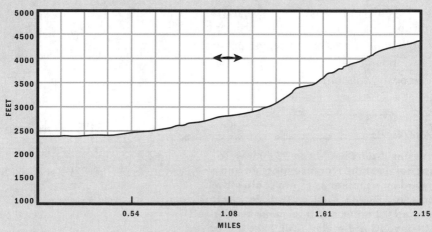

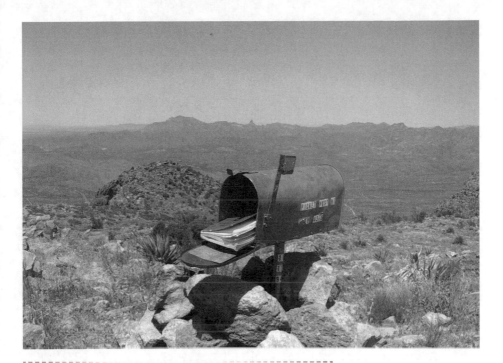

A beat-up mailbox holds the summit log atop Picketpost Mountain.

and flat, but getting there is tough. Despite being relatively short, this trail packs in plenty of elevation gain. Some route-finding and scrambling skills are also necessary in order to navigate a steep section in the chute. Hardy hikers who conquer this mountain love the challenging ascent and usually return to Picketpost Mountain regularly.

The name Picketpost comes from the fact that General George Stoneman built a military camp at the base of the mountain in 1870. The settlement guarded by this outpost eventually grew into the town of Superior just a few miles east of the mountain. Stoneman also commissioned the construction of a mule trail that ran from the outpost at the base of Picketpost Mountain, through the Queen Creek basin, and eventually to an area known today as "Top of the World." Although the soldiers soon abandoned the area, the mule trail still remains as a reminder of the region's history.

From the end of the large trailhead parking lot, find a metal sign describing the Arizona Trail, which stretches from the Mexican border to the Utah border. The first part of the hike follows the Arizona Trail south on an old jeep track named Alamo Canyon Road. Don't be fooled by the flat and inauspicious beginning; there's plenty of fun on the way. At 0.2 miles, pass a mound of lichen-encrusted volcanic tuff. These greenish porous rocks are a fairly common sight in nearby mountains. Follow the road until it parallels a dry creek bed at 0.4 miles. Look for a cairned left turn here, and leave the Arizona Trail to

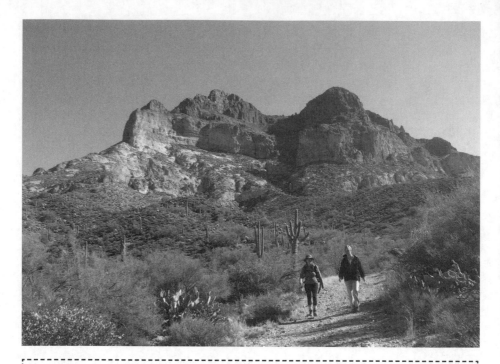

Laurie McGill and Kendra Carver descend from Picketpost Mountain on a segment of the Arizona Trail.

join a smaller dirt road, which crosses the creek bed and heads up toward the mountain.

The trail begins to climb southeast toward the foothills, gently at first but more steeply at 0.7 miles. The road soon ends at a flat area next to an old abandoned mineshaft, which has since been covered to prevent injuries. A rather abused sign marks the trail's continuation, which ascends steep switchbacks up a grassy slope. Typical desert plants like chollas, ocotillos, and jojobas line the trail. In late spring, however, look for bright orange blossoms of the desert mariposa lily, which thrives here. Bearing three delicate and colorful petals, these flowers resemble butterflies, thereby earning their Spanish name.

One mile from the trailhead, you'll reach a mound where you can catch your breath. At 2,800 feet, the view toward the valley below is already quite good. You can visually retrace your approach through the foothills. US 60 lies in the distance, and the Superstition Mountains frame the horizon. The trail bends south next to a ravine and then climbs a rocky ridge where wildflowers grow in abundance after a wet winter.

A fork in the trail appears near 1.3 miles. Take either branch uphill, clamber over the rocks above, and then veer right. What follows is a section of incredibly steep hills, some bare rock, and slippery rocky inclines. The trail bends to the right and hugs the cliff walls. At 1.5 miles you must cross an exposed narrow ledge on the side of a cliff. It's an easy traverse, but be careful with your footing and don't look down. Also, make a mental note that upon returning, you need to keep far to the right after crossing this ledge. Otherwise, you'll drop too low too soon and end up stranded by steep drop-offs.

Enter a narrow chute soon after crossing the scary ledge, and try to remember this spot so you know where to leave the chute later. You are not in the chute for very long, but ascending the deep gully can be tricky in a few places where the trail goes over boulders. Leave the chute at 1.6 miles, where the trail breaks left, and then climb up a smooth bowl into the upper basin. With all the difficult parts behind you, take time to enjoy the scenery as the gully opens wider. Agave stalks dot the hills, and a vertical cliff wall frames the left side of the gully below.

Proceed uphill on switchbacks toward the upper plateau. The trail is still steep, but no longer technical. It eventually reaches a level plateau at 2 miles from the trailhead. Cross the high plain and then turn left at a fork to reach the summit just shy of 2.2 miles from the trailhead. At 4,375 feet, the top of Picketpost Mountain offers an incredible view of the Superstition Mountains and Weaver's Needle. The town of Superior lies to the east, and an expansive wilderness stretches across the southern horizon.

An old mailbox stands proud on the summit, propped up by piles of rocks. The red flag on its side has been raised, but I doubt the postal service ever visits. Inside the mailbox, you'll find a log book where you can leave some words of wisdom for fellow hikers. There are also some drawings and mementos, but the most interesting thing is the inscription on the inside of the mailbox door. Apparently the previous owner of the tattered mailbox got tired of having it knocked down all the time, so he brought it up here for a safe retirement! It's a cute story worth reading.

Take plenty of time to enjoy the scenery from the summit of Picketpost Mountain before retracing your steps. On the way back, remember to leave the chute at the place where you entered, and stay to the right after crossing the scary ledge. If you do end up straying too low too soon, climb back up instead of trying to make an unsafe cliff traverse.

Update: As of early 2009, a new segment of the Arizona Trail has been constructed adjacent to the old Jeep road. The first 0.4 miles of this hike now follows the new Arizona Trail through Sonoran desert foothills. When the trail intersects a small dirt road near the base of Picketpost Mountain, turn left onto the dirt road to begin your ascent.

NEARBY ACTIVITIES

The Boyce Thompson Arboretum (page 135) at the base of Picketpost Mountain is one of the most unique botanical gardens in the southwest. The Superstition Wilderness northwest of Picketpost Mountain offers many other hiking opportunities.

33   REAVIS FALLS

IN BRIEF

A 140-foot-tall waterfall nestled deep in the Superstition Wilderness is the ultimate destination on this hike, but the journey to the falls is equally rewarding. Superb views of Apache Lake and the surrounding mountains abound on this scenic hike.

DESCRIPTION

Free-flowing water is always hard to find in the deserts around Phoenix, so it is difficult to believe that a 140-foot-tall waterfall exists in the Superstition Wilderness. Reavis Falls proves doubters wrong, however, with a spectacular cascade only miles from Phoenix. Fed by mountain springs deep within the Superstition Wilderness, Reavis Creek meanders around high plateaus and through deep valleys. At one particular spot in the shadows of Castle Dome, Reavis Creek tumbles down a sheer cliff to form a spectacular waterfall. The amount of water in the creek may vary with the seasons and with rainfall. Sometimes it is a mere trickle; but when conditions are right, Reavis Falls sends a powerful torrent of water tumbling over the cliff.

GPS Trailhead Coordinates

UTM Zone 12S
Easting   0478888
Northing 3712824
Latitude N33°33.398'
Longitude W111°13.687'

Directions ⟶

Drive east on US 60, and exit onto Idaho Road. Follow Idaho Road north 2.25 miles to SR 88. Turn northeast onto SR 88, Apache Trail, and follow it 29 winding miles. Past mile marker 227 look for a sign that reads "Reavis Trailhead" and turn right onto FR 212. Drive 2.9 miles on FR 212 to the large trailhead parking lot.

Note that FR 212 and portions of SR 88 are dirt roads, which are normally passable by most cars. However, during the rainy season, deep ruts may develop, requiring a high-clearance vehicle.

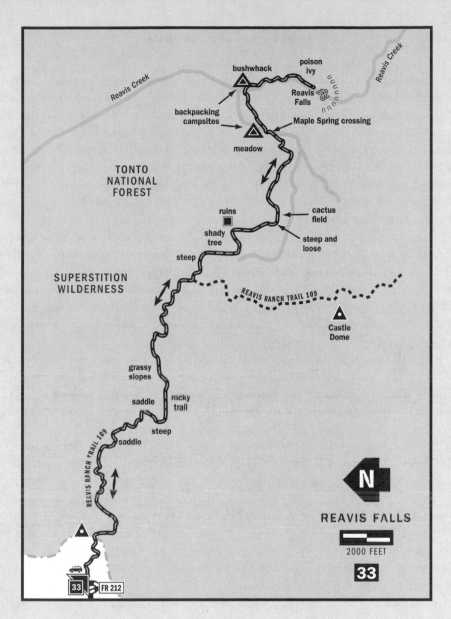

poison
ivy

bushwhack

Reavis Creek

Reavis Creek

Reavis
Falls

backpacking
campsites

Maple Spring crossing

meadow

TONTO
NATIONAL
FOREST

ruins

cactus
field

shady
tree

steep and
loose

steep

SUPERSTITION
WILDERNESS

REAVIS RANCH TRAIL 109

Castle
Dome

grassy
slopes

rocky
trail

saddle

steep

saddle

REAVIS RANCH TRAIL 109

N

REAVIS FALLS

2000 FEET

33

FR 212

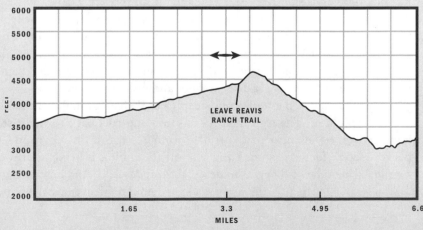

6000
5500
5000
4500
4000
3500
3000
2500
2000

FEET

LEAVE REAVIS
RANCH TRAIL

1.65   3.3   4.95   6.6

MILES

Getting to the falls isn't easy, however. Your adventure begins with the drive to Reavis Trailhead, which traces historic Apache Trail along 30 miles of twisting and winding mountainous curves. Upon arrival at Reavis Trailhead, enjoy a bird's-eye view of Apache Lake while mentally preparing for the 13-mile hike. To reach the falls, you must descend 1,625 feet into a deep valley. Hiking down-first adds a degree of difficulty not normally encountered on a mountain hike. It requires prior knowledge of your hiking ability. The bulk of the uphill toil remains for the return trip, and you can't simply turn around when you are tired. Once you are in the canyon, you must climb out.

Dire warnings aside, the hike and the falls are definitely worth the effort. Begin by heading east on Reavis Ranch Trail 109, which is sometimes called Reavis Trail. Wide and smooth, Reavis Ranch Trail is really an old dirt road that winds through the rolling hills toward Reavis Ranch. Dense patches of chia flowers often line the trail in spring, which is also the best time to visit Reavis Falls. Patches of Mexican gold poppies add some contrasting color, while delicate sego lilies bloom in April.

At 0.4 miles the trail rounds a bend and opens a northeastern view where Apache Lake and the Apache Trail can be seen in the distance. To the east, rolling hills and distant mountains stretch out for as far as the eye can see. The trail levels out and actually descends slightly as it traces a wide basin. Enjoy the wide-open views as the trail carves a path over the hilltops.

The first 2 miles of the hike are relatively flat. Then you'll climb a moderately steep hill to a saddle at 2.2 miles from the trailhead. Another high basin comes into view with the tip of Castle Dome in the distance. The trail turns left and traces the basin at roughly 4,000 feet, with expansive views of nearby mountains. Behind you, Fish Creek Mountain, Black Cross Butte, and Four Peaks line the horizon. On a clear day, you can even see Camelback Mountain in the center of town. At 2.4 miles the trail becomes notably rougher and rockier. Tall grasses blanket the hillside and sway back and forth with the slightest wind. The entire scene looks quite out of place in Arizona.

At exactly 3.5 miles from the trailhead, and with Castle Dome directly ahead, find an obvious spur trail that heads uphill to the left. Leave the Reavis Ranch Trail at this point and branch onto a nameless trail. Steep and rocky, the next quarter mile requires significant work. Hike up the narrow grass-lined trail to a wide saddle at 4,675 feet, the high point on this hike. An expansive valley with a deep ravine comes into view. Don't panic, but your destination is the bottom of the ravine! Try not to get discouraged, and just keep going.

Crossing the saddle, the trail drops steeply but then eases slightly at 4 miles from Reavis Trailhead. The trail then turns south and cuts back to the east. A lone juniper tree stands next to the trail, forming a natural campground for backpackers. Look for some stone ruins just off the trail as it bends southward along a ridge. Then the trail begins to descend. And descend. And descend some more. Watch your footing on the loose rocks—there are plenty of prickly pear

A hiker rests at the base of Reavis Falls in the heart of Superstition Wilderness.

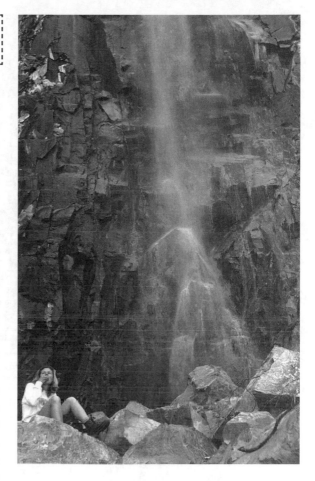

cacti to break your fall if you are not careful.

Turn left and hike around the northern side of Lime Mountain where hackberry, juniper, and manzanita bushes provide some shade. Then descend some more via steep switchbacks to reach the flat meadow of Cedar Basin at 5.5 miles. There are some concrete slabs here, perhaps remnants of an old shelter. Today, backpackers use this spot as a campground. A bit farther along the trail, cross Maple Spring and continue past thick bushes and some malnourished cacti. Then pass through some hop bushes and grassy meadows to ascend a thin ridge. Cross the ridge and descend yet another steep and slippery hill to reach Reavis Creek at 6 miles from the trailhead. On the other side of the creek, natural campsites treat backpackers to a creek-side home away from home.

Now the fun truly begins. Turn right and follow the creek upstream. The trail fades and reappears, crosses over the creek several times, and goes over boulders and fallen logs. When in doubt, look for cairns or just bushwhack up the creek. There are no established trails here, so you'll have to be creative. Watch out for poison ivy, which grows rather well in the shady woods next to the water.

After 0.6 miles of bushwhacking and boulder-hopping, you'll finally see Reavis Falls over the treetops. As you get closer, the falls become more impressive. There used to be a pool at the base of Reavis Falls, but a giant rockslide in January of 2004 buried it under tons of rubble. Nevertheless, seeing the awesome 140-foot waterfall in the middle of the Superstition Wilderness is worth the effort.

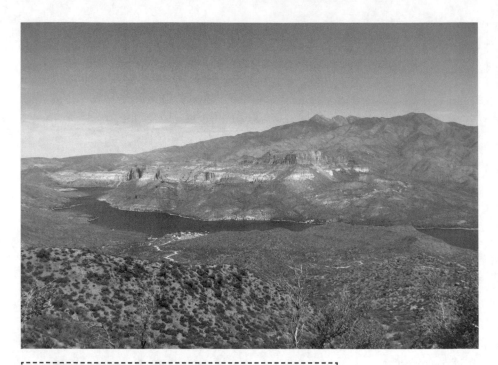

A view toward Four Peaks and Apache Lake from the Reavis Trailhead.

Tall cliffs and rocky slopes encircle Reavis Falls, forming a secluded alcove at the head of the canyon. It's an ideal place to have a picnic or just enjoy the scenery. Rest well because climbing out of the canyon is a lot tougher than entering it. Return the way you came.

NEARBY ACTIVITIES

Apache Lake and Canyon Lake are popular destinations for water sports. The Superstition Wilderness holds a treasure trove of trails; many hikes in this book are based in the Superstitions. Boulder Canyon (page 130), Reavis Ranch (page 177), Rogers Canyon (page 182), and Fish Creek (page 144) are just some of the trails nearby.

REAVIS RANCH VIA
ROGERS TROUGH TRAILHEAD
34

IN BRIEF

Reavis Ranch lies high in the remote Superstition Wilderness among tall pines and adjacent to a perennial creek. It's a popular destination for backpackers, especially in fall when the apple orchard bears fruit. A scenic but long hike is the only way to access Reavis Ranch, ensuring its preservation from overuse.

DESCRIPTION

In 1874, Elisha M. Reavis, an eccentric recluse remembered as the "Hermit of Superstition Mountain," constructed his home in a mountain meadow deep in the wilderness. He became the first Anglo settler in the Superstitions and established a farm next to the perennial creek that bears his name today. The creek fed a 140-acre ranch and nourished the fruits and vegetables that Reavis cultivated on his property. He would cart the produce down long, winding hills to sell them in nearby mining communities. In the winter of 1896 Reavis died along the trail while making one of his

KEY AT-A-GLANCE INFORMATION

LENGTH: 15 miles
ELEVATION GAIN: 940 feet
CONFIGURATION: Out-and-back
DIFFICULTY: Moderate to difficult
SCENERY: Pine forest, high desert, Superstition Wilderness, Reavis Ranch, Reavis Creek
EXPOSURE: Significant shade in the pine forest
TRAFFIC: Light
TRAIL SURFACE: Gravel, rock, riverbed, packed dirt, grass
HIKING TIME: 8 hours
WATER REQUIREMENT: 4–5 quarts
SEASON: Year-round; hot in summer
ACCESS: Sunrise to sunset; free parking; camp at large
MAPS: USGS Iron Mountain, Tonto National Forest map
FACILITIES: None
DOGS: Yes
COMMENTS: Reavis Ranch is a popular backpacking destination. For more information, visit www.fs.fed.us/r3/tonto/wilderness/wilderness-superstition-index.shtml.

Directions

Drive east on US 60 past mile marker 214 to Queen Valley Road. Turn left onto Queen Valley Road, reset your trip odometer, and drive 1.7 miles to Hewitt Station Road. Bear right onto the gravel Hewitt Station Road and follow it until the signed turnoff to FR 172 at odometer 4.8 miles. Turn left onto FR 172, cross Queen Creek, and drive through scenic desert foothills to the junction with FR 172A at 14.1 miles. Turn right onto FR 172A and follow the rough dirt road to a T intersection at odometer 17.7 miles. Turn left and continue 0.4 miles to the Rogers Trough Trailhead.

This drive is very scenic but requires a high-clearance vehicle in good weather. Four-wheel-drive may be necessary after storms.

GPS Trailhead Coordinates

UTM Zone   12S
Easting   0483946
Northing   3697915
Latitude   N33°25.335'
Longitude   W111°10.403'

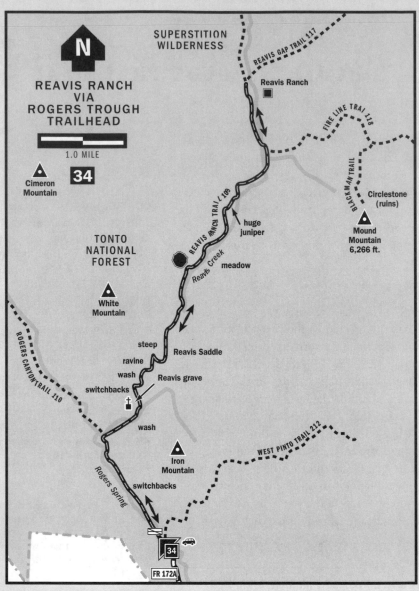

SUPERSTITION WILDERNESS

N

REAVIS GAP TRAIL 117

Reavis Ranch

REAVIS RANCH
VIA
ROGERS TROUGH
TRAILHEAD

1.0 MILE

34

Cimeron
Mountain

FIRE LINE TRAIL 118

BLACKMAN TRAIL

Circlestone
(ruins)

Mound
Mountain
6,266 ft.

huge
juniper

TONTO
NATIONAL
FOREST

REAVIS RANCH TRAIL 109

Reavis Creek

meadow

White
Mountain

steep

ravine

Reavis Saddle

wash

Reavis grave

ROGERS CANYON TRAIL 110

switchbacks

✝

wash

WEST PINTO TRAIL 212

Iron
Mountain

Rogers Spring

switchbacks

34

FR 172A

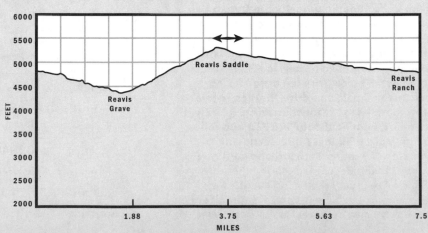

6000					
5500					
5000		Reavis Saddle			
4500					Reavis Ranch
4000	Reavis Grave				
3500					
3000					
2500					
2000					

FEET

1.88   3.75   5.63   7.5

MILES

Dietmar Giebert of Phoenix explores a forested section of Reavis Ranch Trail.

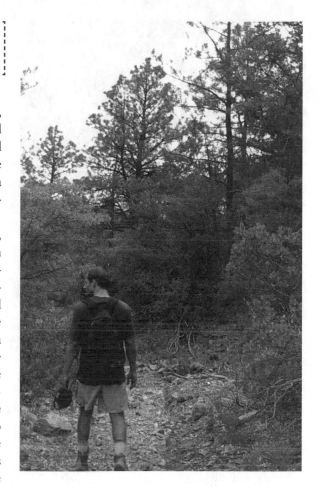

Dietmar Giebert of Phoenix explores a forested section of Reavis Ranch Trail.

countless trips to town, and kind passersby buried him right where they found him. His makeshift grave remains to this day as a reminder of the trail's colorful history.

After Reavis's death, the ranch passed through many hands, with each successive proprietor embellishing it. An apple orchard sprang up, a dirt road came in from the north, and a ranch house was built. The lush meadow high in the mountains became a popular place to visit. Some people had even tried to build a resort here to take advantage of the cool pines and trickling spring. The Department of Agriculture eventually acquired the property in the late 1960s as part of Tonto National Forest and subsequently closed the dirt road.

With cool pine forests, an apple orchard, and a flowing stream, Reavis Ranch has become a mecca for backpackers. The ranch house served as a welcome shelter for hikers and equestrians until a fire leveled it in 1991. The ranch is slowly but surely returning to nature. Today only the apple trees and some rusty farm tools survive as reminders of its domesticated past. The ranch is still a pleasant place to visit, however. Retracing Reavis's footsteps on historic Reavis Ranch Trail 109 transports you back in time, while trekking through the cool pine forest imparts an experience many would not believe possible so close to Phoenix.

Begin this hike from the Rogers Trough Trailhead after a scenic but rough drive through the Superstition Wilderness. A prominent sign indicates that this trail is a segment of the Arizona Trail. The trail runs north parallel to Rogers Creek and soon passes a junction with West Pinto Trail 212. Located at 4,800 feet, the trailside vegetation bears little resemblance to the desert plants near

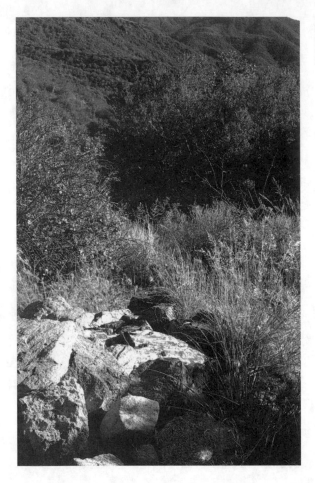

Elisha M. Reavis was burried right along the trail that bears his name today.

Phoenix. Alligator junipers and scrub live oaks dominate the landscape, and the temperature is likely 15–20 degrees cooler than in town.

Pass through a gated fence at 0.3 miles from the trailhead and then follow the obvious trail across Rogers Creek a few times, with Iron Mountain looming over your right shoulder. At 0.5 miles manzanita bushes line the trail as it descends into the canyon. A set of switchbacks near 0.9 miles takes you farther down, and you can't help but think about the return trip and the climb back up. Reach another manzanita patch at the nadir of your descent nearly 1.7 miles from the trailhead. Here, Rogers Canyon Trail 110 forks to the left and eventually leads to some well-preserved Salado cliff dwellings.

Veer right at the Rogers Canyon junction to stay on Reavis Ranch Trail. For the next 0.6 miles, you are generally following the creek bed northeast. Riparian grasses and sugar sumacs have replaced manzanitas as the dominate plant life. At 2.3 miles and just before the trail begins to switchback, a small cairn on the left side of the trail marks an overgrown path to Reavis's grave site. His simple tomb lies atop a small knoll with a view of the surrounding hills, and Reavis would have likely been happy with his final resting place.

Return to the main trail after paying your respects, and then begin climbing switchbacks on the left side of the canyon. Dense patches of sugar sumacs line the smooth trail as you attack the steep hills. This section becomes especially difficult if you are carrying a heavy pack. After a long ascent, the trail reaches Reavis Saddle at an elevation of 5,300 feet where you command an impressive view back down the canyon.

On the high plateau, the scenery changes suddenly from high desert to forest. A convenient fallen tree next to the trail makes an excellent bench on which to rest. As you hike farther north, the trail gently descends and then enters a thick forest of pinyon pines and alligator junipers. The scent of pine needles fills the air, and you'd swear you were in Flagstaff if you hadn't just hiked up from Rogers Trough.

Reavis Ranch Trail remains relatively flat for the remainder of the hike. It crosses a dry creek several times atop the plateau and traverses a large meadow at 5.2 miles from the trailhead. A quarter mile farther, you encounter a flowing Reavis Creek, which is fed by an underground spring. Tiny blue butterflies dance around the water in a wide-open meadow blanketed by tall grasses, an idyllic scene in a pristine wilderness.

Pass a gigantic alligator juniper at 5.8 miles, and then cross the creek twice at 6.3 and 6.5 miles from the trailhead. Fire Line Trail 118 merges in from the right at 6.8 miles. After you pass that trail junction, it's only a half mile or so to Reavis Ranch.

Probably the first obvious sign of the Reavis property is an old well to the left of the trail. Some rusty remnants of farm machinery lie strewn about the grasses. A large sunken meadow sits to the right of the trail and holds a horse corral, while Reavis Creek flows east of the meadow. Allow plenty of time to explore the large property. If you happen to be here in autumn, be sure to sample the plentiful crop of apples from the orchard on the northern end of the ranch.

At 7.5 miles from the trailhead, reach the junction with Reavis Gap Trail 117 and the turnaround point for this hike. The Arizona Trail follows Reavis Gap Trail eastward as it cuts across the meadow. Should you continue north on Reavis Ranch Trail, you'll eventually reach the Reavis Trailhead near Apache Lake after 10 miles. If you are staying the night, consider taking a detour to visit Circlestone. Otherwise, retrace your steps for a 15-mile round-trip hike.

NEARBY ACTIVITIES

The Superstition Wilderness contains hundreds of miles of trails. A popular side trip from Reavis Ranch, Circlestone (page 139) offers panoramic views and ancient ruins. Rogers Canyon (page 182), along the way to Reavis Ranch, holds a well-preserved Salado cliff dwelling. North of Reavis Ranch, a spur trail takes visitors to Reavis Falls (page 172), a tall waterfall hidden in the wilderness.

35 ROGERS CANYON TRAIL

KEY AT-A-GLANCE INFORMATION

LENGTH: 9 miles

ELEVATION GAIN: -1,133 feet

CONFIGURATION: Out-and-back

DIFFICULTY: Moderate

SCENERY: Rogers Canyon, Salado cliff dwellings, mountain stream, rock formations

EXPOSURE: Significant shade

TRAFFIC: Moderate

TRAIL SURFACE: Rock, packed dirt, gravel, streambed

HIKING TIME: 5 hours

WATER REQUIREMENT: 3 quarts

SEASON: Year-round; hot in summer

ACCESS: Sunrise to sunset; free parking; camp at large

MAPS: USGS Iron Mountain

FACILITIES: None

DOGS: Yes

COMMENTS: Ancient cliff dwellings are a bonus on this already scenic hike. For more information, visit www.fs.fed.us/r3/tonto/ wilderness/wilderness-superstition-index.shtml.

GPS Trailhead Coordinates

UTM Zone   12S

Easting   0483946

Northing   3697915

Latitude   N33°25.335'

Longitude W111°10.403'

IN BRIEF

Scenic Rogers Canyon makes the long and rough drive to Rogers Trough Trailhead worthwhile. Shady streamside trails, beautiful deep canyons, and well-preserved Salado cliff dwellings make this hike a must for any outdoor enthusiast.

DESCRIPTION

The rugged Superstition Wilderness never ceases to amaze me because within its confines are some of the finest hikes in Arizona. The charming spring and sheer cliffs in Rogers Canyon typify the natural beauty of the region, and many consider it a hidden gem within the wilderness. Add a scenic drive to the trailhead and the mystique of ancient cliff dwellings, and you have an experience you won't soon forget.

The long drive to Rogers Trough Trailhead passes through gorgeous canyons, sandy wash crossings, and mountain vistas, setting the proper frame of mind for this excursion.

Directions

Drive east on US 60 past mile marker 214 to Queen Valley Road. Turn left onto Queen Valley Road, reset your trip odometer, and drive 1.7 miles to Hewitt Station Road. Bear right onto the gravel Hewitt Station Road and follow it until the signed turnoff to FR 172 at odometer 4.8 miles. Turn left onto FR 172, cross Queen Creek, and drive through scenic desert foothills to the junction with FR 172A at 14.1 miles. Turn right onto FR 172A and follow the rough dirt road to a T intersection at odometer 17.7 miles. Turn left here and drive 0.4 miles to the Rogers Trough Trailhead.

This drive is very scenic but requires a high-clearance vehicle in good weather. Four-wheel-drive may be necessary after storms.

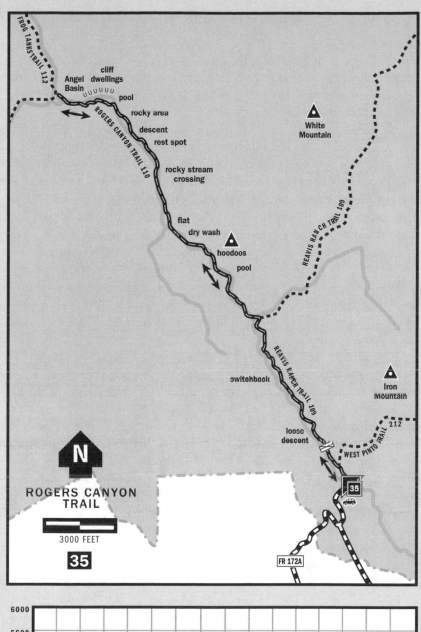

FROG TANKS TRAIL 112

cliff
dwellings
Angel
Basin
ᴜᴜᴜᴜᴜᴜ pool
ROGERS CANYON TRAIL 110
rocky area
descent
rest spot
rocky stream
crossing

flat
dry wash
hoodoos
pool

White
Mountain

REAVIS RANCH TRAIL 109

switchback

REAVIS RANCH TRAIL 109

Iron
Mountain

212
WEST PINTO TRAIL

loose
descent

35

N

ROGERS CANYON
TRAIL

3000 FEET

35

FR 172A

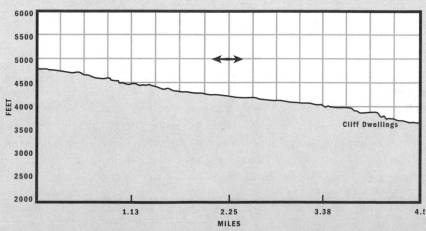

6000
5500
5000
4500
4000
3500
3000
2500
2000

FEET

Cliff Dwellings

1.13   2.25   3.38   4.5
MILES

When you arrive at the trailhead, the outdoor experience gets even better. At its finest, Rogers Canyon offers a winding hike through colorful fall leaves. Ample shade and the trickling sound of water along this trail make it a desirable destination regardless of season.

From the wide parking area at Rogers Trough, head north on Reavis Ranch Trail 109. The 4,800-foot elevation here discourages most desert plants. Instead, junipers and other evergreens dot the hills, and thick grasses cover the ground. The trail follows Rogers Spring, which feeds large deciduous trees such as the Arizona sycamore. At 0.1 mile, pass the junction with West Pinto Trail 212, which branches off to the east. Continue along the Reavis Ranch Trail and pass through a gated fence at 0.3 miles. The trail becomes sandy here as it crosses the spring.

A half mile into the hike, you'll descend a steep, slippery slope. Thickets of manzanita bushes line the trail, their silky-smooth red bark contrasting with silver-green leaves. Cross the spring again, and then climb out of the canyon to a high ledge where an expansive view opens before you. Iron Mountain towers above you to the right. The trail drops off steeply again and returns to the streambed at 0.9 miles.

Hike the next half mile near the spring and among giant sycamore trees with their signature white bark. Pass a bend in the trail where there's a rocky drop-off on the left, and then dive into another patch of cool shady manzanita. At 1.7 miles veer left onto Rogers Canyon Trail 110, which begins with a thick forest of manzanitas and live oaks.

As you enter Rogers Canyon, crisscrossing the spring and passing sycamores and sugar sumacs, the scenery steadily improves. Thick brush surrounds the trail, and rocky ridges top both sides of the canyon. In rainy seasons many stream crossings take you past small cascades where the water tumbles a few feet into shallow pools. When hiking next to the spring, you often walk under shady trees with views of oddly shaped hoodoos along the ridge tops. Near 2.7 miles you'll reach a flat section parallel to the spring, where you have a head-on view of a massive jagged mountaintop.

Roughly 3.3 miles into the hike, cross the spring again at a rocky spot and then climb up its right bank. Soon, a clearing opens with views of yellowish volcanic tuff on the hills framing the canyon. The trail can be a little hard to find here, but it goes along the right side of the spring. The streamside rocks and clearings near this stretch make great rest stops. Then the trail descends again through rough terrain. Watch out for thorny catclaw acacias tearing at your clothing.

Entering the depths of Rogers Canyon, the trail undulates, passing over rocky areas that require a bit more effort and attention. Thankfully, the scenery continues to improve. At 3.7 miles cross a rocky mound where you have an open view straight into the canyon. Continuing next to the spring and seasonal pools, look for the cliff dwellings ahead; they are on the right bank about 100 feet above the canyon floor.

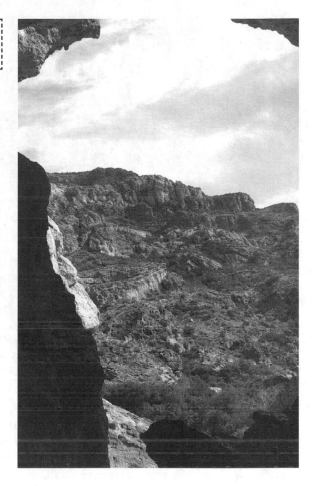

Ancient Salado cliff dwellers enjoyed this view of Rogers Canyon from their hermitic home.

At 4.1 miles a cairned turnoff takes you across the spring and up a steep slope to the cliff dwellings. In the 1300s the Salado people built many such dwellings in canyon walls and caves throughout the region. Judging by the location of this particular settlement, they picked a very scenic and strategic place to live. Taking advantage of natural shelter provided by the canyon walls, the Salado crafted several multistory homes and common living quarters into deep caves. From these ruins, you command a gorgeous view both up and down the canyon, making this spot an ideal picnic setting. Note the large plaque reminding hikers to keep off the walls and to protect the fragile buildings. The most important structure in this cliff-dwelling complex is located high up in the rocks and requires a little light scrambling to visit. Please leave everything as you found it.

Most people turn back after reaching the ruins, but it is worthwhile to hike another five to ten minutes to visit Angel Basin. Backtrack to the main trail and continue west along the Rogers Canyon Trail. Hike through thick thorny brush to a clearing approximately 4.3 miles from the trailhead. Head toward the large open basin directly in front of you, and reach the signed junction with Frog Tanks Trail 112 at 4.5 miles. This is Angel Basin, a favorite destination of backpackers and campers. A ring of scenic mountains surrounds the wide-open plain, which is covered in deep soft grass. In front of you looms a mound topped by massive boulders, perched like a castle overlooking its domain. A narrow vertical gap serves as the doorway to the castle, and there's even a rock in the shape of a dog guarding the entrance.

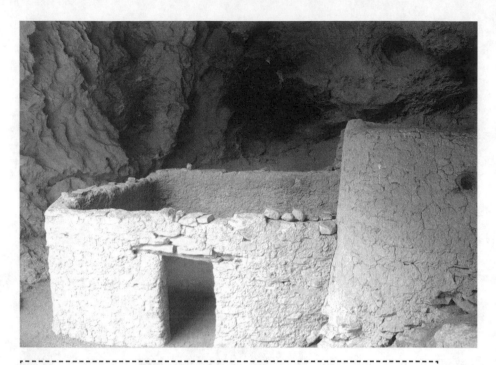

Visit this well-preserved Salado cliff dwelling deep within Rogers Canyon in the Superstitions.

Rogers Canyon Trail continues westward and terminates in JF Trail 106. If you have a shuttle vehicle, you can take JF Trail to the Woodbury Trailhead at the end of FR 172. However, most hikers are content with seeing Angel Basin and the cliff dwellings. Rest here, and return the same way. Remember that the hike out of Rogers Canyon gains over 1,000 feet with the toughest climb near the end, so save some gusto for the last mile.

NEARBY ACTIVITIES

Rogers Canyon lies in the heart of the Superstition Wilderness, home to many hikes in this book, including Siphon Draw (page 187), Boulder Canyon (page 130), Peralta Canyon (page 162), and Lost Goldmine (page 153). Farther out on US 60, Picketpost Mountain (page 167) and Boyce Thompson Arboretum (page 135) offer other hiking opportunities.

SIPHON DRAW TRAIL* 36

IN BRIEF

Siphon Draw Trail and the Flatiron capture the rugged beauty of the Superstition Mountains and package the essence of this wondrous wilderness into a short but very challenging hike.

DESCRIPTION

The Superstition Wilderness offers arguably the best hikes near Phoenix. With a rich and storied history and hundreds of miles of trails running through a land of stark contrasts, the Superstitions draw visitors of all types. Hikers especially enjoy its diverse scenery and challenging trails. Siphon Draw Trail 53 ranks high on most people's lists because it is readily accessible and packs so much scenery into a relatively short 6-mile hike.

Along Siphon Draw Trail, fields of wildflowers cover gentle foothills during spring. Strange rock formations frame the canyon, and the Flatiron, a massive yet smooth protrusion of rock, looms over the trail. A seasonal waterfall delights timely visitors. Views from Siphon Draw and especially atop Flatiron are unparalleled. However, the upper half of the canyon remains raw and rugged, requiring much scrambling and plenty of sweat and toil to explore fully. If you like mild switchbacks, this hike is not for you. There are no switchbacks, and the elevation

 KEY AT-A-GLANCE INFORMATION

LENGTH: 6 miles (optional climb to summit, add 0.4 miles)
ELEVATION GAIN: 2,625 feet (optional climb to summit, add 300 feet)
CONFIGURATION: Out-and-back
DIFFICULTY: Moderate to the waterfall, very difficult to the Flatiron
SCENERY: Superstition Mountains, Flatiron, seasonal waterfall, city panoramas
EXPOSURE: Mostly exposed; some early-morning shade
TRAFFIC: Moderate to heavy
TRAIL SURFACE: Rock, gravel, boulders, scrambling, climbing
HIKING TIME: 5 hours
WATER REQUIREMENT: 3 quarts
SEASON: Year-round; hot in summer
ACCESS: Sunrise to 10 p.m.; $6 per vehicle entrance fee
MAPS: USGS Goldfield
FACILITIES: Restroom, water, picnic area, campground, ranger station
DOGS: Yes, but not recommended for trail above the waterfall
COMMENTS: Spectacular climb to a spectacular vista point at the Flatiron. Call (480) 982-4485 for details, or visit www.azstateparks.com/Parks/LODU/index.html.

Directions ———————————————➤

Drive east on US 60 and exit onto Idaho Road. Drive 2.25 miles north on Idaho Road to SR 88, the Apache Trail. Turn northeast onto SR 88, and continue 5 miles to the entrance of Lost Dutchman State Park. Pay the entrance fee and then follow the signs to the Siphon Draw Trailhead in the Saguaro Day Use Area.

GPS Trailhead Coordinates

UTM Zone 12S
Easting   0455450
Northing 3702110
Latitude N33°27.558'
Longitude W111°28.801'

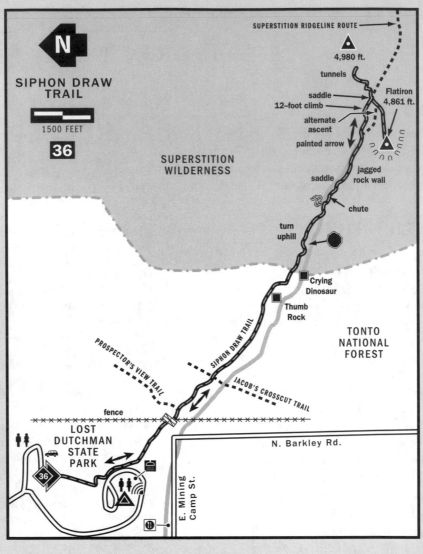

N

SIPHON DRAW
TRAIL

1500 FEET

36

SUPERSTITION
WILDERNESS

SUPERSTITION RIDGELINE ROUTE

4,980 ft.

tunnels

saddle
12-foot climb
alternate
ascent

painted arrow

Flatiron
4,861 ft.

saddle

jagged
rock wall

chute

turn
uphill

Crying
Dinosaur

Thumb
Rock

TONTO
NATIONAL
FOREST

PROSPECTOR'S VIEW TRAIL

SIPHON DRAW TRAIL

JACOB'S CROSSCUT TRAIL

fence

LOST
DUTCHMAN
STATE
PARK

36

N. Barkley Rd.

E. Mining Camp St.

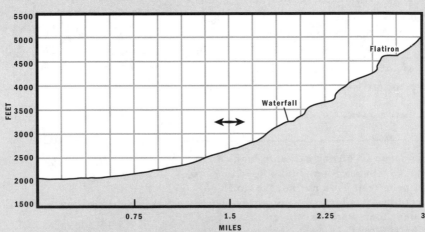

5500

5000

4500

4000

3500

3000

2500

2000

1500

FEET

Flatiron

Waterfall

0.75   1.5   2.25   3

MILES

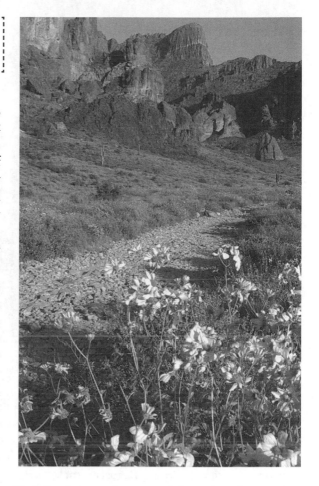

Brittlebush bloom next to Siphon Draw Trail at the base of Superstition Mountains.

profile rises exponentially, something I wish the stock market indexes would do. Perhaps the challenge of conquering Siphon Draw is part of its mystique, and those who succeed are duly rewarded.

The trailhead for Siphon Draw lies inside Lost Dutchman State Park—the state park closest to Phoenix—although most of the trail stretches beyond park boundaries into Tonto National Forest. The park is named after the legend of the Lost Dutchman, actually a German prospector named Jacob Waltz, who purportedly stashed gold in these mountains in the late 1800s. He left a legacy of maps and fantasies of treasures, but no one has ever found gold.

Because of Siphon Draw's popularity, park officials recently relocated the trailhead from a small parking lot near the campground to the larger Saguaro Day Use Area. Begin at the signed trailhead at the western end of the parking lot. The first part of the hike follows the Discovery Trail, a gentle stroll among desert plants along a path with interpretive signs. Turn left at a signed junction just before a wooden bridge to access the Siphon Draw Trail, and you'll soon pass the campground restroom and shower building. At 0.5 miles turn left again and head toward the mountains on a bed of crushed rock.

Siphon Draw Trail heads southeast into the Superstition Mountains, passing a fence and equestrian guard as it enters Tonto National Forest. Climbing gently up a wide path, cross the intersections with Prospector's View Trail and Jacob's Crosscut Trail. Note the trailside remnants of a bunker, which was part of nearby Palmer Mine. During certain springs these foothills display a gorgeous blanket of golden brittlebush flowers. Poppies, lupine, and globe mallows also add a dash of vibrant color.

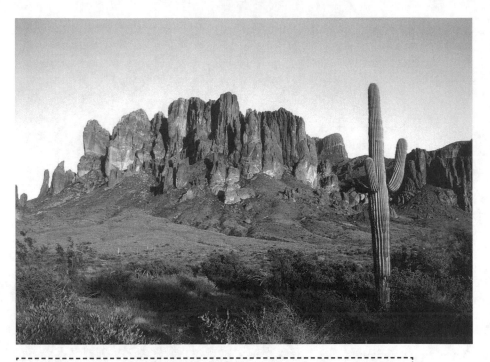

Praying Hands and the Flatiron flank the Superstition Mountains along Siphon Draw Trail.

As the trail enters Superstition Wilderness and approaches the canyon, it gets progressively steeper. At 1.6 miles from the trailhead, look to your right for a large protruding boulder in the shape of a thumb. Some call this formation Thumb Rock. The trail continues to slope up as you enter the mouth of the canyon. Notice the Crying Dinosaur rock formation across the canyon. Near 1.8 miles the trail makes a surprise left turn uphill toward the canyon wall and hooks around a large boulder. Deeper into Siphon Draw the trail dives into a wooded wash but shortly emerges into a large bowl of smooth rock. After seasonal rains, a thin waterfall cascades down the cliff face and empties into the bowl, providing an ideal backdrop for a picnic.

The official trail ends at the waterfall, but there's so much more to Siphon Draw. Who can resist? Just be aware that the next mile covers very rocky terrain on insanely steep slopes and gains over 1,500 feet. Climb out of the bowl right of the waterfall and up a narrow chute directly ahead. After a bit of slipping and sliding on a gravelly hill, you'll reach a narrow saddle with an awesome view of Flatiron directly above. Take time to admire the view behind you and to survey the route ahead. The correct path drops down from the saddle and heads straight up Siphon Draw, which is the first major drainage left of the Flatiron.

Scrambling skills are a must as you go beyond the saddle. White paint dots guide your way, but forest rangers sometimes remove them to preserve the wilderness. When in doubt, stay inside the main drainage of Siphon Draw and avoid the temptation to drift right. If faced with a difficult climb, look for ways around it. You can often bypass it all together or leverage a nearby tree limb. Remember, however, that climbing down upon your return is more difficult than climbing up.

There are three tricky spots that deserve special mention. The first is a jagged wall of granite not far from the saddle. When you reach this wall, simply climb over it. The rock surface has plenty of good footholds. The second tricky area is about halfway up the canyon. Look for a painted white arrow telling you to climb up and turn left around a large boulder. If you turn right here, you end up on a slope of loose scree. It is possible to get to the top that way, but it's fairly miserable. The final tricky spot is a 12-foot wall just before you reach the high plateau. Tackle this climb by using the stepping-stones in the crevice to the right.

Beyond the final climb, emerge from Siphon Draw to reach a ledge level with the top of Flatiron. Strangely eroded rock formations called hoodoos cap the mountaintops. Head right for a quarter mile to visit Flatiron, a large and incredibly flat area covered with strawberry hedgehogs that display bright purple flowers in April and May. Leave the trail and walk west to the cliff's edge where you can admire dizzying views of the valley below.

If you are not too tired, consider taking a 15-minute detour to visit the summit. Backtrack to the point where the trail emerges from Siphon Draw. Continue straight uphill to a saddle point where you can access the Superstition Ridgeline route (page 192). Turn left at the saddle toward the hoodoos, and look for a smooth slope on the right side of the small basin. Ascend this slope and follow a narrow brushy track to an angled slab of rock wedged between boulders. Climb over the slab and then duck through the first rock arch. Turn left and then right to reach the second rock tunnel. Crawl through the opening and immediately climb up the boulder on the left. Follow the trail all the way to the summit.

This unnamed 4,980-foot summit is the tallest point on the western end of the Superstitions. From its peak you can look into the heart of Superstition Wilderness and see Weaver's Needle, view the distant Four Peaks, and survey the ridgeline all the way to Superstition Peak, the tallest point on the eastern end. You can spend hours up here exploring the nooks and crannies among the hoodoos. When satisfied, return by descending Siphon Draw. Be careful not to loose rocks on hikers below as you climb down the steep gully.

Update: Lost Dutchman State Park is scheduled to close on June 3, 2010. Alternate access to the Siphon Draw Trail will be available via First Water Road (1 mile northeast of Lost Dutchman State Park on SR 88) and Jacob's Crosscut Trail, which adds 2 miles each way to the hike. For updates about the park's possible reopening, visit **www.pr.state.az.us**.

37 SUPERSTITION RIDGELINE*

KEY AT-A-GLANCE INFORMATION

LENGTH: 11.7 miles

ELEVATION GAIN: 2,790 feet (4,850 feet accumulated gain)

CONFIGURATION: One-way

DIFFICULTY: Very difficult

SCENERY: Superstition Mountains, Flatiron, Weaver's Needle, mountain panoramas, canyons, seasonal waterfalls

EXPOSURE: Mostly exposed; some shade in canyons

TRAFFIC: Light

TRAIL SURFACE: Rock, gravel, boulders, scrambling, climbing

HIKING TIME: 8–12 hours

WATER REQUIREMENT: 4 quarts

SEASON: November–April; not recommended in summer

ACCESS: Sunrise to sunset; $6 entrance at Lost Dutchman State Park, free at Carney Springs

MAPS: USGS Goldfield and Weaver's Needle, Tonto National Forest map

FACILITIES: Lost Dutchman: restroom, water, picnic area, camping, ranger station; Carney Springs: none

DOGS: Not recommended because of climbing and scrambling

COMMENTS: This is the most difficult hike in the Phoenix area.

GPS Trailhead Coordinates

UTM Zone 12S

Easting 0466290

Northing 3693930

Latitude N33°23.159'

Longitude W111°21.786'

IN BRIEF

Crossing the Superstition Ridgeline is one of those feats that you brag about for a long time. This combination hike and scramble challenges even the hardiest of outdoor aficionados and earns its nickname of "Superstitions Death March."

DESCRIPTION

With a nickname like "Superstitions Death March," the ridgeline hike has attained legendary status, the mere mention of this grueling endurance test evoking awe and trepidation. Despite the ridgeline's well-deserved reputation as the toughest hike near Phoenix, most hikers who tackle it love the experience and can't wait to try it again—after a period of recovery, of course. With open views of Weaver's Needle, Superstition Wilderness, and Four Peaks, scenery along the high ridge is nothing short of stunning.

There is no official trail across the ridgeline, but years of use have carved an established

---

Directions

Lost Dutchman State Park: Drive east on US 60 and exit at Idaho Road. Drive 2.25 miles north on Idaho Road to SR 88, the Apache Trail. Turn northeast onto SR 88 and continue 5 miles to the entrance of Lost Dutchman State Park. Pay the entrance fee and then follow the signs to the Siphon Draw Trailhead in the Day Use Area.

Carney Springs: Continue east on US 60 to Peralta Road at mile marker 204. Turn northeast onto Peralta Road and reset your trip odometer here. Follow Peralta Road which eventually becomes a graded dirt road, to a fork at 5.5 miles. Bear left at the fork and continue to a small pull-out at 6.2 miles. A rugged and rocky dirt road to Carney Springs has been fenced off, so park your car at the pull-out.

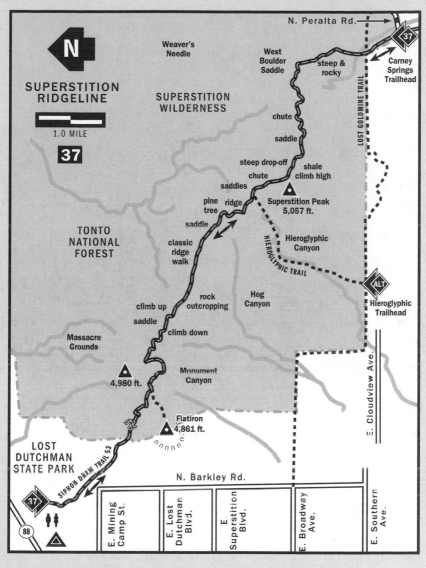

N

SUPERSTITION RIDGELINE

|———— 1.0 MILE ————|

37

Weaver's Needle

West Boulder Saddle

steep & rocky

SUPERSTITION WILDERNESS

chute

saddle

steep drop-off

chute

shale climb high

saddles

pine tree   ridge

Superstition Peak 5,057 ft.

saddle

classic ridge walk

Hieroglyphic Canyon

TONTO NATIONAL FOREST

HIEROGLYPHIC TRAIL

LOST GOLDMINE TRAIL

Carney Springs Trailhead

N. Peralta Rd.

37

ALT

Hieroglyphic Trailhead

rock outcropping

climb up

Hog Canyon

saddle

climb down

Massacre Grounds

4,980 ft.

Monument Canyon

Flatiron 4,861 ft.

E. Cloudview Ave.

LOST DUTCHMAN STATE PARK

SIPHON DRAW TRAIL 53

37

N. Barkley Rd.

E. Mining Camp St.

E. Lost Dutchman Blvd.

E. Superstition Blvd.

E. Broadway Ave.

E. Southern Ave.

88

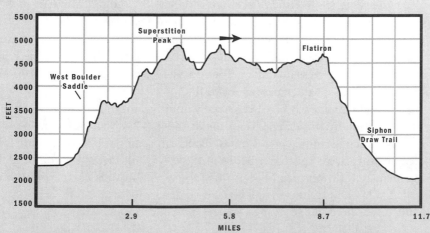

Superstition Peak

West Boulder Saddle

Flatiron

Siphon Draw Trail

FEET

5500
5000
4500
4000
3500
3000
2500
2000
1500

2.9   5.8   8.7   11.7

MILES

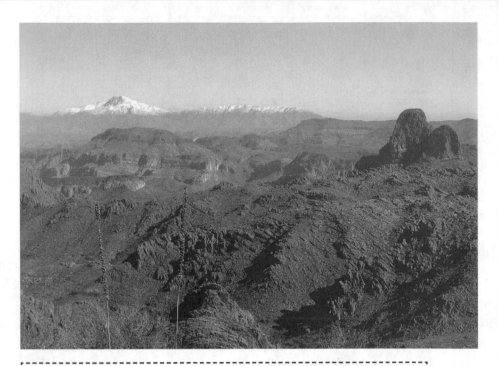

Snowcapped Four Peaks and Weaver's Needle viewed from atop the Superstition Ridgeline.

route marked by cairns. Route-finding and scrambling skills are required for this rigorous hike. Therefore, only conditioned, experienced hikers should attempt the ridgeline, preferably with someone familiar with the route. Because of its difficulty, crossing the Superstition Ridgeline is not recommended during hot summer months. Always tell someone where you are going, and remember to bring plenty of water. Also, leave your four-legged friends at home because they will have trouble with several spots that require climbing.

OK, after so many dire warnings, how can you resist the challenge? You can hike the ridgeline in either direction, though I find going from east to west somewhat easier. Stash a vehicle at Lost Dutchman State Park, and drive around to the Carney Springs parking area. Walk north toward the mountain along an old jeep trail for 0.6 miles, and find a small equestrian guard in the fence that marks the wilderness boundary. Your epic adventure begins here. Cross the fence and head out on the narrow foot trail.

The trail begins gently but turns steeply uphill at 1 mile. Look for a seasonal waterfall in a mountainside crevice in the distance. Climb up ridiculously steep and rocky slopes beginning at 1.3 miles, using cairns to guide your ascent. Take a quick breather at an open intermediate saddle 1.5 miles from the trailhead. In spring many wildflowers can be seen along the way. One particularly interesting succulent indigenous to this region is the rock echeveria or live-forever. Look for its candy-corn-like red and orange flowers clinging to rocky crags.

Resume the torturous climb and reach the higher West Boulder Saddle at 3,680 feet, 1.85 miles from the trailhead. You now have gained 1,350 feet, most of it in only half a mile. Turn around to survey your ascent of the canyon below. The trapezoidal Picketpost Mountain can be seen in the distance. Step around the large boulder at the saddle and catch your first glimpse of the hoodoos atop Superstition Peak.

Turn left at West Boulder Saddle and hike west toward Superstition Peak. The trail mercifully flattens out for a while as you snake around boulders and thick patches of vegetation. Drop into upper West Boulder Canyon, and cross the seasonal Willow Spring at 2.4 miles. Then turn left uphill where the trail flattens out again with a view of Weaver's Needle jutting out above the opposite ridge.

At 2.8 miles cross a small stream in the upper reaches of the basin and begin another steep climb through thick grasses. Then turn left up a rocky chute with a small cairn on top marking the trail, and hike up a rocky ridge with views toward the south. The trail then begins yet another steep and slippery ascent. At these considerably higher elevations, the plants are noticeably different from those lower in the canyon. Sotols and agaves thrive, and banana yuccas display stalks of delicate white flowers in April and May. The climb culminates at a saddle point with huge views of Gold Canyon and Apache Junction to the south. Weaver's Needle stands distinct in the northeast.

Continue up the ridge and down to another saddle. Watch out for the aptly named shindagger, a small but sharp plant that resembles an agave. At 3.6 miles from the trailhead, make your way up a slope of loose shale to find the trail bending to the north and heading toward Weaver's Needle. The trail then bends around the mountain and takes aim at the 5,057-foot Superstition Peak, which upon closer inspection is no more than a pile of hoodoos. The trail can be hard to find here, so look carefully for cairns. When in doubt, head for the tallest peak you see. The correct route skirts Superstition Peak on the right and reaches an obvious saddle just north of the peak, 4.2 miles from the trailhead.

Cross the saddle toward the west, but then go north around the left side of the hoodoos to a large flat area with sheer drop-offs. Look for a cairn near the northern cliff marking your first scary class-3 scramble, which descends a rocky chute. After carefully climbing down, head for the southwestern side of the boulders straight ahead. The trail descends about 50 feet along a steep, loose slope, but then turns north across the base of the boulders. This section requires some scrambling and bushwhacking, but once again, cairns guide your way along a faint path.

Past the scrambling section, a saddle greets you nearly 4.6 miles from the trailhead. Scenic Hieroglyphic Canyon lies to the south. Tackle the uphill to the south of the ridge, and then cross over to the northern side as you bob up and down across several saddles. One of the most challenging aspects of this hike is enduring the undulations along the ridge. Near 5.1 miles, the trail fades once more. You can either veer right and climb up to the top of the ridge, or take a climbing traverse along the southern side of the hill. Look for a lone pine tree on the ridgeline at 5.5 miles. If you lose the trail, head for this pine tree because the trail runs right next to it.

You'll reach a high point on the ridgeline just past the pine tree. From this vantage point, you look down on Weaver's Needle to the northeast and Hog Canyon to the southwest, and see Superstition Peak behind you, and the unnamed peak above Siphon Draw, your destination for the day. Descend from this pinnacle toward a confusing forest of boulders. The trail veers slightly left and squeezes through a crevice before dumping you out on the ridgeline again.

Route-finding becomes much easier now as you pick up the pace along the chiseled ridgeline. The trail tackles the ridge head-on and ducks to the north when it seems impassible, only to return to the ridgeline later. The next mile is a classic ridge walk where you literally hike the spine of the Superstitions. Admire grandiose views to either side of the trail, and look for bright purple blossoms on spiny hedgehog cacti in April.

Near 7.1 miles, the trail comes to a flat outcropping, a scenic overlook into Monument Canyon and a great place to take a quick break. A quarter mile farther, another steep descent awaits. This is the second steep scramble down a rocky, loose chute, but thankfully it is less technical than the first. Dropping to 4,200 feet, you'll reach the final low saddle on the ridge. Climbing up again feels tough, but take comfort in knowing that the worst is behind you.

Regain most of the lost elevation, and draw level with the ridge again. The trail takes a long, flat traverse around the top of Monument Canyon and across the level ledge ahead. At 8.7 miles begin your final ascent, which leads to a high saddle overlooking the famous Flatiron. Those familiar with Siphon Draw breathe a sigh of relief because this is the end of the ridgeline. However, more challenges lurk around the corner. Descending Siphon Draw is no small task.

Refer to the Siphon Draw (page 187) chapter for descriptions on the return to Lost Dutchman State Park, where you should have a shuttle vehicle or a ride waiting. Conquering the Superstition Ridgeline puts you among the most elite of Phoenix hikers and deservedly earns bragging rights for years to come.

Update: Lost Dutchman State Park is scheduled to close on June 3, 2010. Alternate access to the Superstition Ridgeline will be available via First Water Road (1 mile northeast of Lost Dutchman State Park on SR 88) and Jacob's Crosscut Trail, which adds 2 miles each way to the hike. For updates about the park's possible reopening, visit **www.pr.state.az.us**.

NEARBY ACTIVITIES

The Superstition Mountains are home to many hikes detailed in this book. Peralta (page 162), Lost Goldmine (page 153), and Siphon Draw (page 187) trails are just a few examples of excellent hikes in the area. Usery Mountains to the west offer other hiking opportunities.

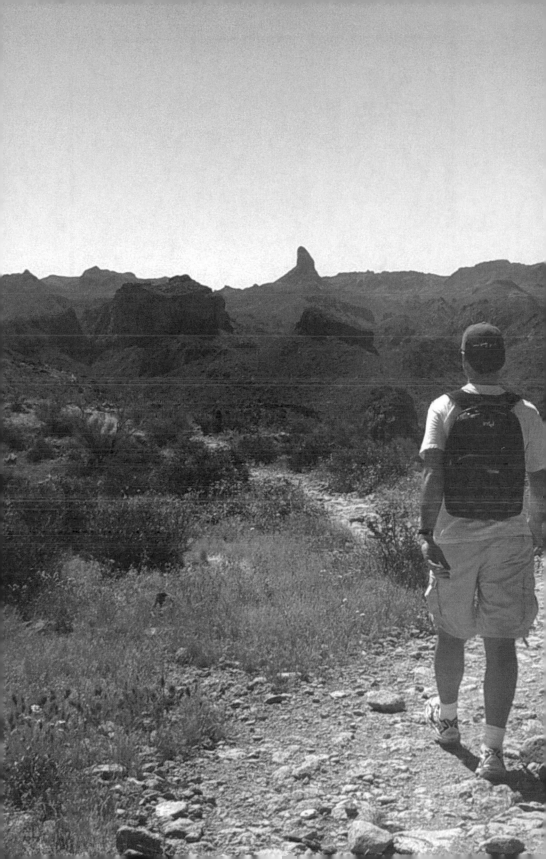

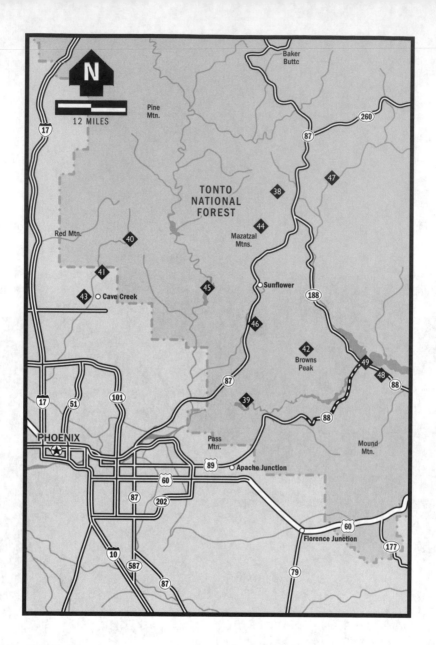

NORTHEAST
INCLUDING CAVE CREEK AND
MAZATZAL MOUNTAINS

38 BARNHARDT TRAIL

KEY AT-A-GLANCE INFORMATION

LENGTH: 14 miles

ELEVATION GAIN: 1,930 feet

CONFIGURATION: Out-and-back

DIFFICULTY: Moderate to difficult

SCENERY: Barnhardt Canyon, waterfalls, Mazatzal Wilderness, Horseshoe Reservoir

EXPOSURE: Mostly exposed, some shade in Barnhardt Canyon

TRAFFIC: Light to moderate

TRAIL SURFACE: Rock, gravel, packed dirt

HIKING TIME: 7 hours

WATER REQUIREMENT: 4 quarts

SEASON: Year-round; hot in summer

ACCESS: Sunrise to sunset; free parking

MAPS: USGS Mazatzal Peak

FACILITIES: None

DOGS: Yes

COMMENTS: The Willow Fire of 2004 damaged much of the forest on the upper reaches of this trail. For more information, visit www .fs.fed.us/r3/tonto/wilderness/ wilderness-mazatzal-index.shtml, or call (928) 474-7900.

GPS Trailhead Coordinates

UTM Zone 12S

Easting 0461120

Northing 3772344

Latitude N34°5.576'

Longitude W111°25.330'

IN BRIEF

Barnhardt Trail takes you on a scenic tour into the heart of Mazatzal Wilderness, offering thrilling views into deep gorges, up rugged mountains, and across picturesque hills. Rocky cliffs and spectacular waterfalls accentuate an already dramatic landscape.

DESCRIPTION

The massive Mazatzal mountain range lies within Tonto National Forest and stretches from the Salt River valley all the way north to Payson. Characterized by a line of tall rocky summits well in excess of 7,000 feet in elevation, most of which are within 60 miles of Phoenix, the Mazatzals offer desert dwellers a convenient escape from the summer heat. The Mazatzal Divide, a north–south watershed along its major axis, separates the Verde River and Tonto Creek valleys and delineates Gila County from Maricopa County.

Many trails crisscross these rugged mountains, but perhaps none offer a better overall hiking experience than Barnhardt Trail 43. In spite of its status as the most popular trail into Mazatzal Wilderness, many Phoenix hikers have yet to discover its charm. The Barnhardt Trailhead access road intersects SR 87, a major transportation vein between Phoenix and Payson. However, most people who pass

Directions

From Loop 202, exit onto Country Club Drive, which is also SR 87 Beeline Highway. Drive north 60 miles on SR 87 to the signed Barnhardt Trailhead turnoff north of mile marker 239. Turn left onto FR 419, a dirt road that is passable by most passenger cars. Follow it west 5 miles to the wide trailhead parking area. Park near the wooden trail map.

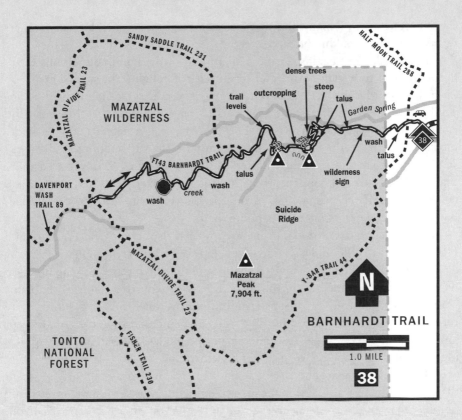

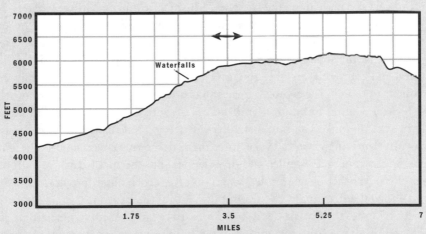

the inauspicious trail sign think it's just another desert trail like many others near town. They couldn't be more wrong!

Barnhardt Trail begins on the plateau east of the mountain, climbs Barnhardt Canyon to a high basin, and terminates at roughly the midpoint of the 29-mile-long Mazatzal Divide Trail, which is also a segment of the Arizona Trail. Along the way, Barnhardt Trail cuts through arguably the most beautiful canyon in the Mazatzals, passes near several seasonal waterfalls, and provides plenty of scenic overlooks from which to admire the surrounding landscape. I should note that the lightning-induced Willow Fire of 2004 devastated more than 100,000 acres of forest in these mountains. Hikers who have been there before can savor the memory of Barnhardt Canyon in its full glory. However, Barnhardt Canyon remains a pleasure to visit.

From the large trailhead parking area, which also serves Y Bar Trail 44 and Half Moon Trail 288, find a wooden sign engraved with a stylized map of nearby trails. Begin by hiking west toward the mountain, staying right at the junction where Y Bar Trail forks south. Initially, large rocks covering the trail challenge your balance, but trail conditions steadily improve once you pass through the forest boundary fence at 0.1 mile. The trail soon enters shady groves of alligator juniper and live oak. A few cacti and agaves lie hidden under the trees, signifying the transition zone between desert and forest.

The trail bends around the hills and begins a moderate but steady ascent that lasts many miles. The slope is mostly moderate, but seemingly unrelenting uphills keep your heart racing and legs burning. As you enter Barnhardt Canyon, the trail carves a path along the steep left hillside, forming a natural ledge at certain bends from which to survey the canyon below. Garden Spring at the bottom of the deep canyon gurgles among enticing pools and inaccessible narrow passages, sending the sound of refreshing water reverberating high up into the hills. Twisted and gnarled layers of sedimentary rock lay exposed across the canyon, a testament to the violent geologic forces that created this rocky wonderland.

Near 1.5 miles Barnhardt Trail makes a sharp bend and begins to ascend switchbacks that take you into a smaller but steeper side canyon. These switchbacks offer amazing views at every outer turn; dense tree cover engulfs the inner bends. Pass a talus at 2.3 miles and dive deeper into the rocky canyon walled by sheer cliffs. Another quarter mile along, look for a rock outcropping from which you command a dizzying view straight down into the canyon.

At 2.7 miles the trail passes a stunning wall of layered sedimentary rock. Just when you think the scenery couldn't possibly improve, some seasonal waterfalls prove you wrong. In winter, spring, and even early summer, cascading waterfalls tumble over the cliffs that line the trail. Depending on the amount of snowmelt, you may see quite a few of them. The biggest one lies near a sharp bend in the trail 3 miles from the trailhead. You'll likely hear rushing water as you walk by. To visit the waterfall, scramble up large boulders to find a secluded rocky alcove where the waterfall tumbles over the cliff from an upper pool. Though reflected

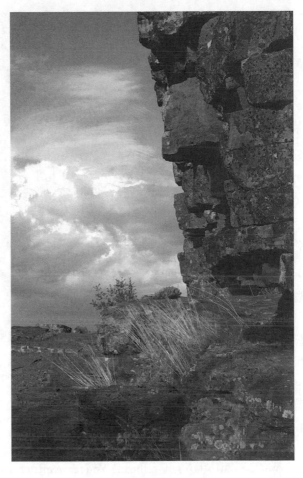

Barnhardt Trail takes a dramatic turn around this view-studded cliff.

sunlight on the upper pool may tempt you, do not attempt to climb the vertical rock face to investigate. Be satisfied with admiring the waterfall from below and return to the trail.

Beyond the waterfall, Barnhardt Trail takes on a completely different character, and understandably, many hikers go no farther. A short ascent beyond the waterfall takes you to an expansive upper basin where damage from the Willow Fire is readily apparent. What was once a forest of beautiful manzanita bushes is now a barren wasteland. In place of shady groves of smooth red bark and lush greenery, eerie stands of manzanita skeletons sprout from the ground like silver and black elk antlers. The trail levels off at a wide bend where some manzanitas and live oaks escaped the fire. From an elevation of 5,870 feet, views of the valley below are amazing. You can look back down Barnhardt Canyon and see the town of Rye in the distance.

Continue hiking west on Barnhardt Trail, which skirts the upper basin at 6,000 feet. The interior of Mazatzal Wilderness appears almost tame compared with the rugged cliffs in Barnhardt Canyon. The trail intersects Sandy Saddle Trail 231 at 4 miles from the trailhead. Stay left and continue following Barnhardt Trail as it crosses a series of dry washes in the wide upper basin.

Near 4.6 miles the trail follows a large dry wash for a short distance. Look for cairns to guide you across. On the other side, enter the remnants of a thick ponderosa pine forest and hike on fallen pine needles and recovering undergrowth. More signs of life appear in the forest at 5.2 miles in the form of lush grasses and small shrubs.

Reach the crest of the Mazatzal Divide at 6.1 miles from the trailhead. This saddle point straddles the county line and affords an excellent view of the

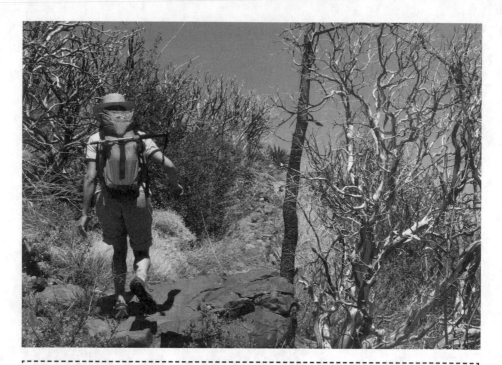

Therese Lohmann of Phoenix hikes through an eerie stand of burned manzanita on the Barnhardt Trail.

surrounding mountains. There's a small trail leading to the right, but make a sharp left turn to stay on Barnhardt Trail. Over the next hill begin a gradual descent with a distant view of Horseshoe Reservoir in the Verde River valley. Barnhardt Trail terminates at the junction with Mazatzal Divide Trail, 7 miles from the Barnhardt Trailhead. You can either backtrack from there or turn south onto Mazatzal Divide Trail and then return via the Y Bar Trail. However, be aware that the Y Bar loop option adds an extra 4 miles and 1,000 feet of elevation gain to your trip.

NEARBY ACTIVITIES

The Barnhardt Trailhead also serves Y Bar Trail and Half Moon Trail. On the opposite side of SR 87 near the town of Gisela, a short hike leads to Tonto Narrows (page 243), a popular swimming hole on Tonto Creek in the Hellsgate Wilderness. Nearby Payson is a popular summertime retreat for Phoenix residents. Farther south on SR 87, many trails lead to other summits in the Mazatzal range, including Mount Peeley (page 230), Mount Ord, and the 7,657-foot Browns Peak (page 220). SR 188, which intersects SR 87 just south of the Barnhardt Trailhead access road, leads to Roosevelt Lake, the largest of the Salt River reservoirs.

BUTCHER JONES TRAIL 39

IN BRIEF

Butcher Jones Trail runs along a section of Saguaro Lake's northern shore, offering many scenic overlooks of the lake and the surrounding mountains. Burro Cove, this hike's destination, commands an impressive view of Four Peaks across the lake.

DESCRIPTION

As the reservoir closest to Phoenix, Saguaro Lake draws plenty of visitors seeking summer fun in the sun. Colorful mountains surround the Salt River basin and add a dramatic backdrop to the lake. While most people go to the lake for water sports, hikers can enjoy a scenic trail along Saguaro Lake's shoreline, especially during the cooler winter months. Butcher Jones Trail 463 provides access to some choice vantage points from which to catch a bird's-eye view of the lake.

Directions _____➤

From Loop 202: Exit onto Country Club Drive, which is also SR 87 Beeline Highway. Drive 22 miles north on SR 87 and turn east onto FR 204, Bush Highway, toward Saguaro Lake. Proceed 3 miles to the signed Butcher Jones turnoff. Turn left onto FR 166 and follow the road until it ends at Butcher Jones Recreation Site. Pay the day-use fee at the automated kiosk and then park near the beach.

From US 60: Exit onto Power Road. Drive north 20 miles on Power Road, which eventually becomes FR 204, Bush Highway, north of town. The Butcher Jones turnoff is 1 mile past the entrance to Saguaro Lake Marina. Turn right at the signed Butcher Jones turnoff and follow the road to the Butcher Jones Recreation Site.

KEY AT-A-GLANCE INFORMATION

LENGTH: 5 miles

ELEVATION GAIN: 175 feet

CONFIGURATION: Out-and-back

DIFFICULTY: Easy

SCENERY: Saguaro Lake, riparian zone, desert, Goldfield Mountains

EXPOSURE: Mostly exposed, but limited shade is available in riparian areas

TRAFFIC: Moderate

TRAIL SURFACE: Gravel, packed dirt

HIKING TIME: 2.5 hours

WATER REQUIREMENT: 1.5 quarts

SEASON: Year-round; hot in summer

ACCESS: Open sunrise to sunset; Tonto Pass and $6 per vehicle required; not sold on site but available in stores and at Forest Service offices.

MAPS: USGS Stewart Mountain

FACILITIES: Restrooms, picnic areas, beach, fishing dock

DOGS: Yes, leashed at all times

COMMENTS: For Tonto Pass info, click www.fs.fed.us/r3/tonto/tp and for trail information, visit www.fs.fed.us/r3/tonto/recreation/rec-hiking-index.shtml.

GPS Trailhead Coordinates

UTM Zone 12S

Easting 0452317

Northing 3715003

Latitude N33°34.525'

Longitude W111°30.869'

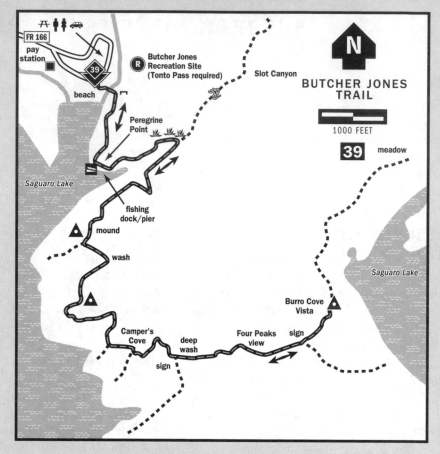

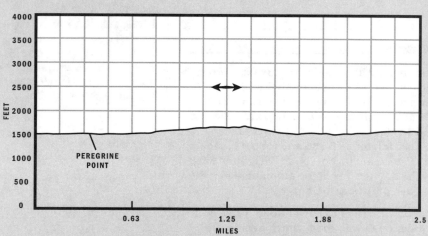

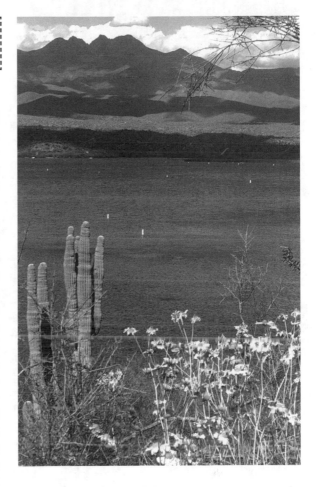

Brittlebush and saguaros accent a view of Four Peaks across Saguaro Lake from Burro Cove Vista.

Fairly easy and well marked, Butcher Jones Trail makes an excellent introductory hike for beginners. The trail's name recalls a 19th-century doctor and rancher whose nickname was "Butcher." I wonder which of his occupations earned him that gruesome moniker. Snaking along a portion of Saguaro Lake's 22-mile shoreline, this scenic trail passes through alcoves, rocky slopes, shady riparian zones, and some Sonoran Desert landscape as it cuts across a peninsula in the lake. Many spur trails branch out to provide waterfront access for fishing, camping, or swimming. Encompassing scenic overlooks of the lake and reflections of distant mountains, views along this trail are nothing short of stunning.

Begin the hike from a signed trailhead near Butcher Jones Beach. Though the sign reads "Saguaro Lake Nature Trail," it marks the correct starting point for Butcher Jones Trail. Diving right into some shady trees, the initial trail segment is paved and has a handrail. Turn right when the first handrail ends. Heading south on the paved Nature Trail next to the water, a few pullouts and benches provide excuses to stop and read the interpretive signs. The paved trail ends at Peregrine Point, where a floating fishing dock protrudes into the lake.

Peregrine Point sits at the tip of a scenic peninsula and is nearly surrounded by water. The Arizona Game and Fish Department stocks the lake with many species of fish, and Saguaro Lake has artificial fish habitats installed on the shoreline near Butcher Jones Trail. Therefore, this fishing dock is a popular destination for anglers seeking walleye, trout, bass, and catfish. It's worth walking out onto the fishing dock for a view from the lake.

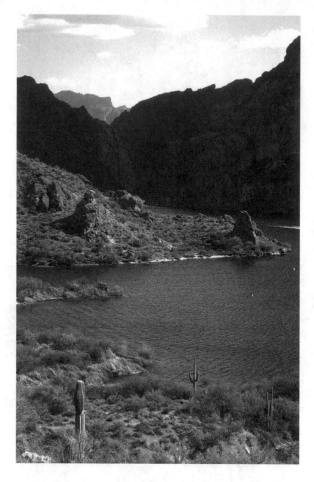

From Peregrine Point pass through a gate and onto a narrow dirt path that hugs the water's edge. The trail follows the contour of Peregrine Cove inland. At the tip of the cove and under shady cover of thick brush, a spur trail runs north while the main trail curves right and heads back out toward the lake. If you feel adventurous, take a small detour up this faint spur trail 0.1 mile to find a seven-foot-tall dry waterfall. If you manage to climb up this rock crevice and continue up the dry creek bed for another 0.1 mile, you'll find a small but charming slot canyon carved through large boulders by eons of occasional runoff. The dry creek bed continues another mile, but further bushwhacking fails to produce any additional interesting sights. After visiting the slot canyon, return to the main trail and resume your hike on the Butcher Jones Trail.

As you hike out toward the lake again, the trail begins to climb a moderate hill. In spring look for wildflowers such as owl clover, lupine, and buckwheat along this hilly section. About a mile from the trailhead is a small mound with an excellent view of the lake and Butcher Jones Beach. The view gets even better at another scenic vista 0.3 miles farther down the trail. Situated 175 feet above the water, this overlook is the highest point on the entire hike. You can see the marina across the lake. Lakeside cliffs to your left frame the distant Superstition Mountains and the Flatiron.

After the scenic overlook, follow the trail as it crosses a dry wash and descends toward the lake. There are several side trails leading to the waterfront. Feel free to explore them, and then return to the main trail. Pass the Camper's Cove junction at 1.7 miles and another signed trail junction at 1.9 miles. Then dip into and cross a large dry wash as you begin to pull away from the lake. Heading inland toward Burro Cove and leaving the noisy motorboats behind, the trail enters a peaceful desert landscape. Saguaros tower over the trail, while chollas, triangle-leaf bursage, and palo verdes dominate the landscape. Immersed in the desert scenery, you might forget that the lake is nearby.

At 2.2 miles, the trail bends north to reveal a head-on view of Four Peaks. Remain on Butcher Jones Trail at the next fork and head for Burro Cove. The lake soon comes into view again, and you realize that the trail's desert section actually cuts across a peninsula in the lake. At 2.5 miles the trail reaches a large flat mound overlooking the lake, with majestic Four Peaks looming on the horizon. Though a faint and sometimes overgrown trail continues to the left and traces the shoreline, the scenic overlook is the recommended turnaround point on this hike. Enjoy the view here before retracing your steps.

NEARBY ACTIVITIES

Usery Mountain Regional Park south of Saguaro Lake offers many excellent hiking trails including Wind Cave Trail (page 123) and Pass Mountain Trail (page 94). Browns Trail to Four Peaks, Pine Creek Trail, and Ballantine Trail are all accessible from SR 87 north of Bush Highway. McDowell Mountain Regional Park (page 90) north of Fountain Hills presents hiking opportunities as well. Nearby Salt River Recreation provides a shuttle service and tube rentals for a relaxing tubing trip down the Salt River.

40 CAVE CREEK TRAIL AND SKUNK CREEK TRAIL

KEY AT-A-GLANCE INFORMATION

LENGTH: 10.4 Miles

ELEVATION GAIN: 1,125 feet

CONFIGURATION: Balloon

DIFFICULTY: Cave Creek Trail: easy; Skunk Creek Trail: moderate

SCENERY: Cave Creek, riparian zone, desert, mountain vistas, Quien Sabe Mine

EXPOSURE: Considerable shade along Cave Creek Trail; Skunk Creek Trail exposed

TRAFFIC: Light

TRAIL SURFACE: Packed dirt, creek crossings, gravel, crushed rock

HIKING TIME: 5.5 hours

WATER REQUIREMENT: 3 quarts

SEASON: Year-round; hot in summer

ACCESS: Open sunrise to sunset; free parking

MAPS: USGS New River Mesa and Humbolt Mountain

FACILITIES: Toilet, campground, picnic area

DOGS: Yes, leashed at all times

COMMENTS: This area suffered significant damage from the Cave Creek Complex wildfire of 2005. For more information, visit www.fs .fed.us/r3/tonto/recreation/ rec-hiking-index.shtml, or call (480) 595-3300.

GPS Trailhead Coordinates

UTM Zone 12S

Easting 0420004

Northing 3759235

Latitude N33°58.344'

Longitude W111°52.000'

IN BRIEF

Cave Creek Trail provides a pleasantly shaded and mild hike along the banks of perennial Cave Creek. Enjoy the classic riparian flora and the trickling water. Then take the hilly Skunk Creek Trail for a workout and to loop back to the trailhead.

DESCRIPTION

The perennial Cave Creek flows through part of Tonto National Forest northeast of Phoenix. Because it supplies water year-round, Cave Creek feeds a riparian oasis and sustains a wide variety of plant and animal life normally not found in the desert. Largely shaded, this area attracts summer hikers aiming to escape the harsh desert environment, and its proximity to town also draws visitors. Hiking Cave Creek Trail 4 is an exercise in serenity and an experience the whole family can enjoy.

If you crave a more challenging hike and prefer not to backtrack, looping back via Skunk Creek Trail 246 satisfies both fancies. The Skunk Creek Trail touts a 1,125-foot elevation gain and takes visitors high above the

Directions

From Loop 101, exit onto Princess Drive and turn east. The road soon becomes Pima Road. Drive north on Pima Road 12 miles and then turn right onto Cave Creek Road. Follow Cave Creek Road 6 miles to the Tonto National Forest boundary. Continue on Cave Creek Road, which turns into FR 24 and eventually becomes a dirt road (suitable for most passenger cars). Go 10 miles down FR 24 to the pay station at Seven Springs Recreation Area. Purchase a parking pass from the automated kiosk, which accepts both cash and credit cards, and continue 0.6 miles to the Cave Creek Trailhead.

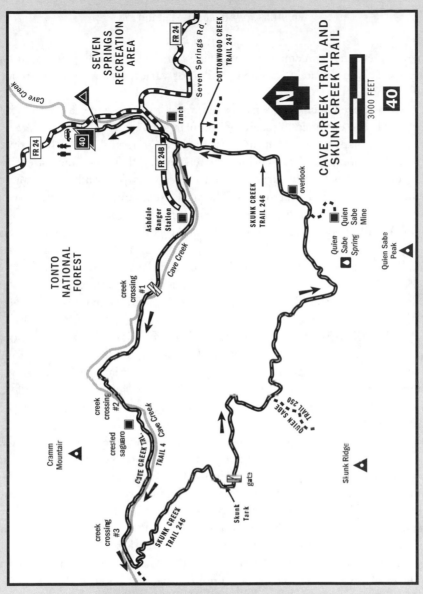

CAVE CREEK TRAIL AND
SKUNK CREEK TRAIL

40

3000 FEET

N

SEVEN SPRINGS RECREATION AREA

FR 24

Seven Springs Rd.

COTTONWOOD CREEK
TRAIL 247

FR 24

Cave Creek

40

ranch

FR 24B

TONTO NATIONAL FOREST

Ashdale Ranger Station

Cave Creek

creek crossing #1

SKUNK CREEK TRAIL 246

overlook

Quien Sabe Mine

Quien Sabe Spring

Quien Sabe Peak

Cramm Mountain

creek crossing #2

crested saguaro

CAVE CREEK TRAIL 4   Cave Creek

QUIEN SABE TRAIL 250

Skunk Ridge

creek crossing #3

SKUNK CREEK TRAIL 246

Skunk Tank

gate

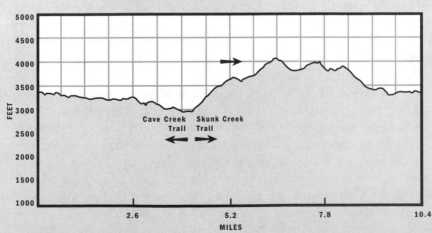

FEET				
5000				
4500				
4000				
3500				
3000				
2500		Cave Creek Trail	Skunk Creek Trail	
2000				
1500				
1000				

2.6   5.2   7.8   10.4

MILES

canyon, where they can enjoy sweeping views of the surrounding mountains and plateaus. This moderately strenuous trail adds variety and a cardio workout to your day hike.

Access Cave Creek Trail 4 from a parking lot just past the campground, 0.6 miles inside the entrance to scenic Seven Springs Recreation Area. A large trail-head plaque maps the trails in the area. Begin by following the trail southward behind the campground. You'll immediately notice that this hike differs from other desert hikes. Shady shrubs shroud the trail as you walk along junipers, Fremont barberry, and lush grasses. The trail runs parallel to the creek, where white-barked sycamores display golden leaves in November.

The trail crosses FR 24B at 0.7 miles and dives into a thicket of trees. Look for a marker for Trail 4, and stay to the right. Climb over a metal stepstool straddling the fence, and then head down toward the creek, where the trail soon intersects Cottonwood Creek Trail 247. At this junction, you can choose to hike the large loop in either direction. I prefer the counterclockwise route. Take the right fork and continue along Trail 4.

The Cave Creek Trail parallels the creek and provides plenty of shade under live oaks. Sycamores and even a few quaking aspen stand closer to the water. Hoof prints in the dirt trail indicate significant equestrian traffic, but the trail is only lightly used. At 1.8 miles, pass through a gated fence and secure the gate behind you. Then make the first of three crossings over Cave Creek by hopping carefully across stepping-stones.

The trail meanders up and down the hills on the creek's left bank where a recent forest fire singed much of the vegetation. As you hike farther downstream, look for the forest of saguaros on opposing slopes which escaped the fire. These giant cacti prefer the warmer and drier environment on sun-drenched southern hillsides. At 2.5 miles, the trail follows Cave Creek southwest and enters a narrow scenic canyon flanked by Cramm Mountain. Watch the shimmering water in the creek flicker in the sunlight as the trail descends back to the creek bed.

Cross the creek a second time at a wide, rocky area 2.9 miles from the trailhead. After crossing the creek, climb up the right side of the canyon and continue west, paralleling Cave Creek. Look carefully beside the trail for a rare cristate or "crested" saguaro, which for yet unknown reasons grows fan-shaped crowns on its branches. This stretch of the creek lies in a narrow canyon, and the rich riparian habitat shelters many animals. Don't be surprised to encounter families of javelina grunting and racing along next to you. Follow the undulating trail until you reach the third and final creek crossing at 4 miles from the trailhead. Then the trail leaves the creek and enters a vastly different landscape. Grass-covered open slopes take the place of dense riparian vegetation. Evergreens such as sugar sumac and juniper replace deciduous trees like the sycamore. Shortly past the creek, find the signed Skunk Creek Trail junction. The Cave Creek Trail continues another 6 miles and ends on FR 48 near the Spur Cross Ranch Conservation Area. To loop back to the trailhead, turn left here onto Skunk Creek Trail, sometimes also called Skunk Tank Trail.

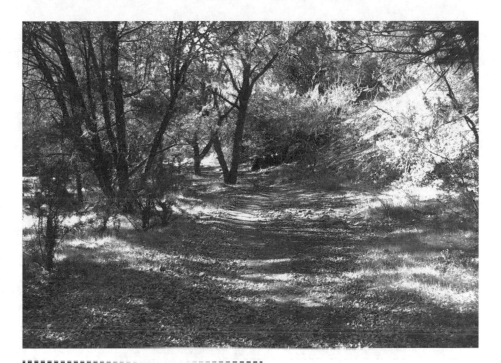

Ample shade entices hikers to the Cave Creek Trail.

Hilly Skunk Creek Trail differs greatly from the creek-side stroll. It turns east and immediately climbs a long series of switchbacks and steep straights to a ridgeline next to Skunk Creek. Don't worry; it doesn't smell like a skunk. The resultant visibility and higher elevation maximize your views in all directions. New River Mesa's flat profile dominates the western horizon, while various hills and distant mountains complete the panorama. The upward gradient remains punishing until the trail crosses Skunk Creek at 3,665 feet 5.3 miles from the trailhead. From there continue along the thankfully gentler uphill trail another quarter mile to Skunk Tank, a seasonal stock tank that catches occasional runoff during the rainy season and remains dry in summer.

Past Skunk Tank, go through a shoddy cowboy fence that requires some effort to close. Then follow the trail east atop broken rock and packed dirt. This section of the Skunk Creek Trail continues to ascend a gentle slope in a shallow basin. Wide-open landscape occupies your entire field of vision, inter- rupted only by skeletons of trailside shrubs charred by the Cave Creek Complex fire of 2005. The only moderately challenging trail segment may be tackling some loose crushed rock at 5.9 miles. The trail bends south and then tops out at a clearing where it meets Quien Sabe Trail 250, which takes off south toward who-knows-where, as its Spanish name suggests. This trail junction is the high- est point on the entire loop at 4,075 feet.

Stay left at the junction and hike east along Skunk Creek Trail, which wanders around the side of Quien Sabe Peak, skirts drainages, drops gently in elevation,

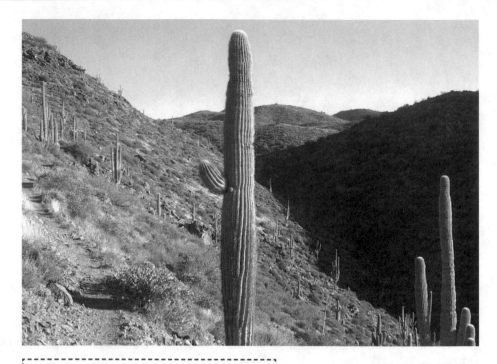

Saguaros dot the landscape along the Skunk Creek Trail.

and then regains it. At 7.7 miles the trail opens up into what looks like a wide jeep road and descends a slope packed with loose rock. Pass Quien Sabe Spring at the bottom of the hill, and then forge ahead toward the east on a high plateau. From here you can see a distant ranch house near FR 24. A 0.2-mile-long spur trail leads uphill to the Quien Sabe Mine at 8.2 miles from the trailhead. Past the mine, the trail finally begins to descend in earnest. Notice an old miner's camp next to the trail where hundreds of rusted tin cans lie strewn under a tree.

Skunk Creek Trail 246 eventually meets Cottonwood Creek Trail 247 at a flat spot 9.3 miles along the loop. Turn left onto the rough Cottonwood Creek Trail toward Cave Creek. Near the creek crossing, the Cottonwood Creek Trail is deeply rutted and bends westward before crossing the creek and joining the Cave Creek Trail at 9.6 miles. Complete the hike by turning east here, and then retrace your steps across FR 24B and back to the Cave Creek Trailhead.

NEARBY ACTIVITIES

The Seven Springs Recreation Area offers creekside camping and picnic areas. The Bronco Trail and historic Sears Kay Ruins are also accessible from FR 24. Elephant Mountain (page 215), in the Spur Cross Ranch Conservation Area, lies downstream from Cave Creek. Nearby Bartlett and Horseshoe Reservoirs provide scenic hikes and opportunities for water sports.

ELEPHANT MOUNTAIN TRAIL

41

IN BRIEF

The relatively new Spur Cross Ranch Conservation Area is the scene of a beautiful hike through undisturbed desert in the shadow of Elephant Mountain. Hiking this trail might make you think you are the first to discover the scenery, and you would not be too far from the truth.

DESCRIPTION

The newest addition to the Maricopa County park system, Spur Cross Ranch Conservation Area clearly shows its raw charm. Upon arrival at the makeshift parking area, you immediately get the sense that this hike is going to be a rugged adventure. Crossing the park boundary on foot, using the primitive self-pay drop box, and seeing the portable toilets and portable office all add to that perception. Though someday these little inconveniences will be replaced with the efficiently managed facilities typical of other Maricopa County parks, they are a small price to pay for the chance to experience Spur Cross in its infancy. The facilities may be rough, but they foretell a hike through pristine desert teeming with abundant plant and animal life yet unmarred by frequent traffic.

KEY AT-A-GLANCE INFORMATION

LENGTH: 9 miles
ELEVATION GAIN: 870 feet
CONFIGURATION: Out-and-back
DIFFICULTY: Moderate to difficult
SCENERY: Pristine desert, Cave Creek, Elephant Mountain
EXPOSURE: Mostly exposed, very little shade
TRAFFIC: Light
TRAIL SURFACE: Packed dirt, gravel, sandy wash, broken rock
HIKING TIME: 4.5 hours
WATER REQUIREMENT: 3.5 quarts
SEASON: Year-round; hot during summer
ACCESS: Sun.–Thu. 6 a.m.–8 p.m.; Fri.–Sat. 6 a.m.–10 p.m.; trails close at sunset; $3 per person entry
MAPS: USGS New River Mesa; park maps are sometimes available at the self-service entrance
FACILITIES: Portable toilets, no water
DOGS: Yes
COMMENTS: No vehicle access inside park boundaries. Parking is 200 yards from entrance. Bring exact change or a checkbook to pay the fee. For more information, visit www.maricopa.gov/parks/spur_cross, or call (480) 488-6601

Directions

Exit Loop 101 onto Scottsdale Road. Drive north on Scottsdale Road 11.8 miles until it Ts into Cave Creek Road. Turn west on Cave Creek Road and follow the winding road 2 miles. Turn north on Spur Cross Road, and take the signed left turn to remain on Spur Cross Road. Then drive 4.1 miles to the Spur Cross Ranch Conservation Area parking lot. The last 1.2 miles are unpaved but suitable for passenger cars.

GPS Trailhead Coordinates

UTM Zone 12S
Easting   0412150
Northing   3750002.
Latitude   N33°53.310'
Longitude W111°57.043'

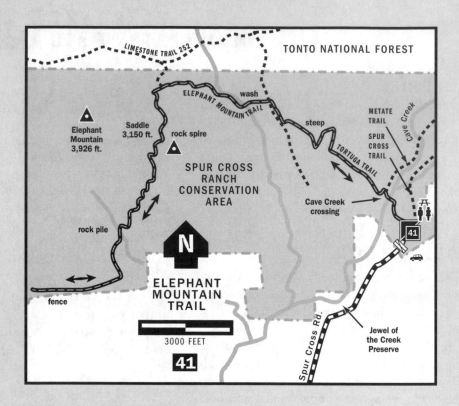

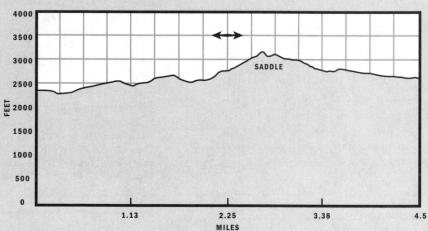

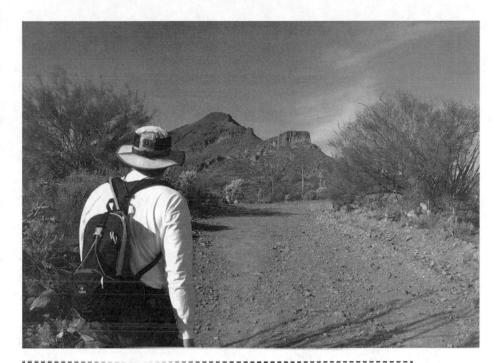

Doug Adamavich of Chandler hikes toward Elephant Mountain along the Tortuga Trail.

As suggested by its name, the Spur Cross Ranch area has a rich history of ranching and even mining. Early settlers of the region found a rich ecosystem along the banks of perennial Cave Creek on which to build their livelihoods. Today there are still many ranches, but the town of Cave Creek and the state of Arizona set aside 2,154 acres of wilderness bordering on Tonto National Forest to create Spur Cross Ranch Conservation Area.

Elephant Mountain is the most prominent feature in the conservation area. A large monolithic hill, this mountain resembles its namesake pachyderm roughly in shape and certainly in stature. The Elephant Mountain Trail carves an S-shaped track around the base of the mountain, offering excellent vistas from many angles. The trail also crosses a high saddle near the elephant's head, giving you an up-close look.

Begin the trek at a covered information kiosk just inside the park entrance. Head northwest on Tortuga Trail, which is really a wide dirt road and serves as a good warm-up for the hike because it begins level and gradually increases in slope. The first trail segment passes through some palo verde and mesquite trees that provide limited shade. Then at 0.3 miles the trail crosses Cave Creek just downstream from the Cottonwood Creek confluence and turns up a gentle hill. The foundations of a masonry building lie in ruins next to the trail.

At 0.8 miles Tortuga Trail levels out and reveals a scenic head-on view of Elephant Mountain. A bit farther the trail crosses an arroyo before resuming its climb. At this point, the dirt road deteriorates into a steep, rough pile of rocks. Huff and puff your way to the top of this hill, where you will find an obvious trail junction. Veer right here and hike along the service road toward the national forest boundary for another 250 yards to Elephant Mountain Trail's true beginning, 1.5 miles from the park entrance.

Leave the service road and turn west onto Elephant Mountain Trail, a narrow footpath that at times passes dangerously close to some prickly chollas. Soon a giant basin opens up in front of you, and the trail descends steeply into it. Watch your step on the slippery gravel while hiking down the 150 feet. At 1.75 miles from the park entrance, the trail intersects a sandy and rocky dry wash at the bottom of the basin. Follow cairns and footprints 0.3 miles as the trail zigzags through the dry wash.

Eventually, the trail leaves the dry wash at a signed point of egress. Follow the loose, steep trail uphill as it draws near a fence indicating the boundary between the park and Tonto National Forest. Continue west parallel to the fence in the shadows of the huge rock spire that makes up the elephant's upturned trunk when viewed from the south. The flat tops of Black Mesa and New River Mesa can be seen to the north across the fence. At 2.3 miles pass a small trail junction. This spur trail cuts across the fence into Tonto National Forest, where it joins Limestone Trail 252. Stay to the left here and remain on Elephant Mountain Trail.

After the trail junction, turn south and aim straight for the saddle between the rock spire and the head of Elephant Mountain. This ascent gets increasingly steep. Even the plants notice the elevation change—you begin to see some yuccas, hop bush, and ocotillos in lieu of dense palo verde trees down by the dry wash. Continue fighting your way up the punishing hill beside the rock spire's sheer northern face. This climb is the most strenuous part of the entire hike, but thankfully it is reasonably short.

Located 2.7 miles from the park entrance, the 3,150-foot saddle commands a splendid view toward the town of Cave Creek and Black Mountain (page 76) to the southeast. Take a well-deserved break here to enjoy the scenery and the cool breezes rushing through the saddle. Notice a series of small rock walls constructed of piled stones on top of the spire to the east of the saddle. Many mysterious ruins like this one exist in central Arizona. Table Top Mountain (page 310) holds a nearly identical wall on its summit. Though it is tempting to climb up for a closer look, a sign prohibits entry into the area.

Many hikers feel content with getting this far and turn back at the saddle. Should you choose to press on, the remainder of the trail rewards your efforts with impressive profiles of Elephant Mountain from its photogenic southern side and a scenic tour through a variety of desert microclimates, each with unique characteristic geology and flora. Follow the trail south over the saddle as it quickly descends through a layer of chalky loose dirt. As is the case with typical desert hills, the sunny southern slopes host many species of warmth-loving cacti. The teddy bear cholla does especially well here. Watch for clusters of prickly branches littered about the trail.

Continue hiking along the slope to a ridge crest at 2.9 miles where on a clear day you can see Superstition Mountains and Weaver's Needle to the southeast. Turn around and look closely at the head of Elephant Mountain. Notice the strangely striated sedimentary rock that decorates the rugged cliffs like wallpaper. A quarter mile farther, pass a relatively flat landing covered with teddy bear chollas. Then turn southwest onto rough igneous rock indicative of ancient volcanic activity. The trail is a bit overgrown here from infrequent use, but the path remains fairly obvious. Few hikers venture this far along the trail, but their absence is your gain because the desert environment remains pristine and unspoiled. It's hard to believe that the Spur Cross Ranch area nearly became home to condos and golf courses before state and municipal governments preserved it in 2001.

The trail continues mostly southward as it gently descends the hillside. At 3.5 miles cross a dry wash littered with large boulders. There's nothing but mountains and saguaros as far as the eye can see. Walk a bit farther and pass the remnants of an old fence. As the trail flattens out on a high basin, it bends toward the west and traverses the drainage south of Elephant Mountain. The flora changes dramatically here. An eerie field of dead grasses, dead mesquite branches, and dead cacti surrounds you. You might even find some skeletons of unfortunate critters next to the trail. Follow the trail as it runs parallel to the park boundary, marked by a fence barely visible to the south. At 4.3 miles the small trees and brush seem to be thriving again. Mesquites, acacias, and palo verdes line the trail covered in large volcanic rock.

Elephant Mountain Trail officially ends at the park boundary, 4.5 miles from the entrance. A sign and a loosely gated fence demarcate the transition between the park and state trust land. Though the path continues southward, you need a special permit to explore beyond the fence. Therefore, enjoy the solitude and the view of Elephant Mountain before returning via the same trail.

NEARBY ACTIVITIES

Cave Creek Trail (page 210) runs along its namesake creek just north of Spur Cross Ranch Conservation Area. Black Mountain (page 76) offers a good hike in the town of Cave Creek. Nearby Cave Creek Recreation Area hosts many hiking trails, including Go John Trail (page 225) and Overton Trail.

42 FOUR PEAKS: BROWNS PEAK

KEY AT-A-GLANCE INFORMATION

LENGTH: 5 miles

ELEVATION GAIN: 1,957 feet

CONFIGURATION: Out-and-back

DIFFICULTY: Moderate to Browns Saddle; very difficult from there to the summit

SCENERY: Roosevelt Lake, Four Peaks Wilderness, forest, mountain vistas

EXPOSURE: Partially shaded

TRAFFIC: Light

TRAIL SURFACE: Packed dirt, gravel, scree, and exposed scramble near the summit

HIKING TIME: 4 hours

WATER REQUIREMENT: 2.5 quarts

SEASON: Spring–fall (may be snowy in winter)

ACCESS: Sunrise to sunset; free parking

MAPS: USGS Four Peaks

FACILITIES: None

DOGS: Yes

COMMENTS: Most of the trail is moderately difficult. There's an exposed class-4 scramble near the summit. For more information, visit www.fs.fed.us/r3/tonto/wilderness/wilderness-4peaks-index.shtml.

GPS Trailhead
Coordinates

UTM Zone   12S

Easting   0468753

Northing   3729341

Latitude   N33°42.321'

Longitude   W111°20.273'

IN BRIEF

Browns Peak, the tallest of Four Peaks, is the highest point in Maricopa County. Hike through its oaks and pines in summer for a cool escape from the desert heat. The thrilling scramble to the summit is a heart-pounding and palm-sweating adventure.

DESCRIPTION

Phoenix hikers often escape to Flagstaff or the Mogollon Rim to hike the cool pines in summer. Many are surprised to learn that such a hike can be found much closer to home in the Four Peaks Wilderness. The jagged ridgeline of Four Peaks guards the eastern skyline of Phoenix. Often after winter rains in the Valley of the Sun, a coat of fresh snow caps the four summits like alpine glaciers, making it seem quite out of place among the desert scenery. For that reason, most people also think Four Peaks is farther away than it really is. The

Directions

High-Clearance Vehicles: From Loop 202, exit onto Country Club Drive (SR 87). Drive north on SR 87 about 25 miles to mile marker 204. Turn east onto Four Peaks Road (FR 143). Proceed cautiously 18 miles on the rough dirt road to the FR 648 junction. Turn sharply south and go 1.8 miles down FR 648 to the Lone Pine Trailhead.

Passenger Cars: Continue 30 miles on SR 87 to SR 188. Turn southeast onto SR 188 and drive 20 miles to El Oso Road, which is the other end of FR 143. Turn west onto El Oso Road and proceed 9 miles on the relatively smoother dirt road. Turn southeast toward Lone Pine Trailhead at a signed junction and drive 1 mile to the FR 648 junction. Turn south and follow FR 648 to the Lone Pine Trailhead, 1.8 miles further.

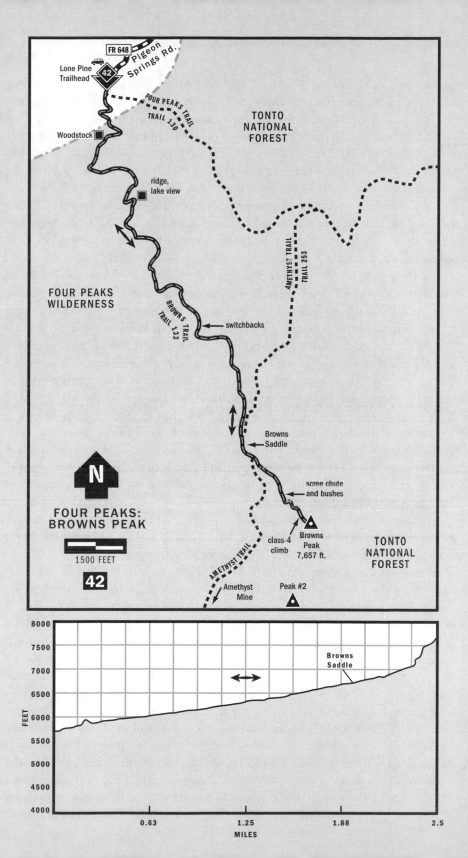

highest point in Maricopa County at 7,657 feet, Browns Peak is the northernmost and tallest of the four summits and is easily doable as a day hike from Phoenix.

To reach the summit of Browns Peak, hike the pleasant and scenic Browns Trail from Lone Pine Trailhead to Browns Saddle, and then scramble up a gully of scree and boulders for a stunningly beautiful panoramic view. The first adventure of the day, however, is getting to the Lone Pine Trailhead deep in the Mazatzal mountain range. The most direct route from Phoenix is via Four Peaks Road, a 20-mile-long twisty and mountainous suspension durability test. I have tried and some have even succeeded in negotiating this road in a passenger car (hopefully a rental), but doing so is not advisable. Although four-wheel drive is not necessary, having a high-clearance vehicle would certainly prevent knuckle fatigue from gripping the steering wheel too tightly during this drive. For those who don't have an off-road vehicle or a friend who owns one, take the more reasonable El Oso Road from the eastern side of the mountain. While this route requires a long detour, it should be passable by all but low-slung sports cars.

At 5,700 feet, the Lone Pine Trailhead sees temperatures 20 degrees cooler than the valley floor, a welcome change during hot summer months. You notice the difference as soon as you step out of the car. The air is crisper and more fragrant. Breathing seems easier, too. Look for a sign that reads "Browns Tr. 133" near the end of the parking lot and begin hiking up the well-maintained trail. Live oaks and ponderosa pines provide ample shade as you begin the climb. The trail snakes around the woods, passing oddly shaped rocks and occasional fallen trees. A quarter mile from the trailhead, find a rock that resembles Woodstock, Snoopy's tiny friend from the Charlie Brown cartoon, or perhaps a profile of Barney the purple dinosaur's head.

Continue up the switchbacks and follow the trail as it climbs higher. Notice the manzanita bushes trailside. They have distinctively red and silky-smooth bark. Blooming in April and May, they have delicate pink flowers that resemble decorative lightbulbs hanging upside down. At 0.7 miles the trail reaches the top of a ridge where you can see Roosevelt Lake and the Sierra Ancha Mountains to the east. Unfortunately, you can also see the devastation caused by the Lone Fire of 1996, when a carelessly discarded cigarette butt destroyed much of the forest.

Browns Trail snakes up some more switchbacks and takes a turn toward the eastern side of the mountain. The slope is never unreasonably steep, but its consistently ascending grade quickens the pulse. Once the trail straightens out a bit, it also levels off considerably. Hike a gentle traverse along the eastern slope through Gambel oaks. This stretch is especially scenic in fall when the leaves change colors. At 2 miles from the trailhead, Browns Trail merges into the Amethyst Trail at a signed junction. Follow the continuation of the Amethyst Trail a short distance to Browns Saddle, a wide vista point where you can take a rest and enjoy the sweeping views. You can see Saguaro Lake to the southwest and the city of Phoenix in the distance. The Superstition Mountains loom on the southern horizon. From Browns Saddle, the Amethyst Trail continues south

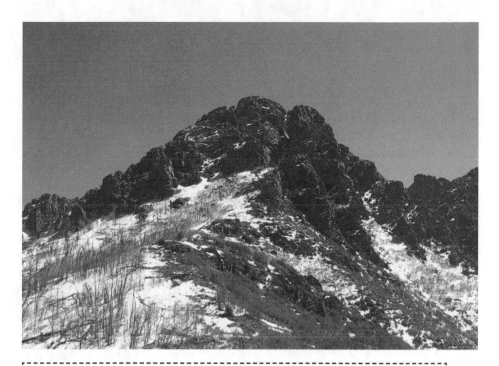

Rugged and inhospitable, Brown Peaks (tallest of Four Peaks) looms over the wintry landscape.

along the western flank of Four Peaks and eventually ends at the Amethyst Mine, a privately owned and inaccessible mine where some of the finest purple amethyst gemstones in the world are extracted from these rugged hills.

The hike to Browns Saddle has so far been moderate and nontechnical. Though Browns Peak beckons to you from above, the scramble to its summit is definitely difficult and not for the faint of heart. Only experienced and conditioned hikers should attempt the daunting climb to the top. In addition to steep inclines and loose scree, there's a section of exposed class-4 scrambling up a rock wall. The route to the peak can also be packed with snow in winter and early spring and should not be attempted under icy conditions.

To scale Browns Peak, break away from the Amethyst Trail at the saddle and start climbing southeast along a faint trail. Look up to find a long, vertical crevice on the western side of the rocky mountain top. That's the scree chute you need to scale. The faint trail eventually peters out and you are left to scramble over large boulders. Find your way into the chute by picking a route over the boulders and through some shrubs. Once atop the scree, slog your way straight up the chute. At one point you will have to scoot to the right along a thicket of bushes next to the cliff to continue. It's important to turn and look back at these bushes from which you emerged. Remember this spot because, when descending, you may find cairns unreliable, and you do not want to overshoot this point of egress. When you reach an imposing 15-foot rock wall, climb up carefully. The hand and foot holds are

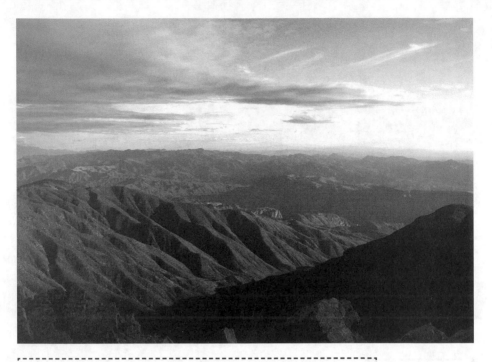

At 7,657 feet in elevation, Browns Peak towers over all else in Maricopa County.

solid, but there is considerable exposure. A fall here would certainly ruin your day. Continue climbing until you come to a spot where it seems you can no longer continue. Look for a cairn on the ledge above your head and to the left. Scramble up the final few boulders to the summit of Browns Peak.

Once your heart has stopped racing from the climb, soak up the breathtaking panorama from the Everest of Maricopa County. On a clear day you can see 100 miles. Off in the distance, Phoenix looks almost small from this vantage point. The Superstitions, Roosevelt Lake, and the Mogollon Rim can all be seen from the 7,657-foot summit of Browns Peak. Descend the way you came, and be extra careful while climbing down the scree chute. For a little variety you can choose to return via the Amethyst Trail at the junction just below Browns Saddle. The Amethyst Trail eventually dead-ends into the Four Peaks Trail. Turning left onto the Four Peaks Trail takes you back to the Lone Pine trailhead.

NEARBY ACTIVITIES

The Mazatzal mountain range provides ample hiking opportunities. The Four Peaks Trail from Lone Pine Saddle meanders around the base of its namesake peaks and eventually connects with the Vineyard Trail (page 252) near Roosevelt Lake. Mazatzal Divide Trail runs nearly 30 miles along the ridge of the Mazatzals. Tonto National Monument is 15 miles south of El Oso Road on SR 188.

GO JOHN TRAIL

IN BRIEF

Go John Trail is one of the best moderate loop trails you can hope for. Scenic hills surround the Cave Creek Recreation Area, and the undulating hike contains just enough ups and downs to keep you on your toes.

DESCRIPTION

Part of Maricopa County's regional park system, Cave Creek Recreation Area spans nearly 3,000 acres of mountain preserves north of Phoenix and west of the town of Cave Creek. Go John Trail, the most popular trail in the park, encircles its most prominent feature, a 3,060 foot tall mountain. Contrary to popular belief, however, Go John Mountain is not the mountain at the trail's center. It's actually located outside the park to the east.

The Go John Trail offers an excellent loop hike through scenic landscape typical of the mountains near Cave Creek. This trail touches hills, plains, dry washes, and unique rock formations, and of course showcases plenty of desert flora. However, prepare to share the trail with other hikers, equestrians, and mountain bikers.

Unlike many loop hikes, where the lay of the land makes one route preferable, either direction works well on Go John. I arbitrarily chose to describe this hike clockwise. Begin

KEY AT-A-GLANCE INFORMATION

LENGTH: 5.8 miles

ELEVATION GAIN: 430 feet

CONFIGURATION: Loop

DIFFICULTY: Easy–Moderate

SCENERY: Desert, Elephant Mountain, Black Mesa, city views

EXPOSURE: Mostly exposed, little shade

TRAFFIC: High

TRAIL SURFACE: Packed dirt, gravel, rock

HIKING TIME: 3 hours

WATER REQUIREMENT: 2 quarts

SEASON: Year round; hot in summer

ACCESS: Sun.–Thu. 6 a.m.–8 p.m., Fri.–Sat. 6 a.m.–10 p.m.; trails close at sunset; $6 per vehicle

MAPS: USGS Cave Creek and New River SE; park map available at entrance

FACILITIES: Picnic areas, water, restrooms, riding stables, campground, playground

DOGS: Yes, leashed at all times

COMMENTS: Hilly and scenic loop through Cave Creek Recreation Area. For more information, visit www.maricopa.gov/parks/cave_creek, or call (623) 465-0431.

Directions

Drive north on I-17 and exit onto SR 74, Carefree Highway. Drive east 6 miles on SR 74 to 32nd Street. Turn north onto 32nd Street and continue 1.5 miles to the Cave Creek Recreation Area entrance. Pay the entrance fee at the gate and then proceed 1.3 miles to the Go John Trailhead.

GPS Trailhead Coordinates

UTM Zone 12S

Easting 0407425

Northing 3743872

Latitude N33°49.969'

Longitude W112°0.071'

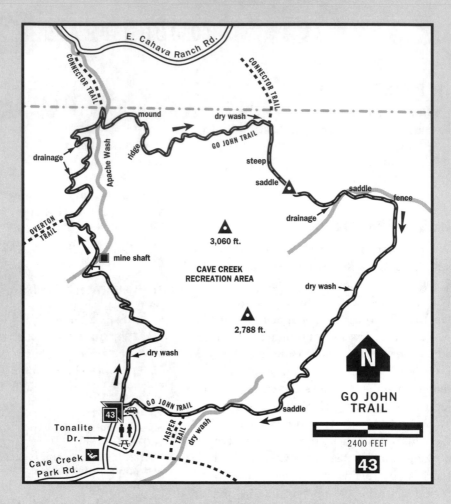

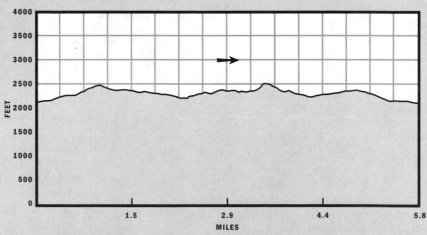

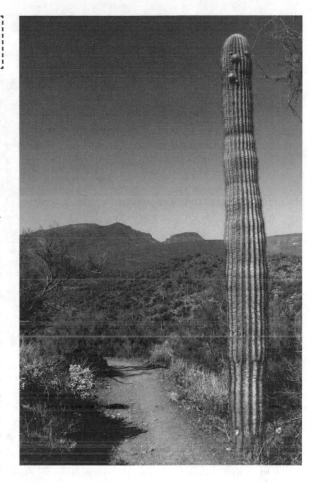

A lone saguaro guards Go John Trail as it heads north toward Elephant Mountain.

by heading north from the trailhead parking lot on a wide, level dirt track lined by chollas, palo verdes, and mesquites. Cross a dry wash at 0.1 mile, and begin a gentle ascent as the trail heads toward a series of switchbacks. The trail bends to the east and then turns northwest with a good view of the city behind you. The climb remains gradual on a smooth, well-maintained trail, which was recently rerouted. The original path can be seen to the left and below the current route. Nearly 1 mile from the trailhead, you reach a 2,450-foot saddle to catch the first glimpse of the mountains and desert wilderness to the north. The distinctive shape of Elephant Mountain lies straight ahead with the tip of Black Mesa just visible behind it. Skull Mesa looms to the right. The trail veers to the west and begins a long hillside traverse. If you are already winded, there's a stone bench here on which to rest.

Pleasant and wide, the smooth packed-dirt trail north of the saddle winds its way through gorgeous desert scenery. Jojoba and staghorn cholla line the trail, while majestic saguaros adorn the slopes. As the trail follows the hillside contour around the first drainage, look back up at the saddle and you'll see a fenced-in area protecting an old abandoned mineshaft. The Overton Trail joins in from the west at 1.3 miles, but continue following Go John Trail northeast, overlooking Apache Wash to your right. The trail meanders in and out of hillside drainages and remains relatively level. Reach the northern boundary of the park at 2.2 miles from the trailhead. Hiking beyond the park and onto state trust land requires a special permit, so the trail makes a hairpin turn back toward the south.

Go John Trail enters Apache Wash shortly after turning back from the park boundary. Seasonal rains collect in the dry wash bed and feed a different

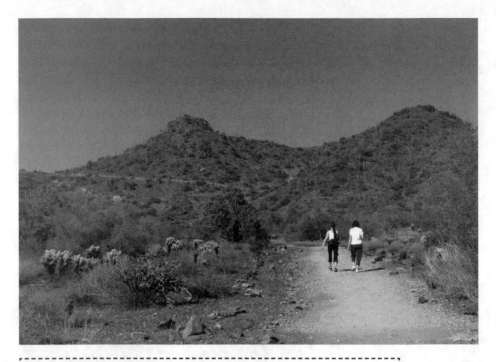

Hikers embark on a clockwise traversal of Go John Trail in Cave Creek Regional Park.

variety of desert plant life, a shady biome of taller brush and small trees. Enjoy momentary shade here, but watch out for prickly cat-claw acacias that tug at your clothing. Almost immediately after entering Apache Wash, climb out and head uphill toward the east.

The northern leg of Go John Trail offers gently rolling hills and open views while roughly traversing the park boundary. Trail conditions become noticeably rockier, narrower, and more rugged. At 2.4 miles survey the open views from the top of a mound. A variety of dense desert vegetation covers the hillside. In the distance, the prominent landmarks Apache Peak and Elephant Mountain provide a frame of reference. Continue hiking eastward through shallow basins, dry washes, and fields of jojoba bushes. Fewer folks share the path here, giving the impression of relative seclusion.

At 3.2 miles another spur trail leaving the park boundary intersects Go John Trail. Turn south here and climb a moderately steep chalky hill for a quarter mile to a 2,515-foot saddle, the highest point on the loop. Admire the view of magnificent Four Peaks on the horizon and the town of Cave Creek below. Shortly after reaching the saddle, look for a small track on the left side of the trail leading to a cluster of sharply protruding rocks. This is a good place to take a quick break and to enjoy the quiet basin.

Continue southeast with Black Mountain (page 76) directly ahead until you drop down into the bottom of the basin. The trail bends toward the east here and follows a brushy, dry creek bed. Jojobas, mesquites, and canyon ragweed encroach on the trail, and a forest of saguaros covers the hill in front of you. Climb out of the dry creek bed at 3.8 miles from the trailhead. Then, a quarter mile farther, turn south for a stretch next to the remnants of a fence, and follow the trail as it bends southwest.

The next mile or so is rather unremarkable as you hike near encroaching housing developments and scrub brush, passing a few dry washes along the way. Some striated layers of flaky sedimentary rock provide a little amusement about halfway through this mile. Pass an open basin covered in teddy bear cholla and white quartz rocks at approximately 5 miles. Then, skirt the side of a hill with the McDowell Mountains to the southeast. The trail reaches a ridgeline at 5.1 miles and crosses over a saddle. From here break west and start heading back toward the trailhead.

Go John Trail slowly creeps downhill and crosses a dry wash at 5.5 miles. Then it meets Jasper Trail, named for the colored quartz that fooled many prospectors into thinking there's "gold in them hills." Notice the mine and slag heap on the hill to the south. After the Jasper Trail junction, continue west a quarter mile to complete the loop hike.

NEARBY ACTIVITIES

The Cave Creek Recreation Area offers horseback riding, camping, and other popular trails such as the Overton. Scenic Spur Cross Ranch Conservation Area to the north presents other hiking opportunities at the base of Elephant Mountain (page 215). Farther north, the Cave Creek Trail (page 210) runs along the perennial spring of the same name.

44   MOUNT PEELEY

KEY AT-A-GLANCE INFORMATION

LENGTH: 5 miles

ELEVATION GAIN: 1,410 feet

CONFIGURATION: Out-and-back

DIFFICULTY: Moderate

SCENERY: Mazatzal Mountains, forest, panoramic vistas

EXPOSURE: Mostly exposed

TRAFFIC: Light

TRAIL SURFACE: Gravel, packed dirt, rock, some off-trail travel required

HIKING TIME: 3.5 hours

WATER REQUIREMENT: 2.5 quarts

SEASON: Year-round; may encounter snow in winter

ACCESS: Sunrise to sunset; free parking

MAPS: USGS Mazatzal Peak, Tonto National Forest map

FACILITIES: None

DOGS: Yes

COMMENTS: The Willow Fire of 2004 damaged portions of this trail.

GPS Trailhead Coordinates

UTM Zone 12S

Easting   0456547

Northing 3762592

Latitude N34°0.289'

Longitude W111°28.275'

IN BRIEF

Follow a section of the Arizona Trail to the top of Mount Peeley, a 7,034-foot peak in the Mazatzal Mountains. Superb scenery from the summit and along the trail rewards hikers, while the high elevation keeps temperatures relatively mild on hot summer days.

DESCRIPTION

The Mazatzal Mountains form a line of rugged peaks and deep valleys in the geographic center of Arizona. This extensive mountain range stretches from the Goldfield Mountains east of Phoenix north to the Mogollon Rim near Payson. Pronounced MAH-zah-tsal but often misspoken as MAT-a-zal, the odd-sounding name was taken from an Aztec word meaning "land of the deer." No doubt many deer roam the forests that cover these mountainsides.

Rising to elevations well in excess of 7,000 feet, a string of tall Mazatzal summits forms a spine along the mountain range and provides a natural boundary for Maricopa, Yavapai, and Gila counties. The most well-known of these giants is of course Four Peaks,

Directions

Take Loop 202 to Country Club Drive, which is also SR 87, Beeline Highway. Drive northeast on SR 87 to the Sycamore Creek and Mount Ord turnoff, which is past mile marker 222. Turn left onto Sycamore Creek Road and drive 1.2 miles to FR 25. Turn right across a cattle guard and then proceed another 1.2 miles to the FR 201 junction. Take the right fork and begin driving uphill on FR 201. Follow FR 201 until it ends at the Peeley Trailhead parking lot 8.3 miles further. FR 201 is a narrow dirt road and has a few rough spots that may require a high-clearance vehicle.

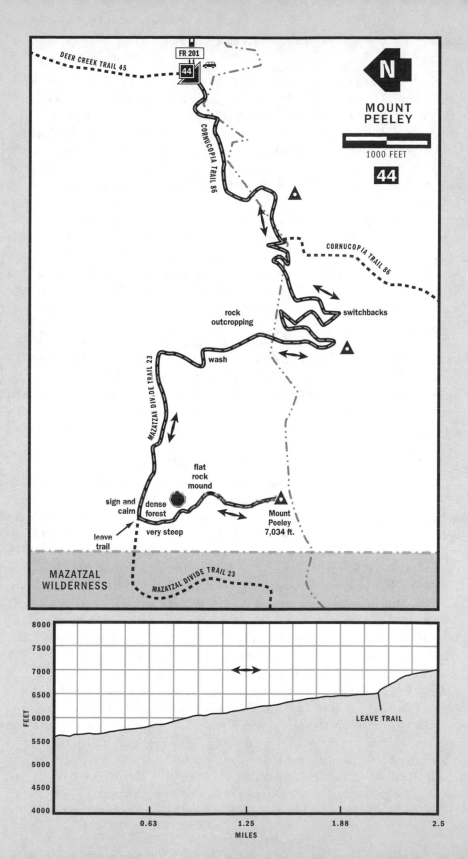

a series of serrated summits that form a unique silhouette against Phoenix's eastern horizon. Hiking Four Peaks requires a long drive on rough roads and some scary scrambling. At 7,903 feet, Mazatzal Peak rises above all others, but there are no established trails near its summit. Mount Ord presents little challenge since you can drive to the top where there's a fire lookout tower. Mount Peeley, on the other hand, provides a reasonable compromise between difficulty and accessibility and allows hikers to pierce the 7,000-foot barrier with just the right amount of effort.

Start your adventure with the scenic drive on FR 201, a narrow forest road that crawls up and down the foothills leading to the Peeley Trailhead. Already at 5,600 feet, you have left behind the desert heat and entered a cooler climate. Find the large Arizona Trail sign, and begin by hiking west on Cornucopia Trail 86. Similar to several other hikes in this book, Mount Peeley requires hiking a section of the Arizona Trail, a system of trails that runs from Utah to the Mexican border.

Cornucopia Trail begins in a nicely shaded forest with manzanitas, pines, and live oaks dotting the hillsides. After a few bends, the trail settles into a mild but steady incline heading southwest. At this elevation colorful wildflowers such as Palmer's penstemon bloom well into June. The trail turns westward again and unveils an open view toward Mount Ord and Four Peaks to the south. At 0.6 miles from the trailhead, reach a signed trail junction and the southern terminus of the Mazatzal Divide Trail.

Mazatzal Divide Trail 23 traces the spine of its namesake mountain range 29 miles. It intersects nearly every other trail in the Mazatzal Wilderness. Thankfully, you don't have to hike the whole thing to access Mount Peeley! Veer right at the trail junction and turn onto the Mazatzal Divide Trail, whose switchbacks demand significantly more from your muscles than the Cornucopia Trail. Lined with sugar sumacs and manzanitas, these switchbacks offer grander vistas with each turn. Soon the tip of Weaver's Needle and the Superstition Ridgeline come into view. To the north, two unnamed peaks topping 7,500 feet rise over the horizon. Mazatzal Peak remains hidden for the time being.

At 1.75 miles from the trailhead, the trail crosses a dry wash and turns away from the canyon through which you have been hiking. The slope lessens somewhat as you round the north slope of Mount Peeley. Evidence of the 2004 Willow Fire is visible. That lightning-sparked blaze destroyed more than 100,000 acres of forests and many pristine trails in the Mazatzals. Fortunately for Mount Peeley hikers, the trail you are hiking skirts the edges of the fire zone.

Along a relatively straight section of trail, look for a cairn and a burnt sign at 2.1 miles from the trailhead. To your left, a dense forest of charred trees covers a very steep hill. To make the ascent slightly more tolerable, walk past the sign about 50 yards and then leave the Mazatzal Divide Trail. Turn left and bushwhack uphill through the thick trees. Despite the lack of a trail, finding a route through the shrub-free forest should be fairly easy. Climbing the nearly 40-degree incline

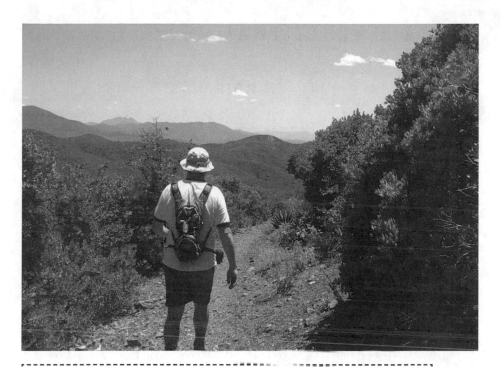

Brian Skerven of Tempe descends the Mazatzal Divide Trail with Four Peaks in the distance.

is anything but easy, however. Take your time as you slog up the steep slope, and make a mental note of your surroundings for the return trip.

After 0.2 miles of arduous ascent, reach a rocky overlook where the forest clears and the hill flattens considerably. Notice the intricate grid-like patterns of reddish mineral deposits on the rocks. Finish your climb in relative ease and reach the wide-open rocky summit of Mount Peeley at 2.5 miles from the trailhead. You can trace the scenic drive along FR 201, admire Saddle Mountain to the southwest, look down upon Horseshoe Reservoir on the Verde River, and sneak a peek at Mazatzal Peak to the north. Remember to slather on some sunblock because solar radiation can be brutal at higher elevations. When satisfied with the view, return to the Mazatzal Divide Trail and backtrack to the Peeley Trailhead.

NEARBY ACTIVITIES

The Peeley Trailhead also serves Deer Creek Trail. Many abandoned mines are sprinkled throughout the hills near Sunflower and provide a fascinating look into the history of the area. Other excellent trails in the Mazatzal Mountains include Barnhardt Trail (page 200), Y Bar Trail, Half Moon Trail, and the Mazatzal Divide Trail. Near the town of Gisela, Tonto Creek tempts hikers and canyoneers with some choice swimming holes. Other hikes accessible from SR 87 include Ballantine Trail via Pine Creek Loop (page 238) and Browns Peak (page 220), the tallest of Four Peaks.

45 PALO VERDE TRAIL

KEY AT-A-GLANCE INFORMATION

LENGTH: 8.2 miles (one way: 4.6 miles)
ELEVATION GAIN: 100 feet (nearly 1,000 feet accumulated gain)
CONFIGURATION: Out-and-back or one-way
DIFFICULTY: Moderate
SCENERY: Bartlett Reservoir, mountain views, desert
EXPOSURE: Completely exposed
TRAFFIC: Light to moderate
TRAIL SURFACE: Gravel, sand
HIKING TIME: 4 hours (one way: 2.5 hours)
WATER REQUIREMENT: 2.5 quarts
SEASON: Year-round; hot in summer
ACCESS: Trails open sunrise to sunset; Tonto Pass and $6 per vehicle required; not sold on site but available in stores and at Forest Service offices.
MAPS: USGS Bartlett Dam and Maverick Mountain; maps on plaques in recreation areas
FACILITIES: Restrooms, picnic area, drinking water, outdoor shower
DOGS: Yes, leashed at all times
COMMENTS: For info on Tonto Pass, click www.fs.fed.us/r3/tonto/tp; for hike info, visit www.fs.fed.us/r3/tonto/recreation/rec-hiking-index.shtml, or call (480) 595-3300.

GPS Trailhead Coordinates

UTM Zone   12S
Easting   0441514
Northing   3745358
Latitude   N33°50.919'
Longitude   W111°37.975'

IN BRIEF

The Palo Verde Trail winds along the shoreline of Bartlett Reservoir, giving hikers an up-close view of the lake and surrounding mountains. Plenty of ups and downs along this trail give your legs and lungs a workout.

DESCRIPTION

Hiking near water is a treat for desert dwellers. Fortunately, Arizona has plenty of lakes, many of which are close to Phoenix. A series of dams on the Salt and Verde rivers provide the water storage necessary to sustain the fifth-largest U.S. city, situated in the middle of a desert. These reservoirs also offer valley residents the means to enjoy water sports. A popular urban myth ascribes to Arizona the distinction of having the highest-per-capita boat ownership of any state in the country. Though this is inaccurate, Arizona does have a relatively high percentage of boat owners.

Bartlett Reservoir near Cave Creek sets the backdrop for this scenic lakeside hike. Palo Verde Trail 512 links Rattlesnake Cove with SB Cove, two recreational areas situated on the lake's western shore. Along this trail,

Directions

From Loop 101, exit onto Princess Drive and turn east. The road soon becomes Pima Road. Drive north on Pima Road 12 miles, then turn east onto Cave Creek Road. Go 6 miles and turn right onto Bartlett Dam Road. Follow Bartlett Dam Road 14 miles to the pay station at Bartlett Reservoir. Purchase a single-vehicle pass (without boat, unless you are actually towing one, of course). Turn left onto SR 459 and then follow signs to Rattlesnake Cove Recreation Site. Take the one-way loop drive and park near the last restroom.

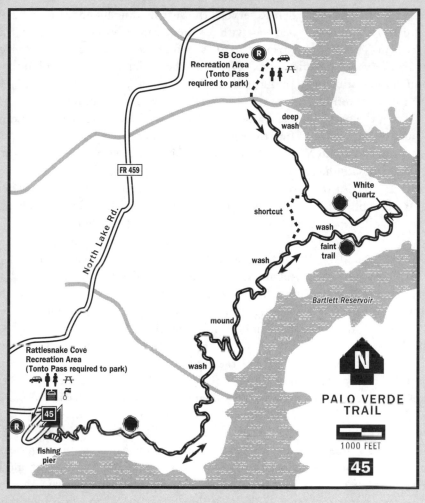

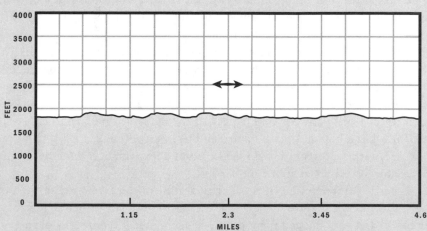

hikers enjoy views of Bartlett Reservoir, the surrounding mountains, and desert foothills. Hike this trail one way with a shuttle car or boat, or just go out and back to make it a longer trip. A small shortcut near the trail's northern end shaves off a mile along the shore, giving you the option to create a balloon hike. Though the trail never gains more than 100 feet at any one stretch, it undulates with the wavy terrain and satisfies those who crave a workout on their hikes.

From the parking lot at Rattlesnake Cove, walk down to the line of ramadas and picnic sites, and find the signed trailhead at the northeastern end. The lake sits inside Tonto National Forest, so the signs you see along the trail are all emblazoned with the Forest Service logo. Hike toward the boardwalk jutting out into the water. At the base of the boardwalk, turn sharply uphill to embark on the gravel trail. At 0.25 miles pass a short peninsula projecting into the lake, and continue following the trail as it traces the contours of the shoreline.

This lakeside trail is surprisingly rugged, with several steep climbs and descents. A good variety of flora lines the trail. Some conspicuous flowers you might encounter include tubular chuparosas, pink fairy dusters, fragrant desert lavender, odd-looking chias, and Mexican gold poppies. Plenty of palo verde trees, jojoba bushes, brittlebush, and various cacti also inhabit these sandy hills.

Cross a dry wash at 0.6 miles and then climb a hefty slope to a rocky hilltop. The trail gradually rounds the tip of the hill with views of Maverick Mountain and SB Mountain across the lake. At 1.1 miles, the trail makes a turn westward atop a scenic mound overlooking the lake. The next 1.5-mile section takes you up and down hills, and in and out of coves. The trail also crosses several dry washes feeding the lake and follows a high ridge with open views of the mountains and surrounding desert.

Near 2.9 miles from the trailhead, drop into a wide, sandy wash with a tall saguaro guarding the opposite bank. The trail forks here. Turning left up the wash shortcuts the hike by 1 mile, while crossing the wash takes you along the scenic lakeshore. You can go either way, but if you wish to make a loop out of the hike, I recommend you take the scenic route first because it is easier to find your way when you're coming down the wash.

Past this fork the trail becomes difficult to follow at times, so look carefully for trail markers in the form of cairns or plastic ribbons tied to tree limbs. At 3.4 miles the trail crosses another wash and passes a patch of white quartz. Then round the end of a wide peninsula near an elbow in the lake and turn uphill toward the west. As you hike across a ridge with the lake to either side, look for a large boulder that oddly resembles the profile of a face. This scenic route rejoins the shortcut trail at a saddle point approximately 0.5 miles from SB Cove, which was named after Sam Bartlett.

From this intersection, turn right downhill if you wish to visit SB Cove. The trail descends a gravelly section and then follows the shoreline toward the recreation area, ending at a point on the beach about 0.2 miles shy of the parking lot. Upon your return from SB Cove, take the shortcut at this trail junction

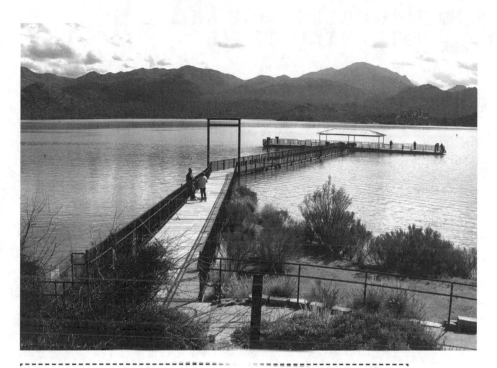

A boardwalk and fishing dock protrude into Bartlett Reservoir from Rattlesnake Cove.

by heading southwest. One-tenth of a mile farther, the trail bends south and enters a wide dry wash. Follow this wash 0.2 miles toward the lake, where it meets the scenic route again at the base of the tall saguaro.

Turn right at the trail junction and follow the common section of Palo Verde Trail back to Rattlesnake Cove. The distance from Rattlesnake Cove to SB Cove along the scenic route is 4.6 miles, while returning via the shortcut measures only 3.6 miles, forming an 8.2-mile circuit. One good thing about hiking next to a lake is having the option to jump in after a hot hike. You can also use the outdoor showers on the side of the restrooms to cool off.

NEARBY ACTIVITIES

Bartlett Reservoir has a shorter lakeside trail called the Jojoba Trail, which also starts at the Rattlesnake Cove Recreation Site, but heads in the opposite direction from the Palo Verde Trail. The scenic Cave Creek Trail (page 210) is located on Cave Creek Road, 10 miles past the Bartlett Dam Road turnoff.

46 PINE CREEK LOOP AND BALLANTINE TRAIL

KEY AT-A-GLANCE INFORMATION

LENGTH: 8.8 miles

ELEVATION GAIN: 1,466 feet

CONFIGURATION: Inverse balloon

DIFFICULTY: Moderate

SCENERY: Desert, Four Peaks Wilderness, mountain vistas, seasonal streams

EXPOSURE: Mostly exposed

TRAFFIC: Light to moderate

TRAIL SURFACE: Gravel, rock, packed dirt

HIKING TIME: 4.5 hours

WATER REQUIREMENT: 3 quarts

SEASON: Year-round; hot in summer

ACCESS: Sunrise to sunset; free parking

MAPS: USGS Boulder Mountain, Tonto National Forest map

FACILITIES: None

DOGS: Yes

COMMENTS: The Ballantine Trail begins at the halfway point on Pine Creek Loop. Hike out and back on Ballantine, and then complete the loop for an inverse balloon. For more information, visit www.fs .fed.us/r3/tonto/recreation/ rec-hiking-index.shtml.

GPS Trailhead Coordinates

UTM Zone 12S

Easting 0454378

Northing 3735942

Latitude N33°45.862'

Longitude W111°29.601'

IN BRIEF

Though Pine Creek Loop and Ballantine Trail offer easy access to a scenic hike, relatively few people bother to explore these trails. Those who do visit this area enjoy stunning boulder-strewn canyons, views of mountains near Four Peaks, and some delightful seasonal springs.

DESCRIPTION

A major transportation artery between Phoenix and Payson, SR 87, Beeline Highway, runs from the low-lying valleys of Phoenix, through the rugged Mazatzal Mountains, to the pine-covered Mogollon Rim. In recent years, this route has grown quickly from a two-lane twisty mountain road into a busy divided highway. Many Mazatzal trails can be accessed via this road, and the Ballantine Trailhead is perhaps the most obvious.

Situated on SR 87 and prominently signed, Ballantine Trailhead sees thousands of vehicles everyday. Despite easy access, however, Ballantine Trail 283, reachable from this trailhead via Pine Creek Loop 280, remains relatively unknown to Phoenix hikers. Those who hike Ballantine for the first time often express their surprise at how pleasant the trail is and their regret at not having explored it sooner. Pine Creek Loop, named for the large seasonal stream north of the trailhead, loops over a hill next to SR 87. Ballantine Trail begins at the farthest point on the loop and extends east into Ballantine

---

Directions

Exit Loop 202 onto Country Club Drive, also known as SR 87 or Beeline Highway. Follow SR 87 north 33 miles to the signed Ballantine Trailhead beyond mile marker 210.

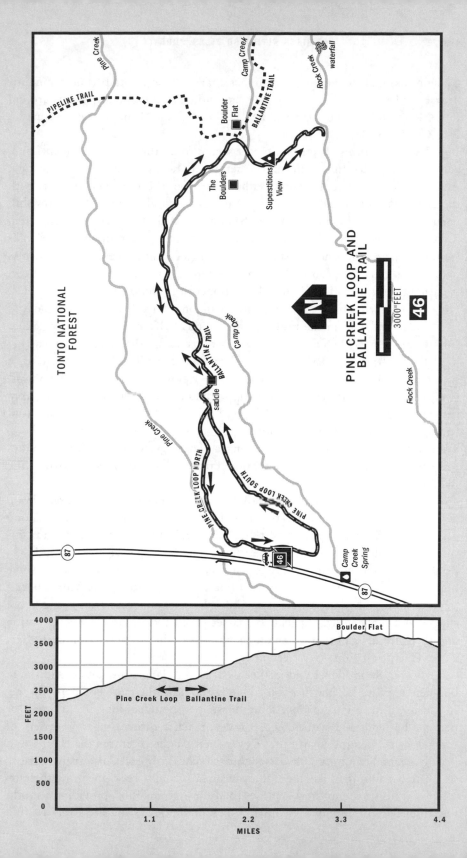

PINE CREEK LOOP AND BALLANTINE TRAIL

46

3000 FEET

N

Pine Creek

Camp Creek

Rock Creek

waterfall

PIPELINE TRAIL

BALLANTINE TRAIL

Boulder Flat

Superstitions View

The Boulders

TONTO NATIONAL FOREST

Camp Creek

Pine Creek

BALLANTINE TRAIL

saddle

PINE CREEK LOOP NORTH

PINE CREEK LOOP SOUTH

Rock Creek

Camp Creek Spring

46

87

87

Elevation profile:

FEET

4000
3500
3000
2500
2000
1500
1000
500
0

Boulder Flat

Pine Creek Loop   Ballantine Trail

1.1   2.2   3.3   4.4

MILES

Canyon, parallel to many other canyons that channel rainfall from mountains near Four Peaks. The continuation of Ballantine Trail eventually wraps around Pine Mountain and ends at the Cline Trailhead about 11 miles from its start on Pine Creek Loop.

The hike in this chapter follows a scenic route through Pine Creek Loop, a portion of Ballantine Trail, and a detour to Rock Creek before returning. Although you can hike the loop in either direction, I recommend you start with the southern half because it's more scenic, and you also save all the downhill parts for the end. From a signed trailhead at the end of the large parking area, begin by turning right onto Pine Creek Loop South. The trail circles the hill's southern tip and turns northeast up its main ridge. Plentiful desert plants such as palo verdes and chollas cover the slopes. When in season, a variety of wildflowers also graces the landscape. Blue dicks, popcorn flowers, phacelias, gold fields, fairy dusters, brittlebush, and many others bloom in a kaleidoscope of colors.

At 0.4 miles from the trailhead and about halfway up the hill, pause to survey the scenery. Behind you, SR 87 swoops across the valley, broadcasting loud tire noise from passing vehicles deep into the hills. Toward the east, a scenic basin opens where seasonal Camp Creek flows down from the high hills. Continue following the ridge among chollas and brittlebushes. At 0.8 miles from the trailhead, you'll reach the highest point on Pine Creek Loop. This 2,785-foot vantage point offers a superb panorama of surrounding mountains and valleys. The trail then proceeds northeast along a flat ridge, with Boulder Mountain towering over the horizon. A quarter mile farther, descend to a saddle where the Ballantine Trail begins.

At 1.4 miles from the trailhead, Ballantine Trail meets the Pine Creek Loop at a well-marked three-way intersection. The northern half of Pine Creek Loop turns back sharply toward the west. Save that trail for the return trip, and continue hiking northeast on the Ballantine Trail. A plaque says it is 3 miles to Boulder Flat, but the true distance is just over 2 miles. The trail first passes some hop bushes and sotols on level ground but soon begins to climb. More charming and noticeably quieter than Pine Creek Loop, Ballantine Trail is also more rugged and challenging. It quickly surpasses Pine Creek Loop's highest elevation and then steadily gains more. An old camp at 1.9 miles from the trailhead offers a convenient rest stop if you need one.

As you climb higher and farther east, a hilly landscape dotted with large boulders appears. The farther you go along the trail, the more boulders you see. If you use a little imagination, some misshapen boulders look like animals or perhaps Easter Island statues. At 2.3 miles, reach a clearing where a variety of cacti flourish. Giant saguaros tower over their smaller brethren the chollas and prickly pears. Stringy ocotillos, though not technically cacti, also thrive here.

Farther into the hike, the trail draws near Camp Creek. In spring the gurgling of trailside Camp Creek replaces road noise from SR 87, providing a soothing ambience for the hike. At other times of the year, you are likely to find

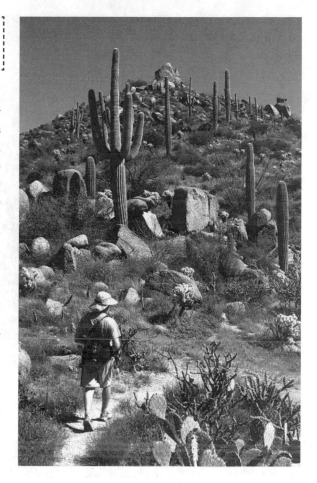

Robert Martin of Phoenix hikes past a scenic bend along the Ballantine Trail.

total silence here. Follow Ballantine Trail as it enters a large open basin studded with stunning boulders and tall saguaros. Near 3.2 miles cross a small oasis fed by a Camp Creek tributary and then resume your eastbound traversal of the wide basin. Notice the large reddish hill to your right seemingly comprised of crumbly piles of rocks. On topographical maps of the area, this hill is labeled "The Boulders," for obvious reasons.

At 3.6 miles from the trailhead, Ballantine Trail climbs to a 3,700-foot saddle guarded by a huge stack of boulders on the left and a lone pine tree on the right. This point is essentially the entry into Boulder Flat, and many hikers make this their turnaround spot. Should you choose to explore further, be aware that there are several confusing and unmarked trail junctions just beyond this saddle. A trail sign explaining your options would be most welcome should the Forest Service see fit to install one here. Ballantine Trail proper goes straight through a wide valley and then continues several more miles before bending south toward the Cline Trailhead. A left fork heading uphill eventually becomes the northbound Pipeline Trail. When the seasonal streams are flowing, however, I suggest you visit Rock Creek by turning right and hiking around The Boulders.

The detour to Rock Creek travels south 0.8 miles from the aforementioned saddle. Though unmarked, the narrow trail is easy to follow. Along the way, capture an awesome southern view encompassing the Flatiron in the Superstitions, SR 87, and the McDowell Mountains. This view is worth the extra effort even if Rock Creek is out of season. When there is water in the mountains, proceed farther and head downhill to where the unmarked trail intersects Rock Creek.

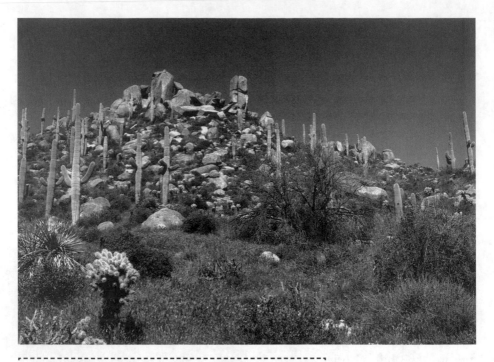

Odd rock formations seem commonplace along the Ballantine Trail.

There you will find a slick-rock area in the stream ideally suited for a picnic.

Return via Ballantine Trail to the three-way intersection with both branches of Pine Creek Loop. Now take the gentle northern route back to the trailhead. This flat 1.4-mile section of trail hugs the hillside above Pine Creek until it reaches SR 87. Though the trail doesn't actually meet Pine Creek, some people bushwhack down to the stream to explore the creek bed. Finally, head south parallel to the road to complete the Pine Creek Loop.

NEARBY ACTIVITIES

Nearby Four Peaks Wilderness contains many miles of rugged and remote hiking trails. Browns Peak, the tallest point in Maricopa County, can be reached via Browns Trail (page 220). Trails such as Barnhardt (page 200), Mazatzal Divide (page 230), and Deer Creek in the Mazatzal Mountains are also accessible via SR 87.

TONTO NARROWS*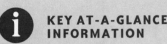

IN BRIEF

Update: As of February 2009, this trailhead has been closed by private land owners with no known alternate access available.

Take a relatively short and easy hike to popular Tonto Narrows, and then forge upstream as far as you'd like for more-secluded swimming holes and fascinating scenery.

DESCRIPTION

Let's face it; Phoenix summers can be brutally hot. When the mercury hits triple digits and beyond, what's a desert hiker to do? Hiking in town doesn't seem like such a good idea. All but the most hard-core hikers have fled for Flagstaff, and the remaining few are forced to rise at the crack of dawn for a go at Camelback, South Mountain, or Piestewa Peak.

You don't have to let the oppressive heat turn you into an air-conditioned hermit. There are plenty of summer hikes within a short drive from town. The best summer trails take you either high into the mountains where it's cooler or down to a stream where you can

KEY AT-A-GLANCE INFORMATION

LENGTH: 2.4 miles (optional canyoneering upstream for as long as you'd like)

ELEVATION GAIN: -90 feet

CONFIGURATION: Out-and-back

DIFFICULTY: Easy to Tonto Narrows, moderate beyond

SCENERY: Tonto Creek, Hellsgate Wilderness, Gisela Mountain, riparian zone, desert

EXPOSURE: Mostly exposed; limited shade near Houston Creek

TRAFFIC: Moderate to heavy

TRAIL SURFACE: Packed dirt, sand, river rock, creek, canyoneering skills required beyond Tonto Narrows

HIKING TIME: 1.5 hours (add swimming time)

WATER REQUIREMENT: 2.5 quarts

SEASON: Year-round; hot in summer

ACCESS: Sunrise to sunset; free parking

MAPS: USGS Gisela, Payson South, McDonald Mountain, and Sheep Basin Mountain

FACILITIES: None

DOGS: Yes

COMMENTS: Escape from the heat by jumping into a cool creek.

Directions

Take Loop 202 to Country Club Drive, which is also SR 87 or Beeline Highway. Follow SR 87 northeast toward Payson 60 miles. After mile marker 239, turn right onto Gisela Road. Drive east on Gisela Road 5 miles, going straight through all intersections, until you come to a T facing a wire fence. Bear left here and follow the road until it ends at the trailhead gate. Parking is limited, so you may have to park along the road. However, take care not to obstruct the roadway because local ranchers need to drive past the gate. A portion of the access road is a graded dirt road passable by most cars.

GPS Trailhead Coordinates

UTM Zone 12S

Easting 0475396

Northing 3775921

Latitude N34°7.538'

Longitude W111°16.050'

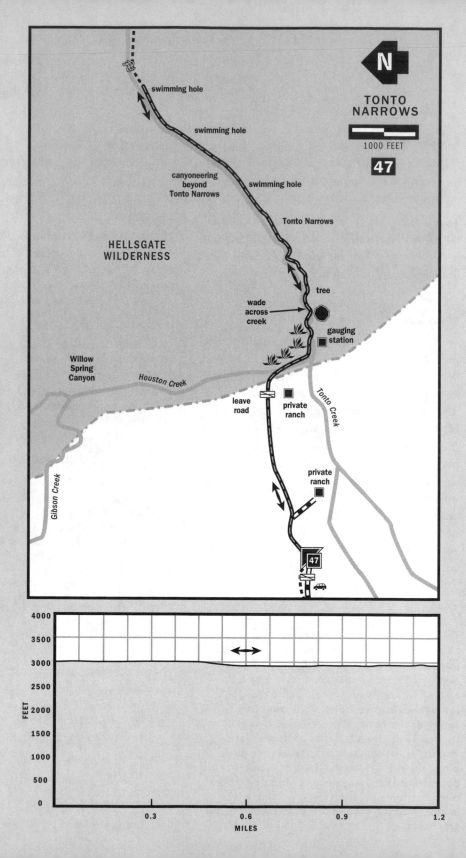

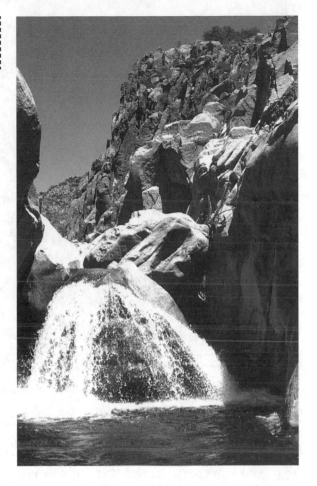

A hidden waterfall nestled in scenic Hellsgate Wilderness upstream from Tonto Narrows.

swim. Tonto Narrows is an excellent example of the latter. With a relatively short and easy access trail, a trip to Tonto Narrows is sure to please the whole family, especially Fido. Remember to take plenty of sunblock and a pair of old sneakers so you can wade into the stream. Sandals also work, but they can expose your toes to underwater hazards.

Tonto Creek originates high on the Mogollon Rim and ultimately empties into Roosevelt Lake on the Salt River basin. Along the way it flows through Hellsgate Wilderness, home of some of the most scenic and remote central Arizona canyons. At a particular section near the community of Gisela, Tonto Creek squeezes through a narrow rocky passage, forming some deep pools ideal for swimming. Locals call this part of the creek Tonto Narrows and pay regular visits to take advantage of its superb swimming opportunities.

The hike to Tonto Narrows begins from a gated fence on a dirt road that serves local ranches. A sign on the fence reminds hikers to keep the roadway clear and free of litter. Cross the fence and then begin hiking east on the wide, level road, which meanders through scenic hills. Gisela Mountain and Neal Mountain stand guard to the right, while typical high Sonoran Desert flora blankets the hills. It's difficult to believe at this point that any water can be found amid all the cacti and prickly bushes.

Stay left at a fork in the road 0.2 miles from the trailhead. Local property owners put up ample signs to keep the public on the right path, so please respect their property. The dirt road soon drops gently into a valley where the road ends at a local ranch a half mile from the parking area. Find a small trail on the left, and leave the road at this point. Once again, there are signs guiding you toward the "Swim Hole."

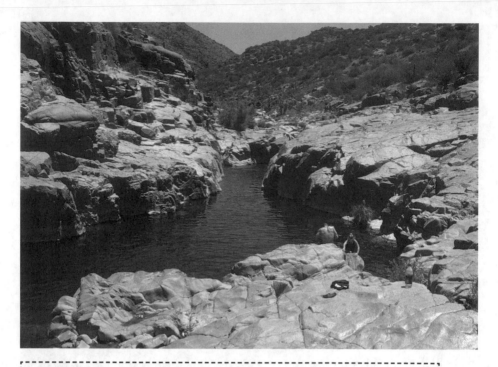

Hikers and swimmers enjoy cooling off in Tonto Narrows, a deep rocky channel on Tonto Creek near Gisela.

Go through a gate with a rather simple but ingenious automatic closer, and then hike down a steep, slippery slope flanked by thorny bushes. Fortunately, this tricky section is fairly short. The trail reaches Houston Creek and follows its right bank down toward Tonto Creek. Fed by perennial streams, riparian bushes like willows and salt cedars grow in abundance here. At 0.7 miles turn left and cross Houston Creek near its confluence with Tonto Creek.

Continue hiking east along the reed-covered sandy banks of Tonto Creek. Notice the gauging station across the river. Soon the sand gives way to an uneven bed of river rock. Take care not to twist an ankle while traversing this rocky field. At 0.9 miles ford the creek and head toward a large tree on the southern bank. From this tree you can turn left upstream to find a large swimming hole fed by Tonto Narrows' outlet. However, if you want to reach the Narrows on foot, look for a small trail behind the tree. Take this trail uphill and hike parallel to the creek's southern bank until you reach the rocks that frame the Narrows.

On a warm weekend you'll likely meet quite a few people at the Narrows, which unfortunately suffers from overuse judging by the amount of trash strewn about the rocks. Despite there being plenty of company and unkempt surroundings, Tonto Narrows is a wonderful place to splash around. Visitors enjoy sunbathing on the rocks, picnicking, or just playing in the water with newfound friends. If you choose to jump off the rocks, make sure the water below is deep enough, and never dive in headfirst.

Casual hikers should make Tonto Narrows their turnaround point. If you are adventurous, consider forging upstream for more-secluded swimming holes and even better scenery. However, venturing beyond the Narrows requires canyoneering skills.

Think of canyoneering as hiking with a splash—just add water. A combination of hiking, scrambling, wading, swimming, and climbing, canyoneering has become an increasingly popular sport among outdoor enthusiasts in recent years. You can learn the basics at Tonto Creek without getting into any technical rope work. However, be aware of some added risks you must assume. The most obvious danger is drowning. If you can't swim 100 yards, do not attempt to go upstream. While Tonto Creek flows at a gentle and predictable rate most of the year, spring snowmelt and seasonal storms can turn the creek into a dangerous river. Even in calm waters you can slip on moss-covered rocks or trap your foot in unseen crevices.

It's never a good idea to venture into the wilderness alone. Bring a friend, preferably someone who is familiar with the terrain and canyoneering. Before venturing upstream, put your valuables inside two layers of zippered plastic bags to keep them dry. Then, follow Tonto Creek deeper into Hellsgate Wilderness. You'll have to hop around boulders protruding from the creek bed, skirt small rapids, wade through shallow pools, and swim through deeper and longer passages. You'll love every minute of it.

Near 1.9 miles from the trailhead, reach a large secluded swimming hole surrounded by towering rocks and flanked by a 12-foot waterfall. This is a stark contrast to Tonto Narrows in that you will almost certainly enjoy this idyllic setting in solitude. It is possible to climb up the waterfall's right side and follow Tonto Creek upstream for many more miles. As a matter of fact, some die-hard canyoneers make a multiday backpacking trip out of traversing Tonto Creek, although in the opposite direction and starting from a point on SR 260 east of Payson. For most day hikers, however, this waterfall makes an excellent final destination before backtracking toward Gisela.

NEARBY ACTIVITIES

The Barnhardt Trail on the opposite side of SR 87 offers an excellent hike into the heart of Mazatzal Wilderness. Nearby Payson is a popular summertime retreat for Phoenix residents. Blessed with higher elevation and many streams that flow from the Mogollon Rim, several hikes near Payson lead to popular swimming holes. Horton Creek, Ellison Creek, Christopher Creek, and Fossil Springs all offer perennial streams in which to swim. Farther south on SR 87, numerous trails lead to tall summits in the Mazatzal range including Mount Peeley (page 230), Mount Ord, and the 7,657-foot Browns Peak (page 220). SR 188, which intersects SR 87 just south of Gisela Road, leads to Roosevelt Lake, the largest of the Salt River reservoirs.

48   TONTO NATIONAL MONUMENT: UPPER CLIFF DWELLINGS

KEY AT-A-GLANCE INFORMATION

LENGTH: 2.4 miles

ELEVATION GAIN: 600 feet

CONFIGURATION: Out-and-back

DIFFICULTY: Easy

SCENERY: Cliff dwellings, Roosevelt Lake, high desert panorama, riparian habitat

EXPOSURE: Partially shaded, open areas can be windy

TRAFFIC: Very light

TRAIL SURFACE: Packed dirt, creek bed, gravel

HIKING TIME: 3.5 hours (guided program)

WATER REQUIREMENT: 1 quart

SEASON: Saturday–Monday, November–April

ACCESS: Tonto National Monument, reservations required; $3 per person entrance fee

MAPS: USGS Windy Hill

FACILITIES: Visitor center, restroom, drinking water, ranger station

DOGS: No

COMMENTS: By guided tour only, 15-person limit, reservations required, call (928) 467-2241, or visit www.nps.gov/tont.

GPS Trailhead Coordinates

UTM Zone   12S

Easting   0489615

Northing   3722523

Latitude   N33°38.656'

Longitude W111°6.760'

IN BRIEF

A lesson in desert ecology featuring several microclimates, a history lesson on the Salado people, and an archaeology lesson, this educational trip to the upper cliff dwellings at Tonto National Monument has it all. The hike and scenic views aren't bad either.

DESCRIPTION

Tonto National Monument is small by national park standards but has plenty to offer visitors in the way of history, scenery, and a memorable hike for the entire family. For an educational outdoor experience, make a reservation for the upper cliff-dwellings tour, pack a picnic lunch, and spend a day learning about the lives of the Salado people who inhabited the area 700 years ago.

Leave extra early for this trip because it requires a considerable amount of time to navigate through the twisting mountain roads of the very scenic Apache Trail. Arriving at the Tonto National Monument visitor center, check in with the rangers to make sure you get on this exclusive tour. They allow only 15

Directions

Take US 60 east and exit onto Idaho Road. Drive north on Idaho Road 2.25 miles and turn northeast onto AZ 88, the old Apache Trail. Follow the scenic Apache Trail 41 miles until it ends at Roosevelt Dam. From the dam, turn southeast onto AZ 188 and drive 4.5 miles to the signed entrance of Tonto National Monument. Note: Half of AZ 88 is a gravel road. Passenger cars should be OK.

For a paved alternative, continue on US 60, traveling 50 miles past Miami, Arizona. Turn northwest onto AZ 188 and drive 27 miles to Tonto National Monument.

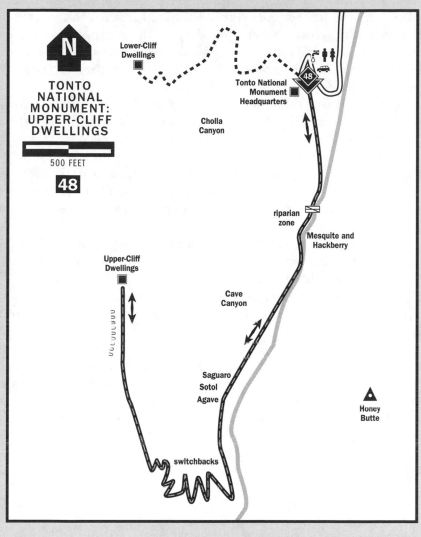

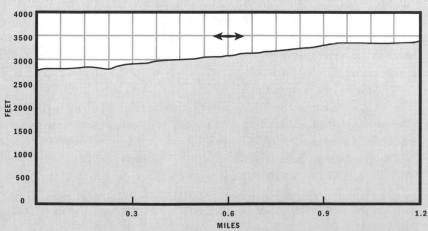

people per day to visit the upper cliff dwellings, and the tour is available only three days a week between November and April. The extremely low traffic on the trail to the ruins makes this trip a pleasant experience every time. Knowledgeable park rangers guide you up the canyon at an easy pace, stopping often to explain various desert features along the way.

The tour begins at the southern end of the parking lot. After some quick, obligatory safety reminders, the group heads out on the lightly used but well-maintained trail. The rangers unlock a gate and lead the group into Cave Canyon, a delightful and pristine desert canyon that sees very little foot traffic. The first lesson in ecology begins here at a riparian habitat next to the creek bed. Standing in the shade of large walnuts and sycamores, you learn about how this surprisingly moist desert environment provides precious water to feed the plants and animals living nearby.

Knowledge of plants and their uses helped the Salado people thrive in this seemingly harsh environment. As the hike progresses, you tour several microclimates. Each of these tiny ecosystems is distinct and supports a specific kind of plant. The colonies of hackberries and dewberries supplied tasty fruits. Clusters of mesquite provided firewood, and their seedpods are an important source of nutrition.

Hike farther up the canyon as the trail zigzags across the creek bed several times. The upper Cave Canyon is drier as the presence of more cacti, agaves, and yuccas indicates a dearth of water. The Salado people made ample use of these important plants. The giant saguaro leaves behind a column of tough spines when it dies, and the Salado used them extensively as construction material for their cliff dwellings. Yucca root can be used to create soap as well as to sooth arthritis, and its fibrous leaves make great weaving material. The juices from agaves can be fermented into an alcoholic drink. Indeed, we still drink it today in the form of tequila.

Approximately a half mile into the hike, the trail leaves the canyon and ascends the western slopes in a series of switchbacks. Even though you are climbing 600 feet to reach the cliff dwellings, the rangers go at a sufficiently slow pace to make the hike an easy stroll. On cold, windy days you might even be itching to go faster in order to keep warm. The switchbacks eventually give way to a long straight traverse toward the cave where the cliff dwellings are located. As you climb higher, Roosevelt Lake comes into view in the distance. The Sierra Ancha Wilderness lies beyond the lake.

The final segment of the hike skims the base of an imposing, overhanging cliff. When the cliff dwellings come into view, you realize how well protected these ancient homes really are. The inhabitants can see for many miles, and the cave shielded their adobe-style homes from the elements. Break out the picnic lunch here, and listen to the park ranger's lesson in archaeology. Admire the Salado people's engineering feat in constructing these elaborate multilevel homes from the raw materials at hand. Crawl around among the ruins and get

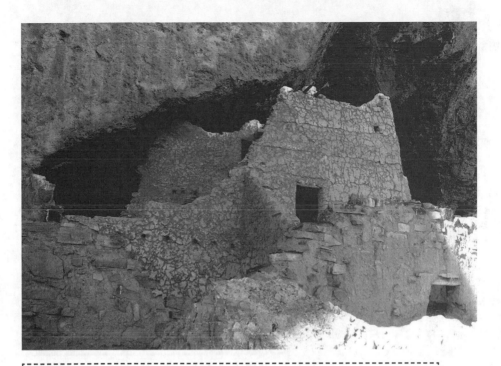

Salado cliff dwellers built this massive 40-room complex high above Tonto Basin in the 1300s.

a sense of how they lived. Close your eyes. Try to imagine being among the ancients nearly a millennium ago, and wonder what kind of legacy we will leave 1,000 years from now.

After the informative tour, take a moment to enjoy the views from the cliff dwellings. The scenic Roosevelt Lake is even more beautiful when framed by one of the windows in a cliff dwelling. Once satisfied that you have learned all you can, descend the mountain at your own pace along the same trail.

49 VINEYARD TRAIL

KEY AT-A-GLANCE INFORMATION

LENGTH: 6.1 miles

ELEVATION GAIN: 1,480 feet

CONFIGURATION: One-way

DIFFICULTY: Moderate

SCENERY: Roosevelt Lake, Apache Lake, Four Peaks, Superstition Wilderness, desert

EXPOSURE: Completely exposed

TRAFFIC: Very light

TRAIL SURFACE: Crushed rock, grass, packed dirt

HIKING TIME: 3 hours

WATER REQUIREMENT: 2.5 quarts

SEASON: Year-round; hot in summer

ACCESS: Sunrise to sunset

MAPS: USGS Theodore Roosevelt Dam

FACILITIES: None at either trailhead. The nearby Roosevelt Lake provides services at the marina and at various picnic areas.

DOGS: Yes

COMMENTS: This secluded trail can be overgrown in places. Wear long pants to protect your legs from prickly plants. For more information, visit www.fs.fed.us/r3/tonto/recreation/rec-hiking-index.shtml, or call (928) 467-3200.

- -

GPS Trailhead Coordinates

UTM Zone   12S

Easting   0485125

Northing   3726136

Latitude   N33°40.609'

Longitude W111°9.668'

IN BRIEF

Striking views of Roosevelt Lake, Apache Lake, and Four Peaks grace this secluded and scenic hike in Tonto National Forest. Vineyard Trail is a segment of the Arizona Trail and also passes the site of historic Camp O'Rourke, where Roosevelt Dam construction workers lived in the early 1900s.

DESCRIPTION

A system of dams and reservoirs along the Salt River valley manages most of Phoenix's water

- -

Directions ⟶

Roosevelt Lake Bridge: **Drive east on US 60 and exit onto Idaho Road. Follow Idaho Road north 2.25 miles to SR 88. Turn northeast onto SR 88, Apache Trail and then follow this scenic but twisty road 44 miles until it ends at the Roosevelt Lake Bridge. Turn left, cross the bridge, and park in the pullout immediately north of the bridge.**

Part of SR 88 is a graded dirt road suitable for most passenger cars. Two alternate routes exist if you prefer smoother and straighter roads. You can continue east on US 60 through the town of Miami and then turn north onto SR 188, or take SR 87 northeast out of Fountain Hills and then turn southeast onto SR 188. Both alternate routes add significant mileage to the approach. However, traveling at highway speeds should shave a few minutes off your total commute time.

Mills Ridge Trailhead: **From Roosevelt Lake Bridge, drive northwest 2 miles on SR 188. Turn west onto FR 429 just north of Vineyard Canyon Picnic Area. Note that there is a subtle left turn on FR 429 shortly after you leave SR 188. Go 4.8 miles down FR 429 until it ends at the Mills Ridge Trailhead. FR 429 is a rough dirt road but should be navigable by most passenger cars in good weather.**

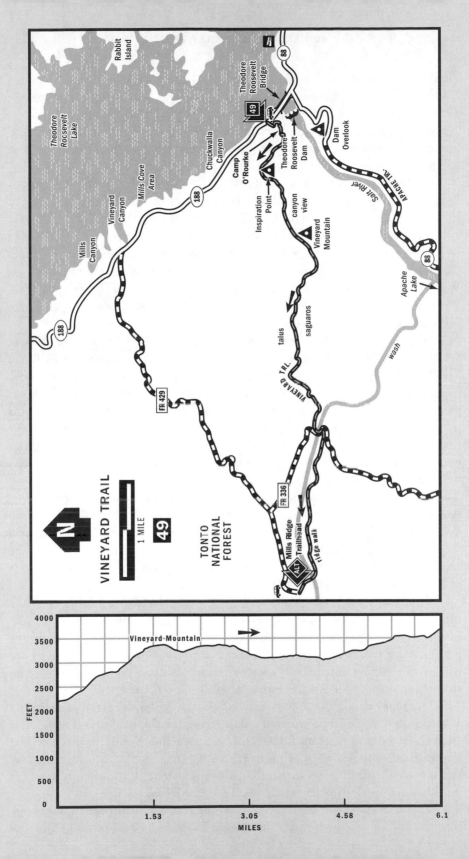

supply. Theodore Roosevelt Lake, commonly known as Roosevelt Lake, is the highest, oldest, and largest of the Salt River reservoirs. Originally constructed in 1911 and expanded in 1996, a large concrete dam located at the confluence of Tonto Creek and the Salt River retains the lake that bears the name of our 26th president. This historic dam was one of the first reclamation projects in the West and provides the backdrop for a picturesque hike in Tonto National Forest.

Vineyard Trail 131 connects Roosevelt Lake with mountains in the Four Peaks Wilderness. The trail begins next to Roosevelt Lake Bridge and ends at the Mills Ridge Trailhead high above Tonto Basin. Along this scenic 6-mile trek, expansive views abound. Hikers can expect dramatic panoramas overlooking two major reservoirs on the Salt River watershed, one of the prettiest bridges in the Southwest, historic Roosevelt Dam, rugged Four Peaks, and the Superstition Wilderness. With so many nearby attractions and as a part of the Arizona Trail, Vineyard Trail receives surprisingly few visitors. You will likely enjoy complete solitude while hiking this trail.

With a shuttle vehicle, you can hike Vineyard Trail in either direction. Starting from Roosevelt Lake Bridge and climbing uphill toward Mills Ridge Trailhead is obviously the more challenging route. The first 1.5 miles yield a heart-pounding workout as you ascend 1,100 feet to Inspiration Point and Vineyard Mountain. The remainder of the trail undulates over rolling hills and winds its way toward Four Peaks. If you don't have a shuttle vehicle, start from the bridge and hike out as far as you'd like before turning around. Even if you traverse the entire trail in both directions for a 12-mile roundtrip, the endless vistas will make it worth your while.

From the pullout immediately north of Roosevelt Lake Bridge, walk across the road to find a trail marker behind the guard rail. Begin by hiking into a small canyon and away from the lake. An interpretive sign at 0.2 miles marks the site of Camp O'Rourke, where dam workers and their families lived in the early 1900s. The population reached 400 near this location, although remnants of the camp are barely visible today.

Continue up the trail and climb some switchbacks to a large flat area offering overhead views of the dam. Before the construction of Roosevelt Lake Bridge in the early 1990s, the dam itself carried SR 188 traffic. An interesting bit of trivia is that the original width of the dam barely accommodates two Ford Model-Ts traveling abreast. It's easy to see why a new bridge had to be constructed in preparation for the expansion of Roosevelt Lake.

From the dam overlook, backtrack 200 feet and follow the trail as it resumes a steep ascent. At 0.7 miles reach a saddle where the slope tapers off for a short stretch and the trail parallels Roosevelt Lake's shoreline. Sotols, yuccas, and hop bushes frame an open view of the northern half of the lake. Much of the lake you see is part of the 1996 expansion, which remained dry for nearly a decade until heavy rainfall in 2005 finally filled the lake to capacity.

Vineyard Trail soon bends away from the lake and again climbs steeply up Inspiration Point. Follow a wide ridge toward an abandoned reflector on Vineyard

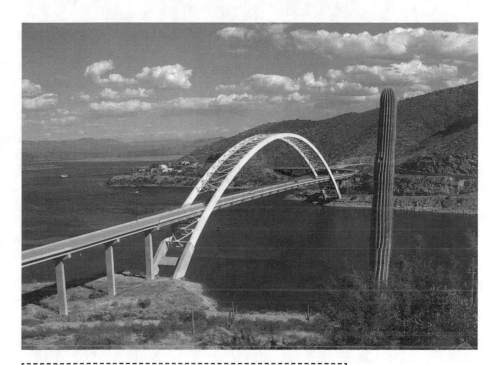

Roosevelt Lake Bridge viewed from an overlook on the Vineyard Trail.

Mountain. The Roosevelt Lake area hosts a wide range of birds and wildlife. Herons, migrating ducks, and other waterfowl flock near the water while hawks and even bald eagles cruise the higher elevations. Birds of prey often perch on the metal framework of the reflector while scouting their next meal.

Past the reflector the trail skirts Vineyard Mountain and the surrounding hills. With most of the hard work behind you, you can now savor the open views of Four Peaks straight ahead and the Superstition Wilderness to the left. Around a bend in the trail at 1.75 miles, the long, narrow Apache Lake comes into view, with the Apache Trail winding along its banks. Though still fairly obvious, the trail becomes somewhat overgrown with tall grasses here. Watch out for hidden cacti and prickly catclaw acacia.

The trail descends slightly while traversing the side of a steep hill. To your left, the Salt River flows through scenic Alchesay Canyon on its way down to Apache Lake. Across the canyon, you can make out the tips of Castle Dome and Mound Mountain in the Superstition Wilderness. This canyon was named after an Apache chief who earned the Congressional Medal of Honor while serving as a scout for the U.S. Army. He also reportedly convinced Geronimo to surrender in 1886.

The trail continues to bend around the hills and remains relatively level. Near 3 miles from the trailhead, the trail descends toward a dense stand of saguaros on a rocky hill and then cuts across a steep talus overgrown with brittlebush and chia. In spring, when the flowers bloom in unison, this area is

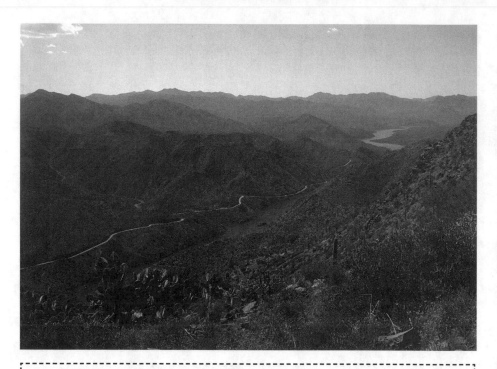

Vineyard Trail overlooks SR88 Apache Trail and Apache Lake as they wind through Salt River Canyon.

especially scenic. Beyond the talus, Vineyard Trail dips into a shallow basin and approaches FR 336. The trail becomes somewhat faint and difficult to follow here. Look for cairns to guide you.

Reach the FR 336 junction at 4.2 miles from the trailhead. Turn left and follow FR 336 as it crosses a dry wash and crests a small hillock. Atop the hill, you'll find an open parking area where a prominent sign directs you to leave the road and head up a gentle ridge. The trail again becomes very faint. When in doubt continue straight up the ridge crest. Follow the ridge 1.5 miles with wide-open views to either side. Vineyard Trail terminates at the Mills Ridge Trailhead at the end of FR 429.

NEARBY ACTIVITIES

Four Peaks Trail 130 connects Mills Ridge Trailhead with Lone Pine Trailhead in the shadow of Four Peaks. Tonto National Monument (page 248) south of the Roosevelt Lake Bridge, showcases prehistoric Salado Cliff Dwellings. Many hikes in the Superstition Wilderness begin from trailheads on or near SR 88. Inspiration Point and Theodore Roosevelt Dam interpretive overlooks on SR 88 provide fascinating facts and up-close views of the dam. Behind the dam, Roosevelt Lake offers ample opportunities for camping, fishing, waterskiing, and boating.

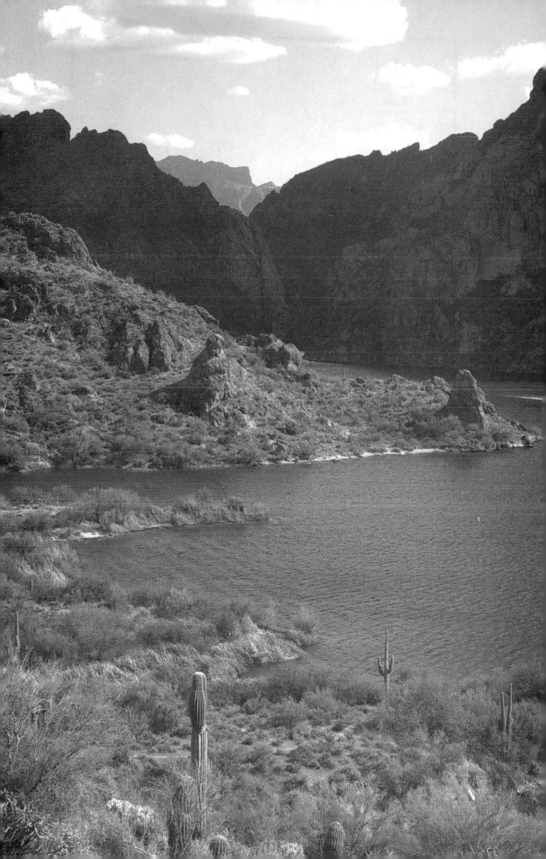

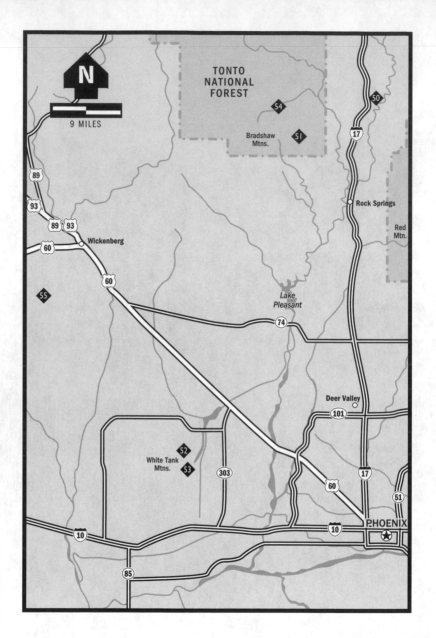

NORTH AND NORTHWEST
INCLUDING BRADSHAW AND WHITE TANK MOUNTAINS

50 BADGER SPRINGS WASH TRAIL

KEY AT-A-GLANCE INFORMATION

LENGTH: 2 miles

ELEVATION GAIN: -100 feet

CONFIGURATION: Out-and-back

DIFFICULTY: Easy

SCENERY: Agua Fria River, Badger Springs Wash, desert riparian environment, pools

EXPOSURE: Mostly exposed

TRAFFIC: Light

TRAIL SURFACE: Sand, creek bed, boulder hopping, shallow river

HIKING TIME: 1.5 hours

WATER REQUIREMENT: 1.5 quarts

SEASON: Year-round; hot in summer

ACCESS: Sunrise to sunset; free parking

MAPS: USGS Joes Hill; map available at information kiosk

FACILITIES: A vault toilet is located on the access road; no water

DOGS: Yes, leashed at all times

COMMENTS: Shallow creek and river crossing may require waterproof shoes or sandals. This area sustained some damage from the Cave Creek Complex wildfire of 2005. For more information, visit www.blm.gov/az/st/en/prog/blm_special_areas/natmon/afria.html, or call (623) 580-5500.

GPS Trailhead Coordinates

UTM Zone 12S

Easting 0398837

Northing 3788034

Latitude N34°13.815'

Longitude W112°5.946'

IN BRIEF

Part of the recently established Agua Fria National Monument, Badger Springs Wash runs a short distance to the Agua Fria River. A sandy trail follows the wash and provides access to Agua Fria's meandering path through an arid high-desert landscape.

DESCRIPTION

Interstate 17, a major north–south transportation vein, connects metropolitan Phoenix and the cool pines of Flagstaff. Drivers who routinely make this two-hour weekend pilgrimage to the high country become intimately familiar with major landmarks along the way. Most motorists habitually develop mental waypoints for Black Canyon City, Sunset Point, and Cordes Junction, the halfway point between Phoenix and Flagstaff. Some can even recall with certainty the point at which I-17 climbs to the top of amazingly flat Black Mesa near Sunset Point. However, very few I-17 drivers know that a large portion of the plateau near Sunset Point belongs to the Agua Fria National Monument and that amid the grassy mesa, a perennial river flows parallel to the freeway.

Directions

Drive north from Phoenix on I-17 past Sunset Point and take exit 256 to Badger Springs Road. Turn east on Badger Springs Road to the Agua Fria National Monument kiosk, where you can pick up a map. Take the dirt road next to the kiosk southeast approximately 1 mile to a large turnaround lined with stones. Parking is available in any of several small pullouts. The trailhead is just southeast of the turnaround. The dirt road has a few dips, but most passenger cars can safely make it to the trailhead.

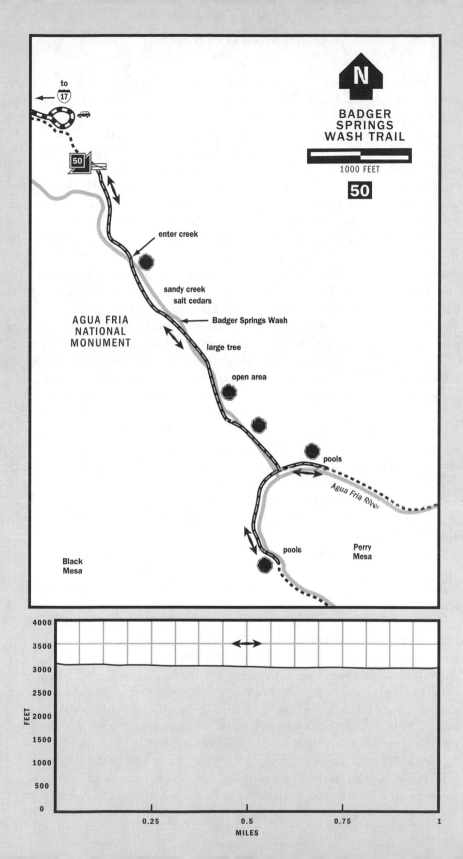

Agua Fria National Monument was created in 2000 and protects 71,000 acres of wilderness east of I-17 between Black Canyon City and Cordes Junction. Agua Fria River, a rare perennial stream and the central feature in this preserve, flows through an indubitably arid landscape, creating a riparian oasis recessed in the canyons and hidden from view of the freeway traffic. For centuries this river has served as the lifeblood of many ancient indigenous people who made their homes here. As a result the Agua Fria National Monument holds one of the highest concentrations of archaeological sites within the state. More than 450 such prehistoric sites, including large stone pueblos with dozens of rooms, exist within the boundaries of the preserve, many of them in jeopardy from the encroachment of modern development. The creation of a national monument attempts to stem careless destruction of the landscape and its cultural assets.

The high-desert plateau and nearby canyons provide the setting for this hike. Being relatively new, this Bureau of Land Management–managed national monument has only one developed trail. The Badger Springs Wash Trail follows its namesake creek, a tributary to the Agua Fria River. Once at the river, hikers can explore the canyon through which the river flows and many small rapids and pools along the way. There's a stark contrast between the mostly dry and seemingly inhospitable canyon and lush grass and trees growing along the riverbanks.

The Badger Springs Trailhead is located roughly 1 mile east of I-17 on Badger Springs Road, safely out of earshot of the speeding freeway traffic. Find a gate and trailhead plaque just east of the large circular turnaround area, and sign the trail log inside a large metal enclosure. The trail begins on a sandy track lined by high-desert brush such as the Fremont barberry, mesquite, and various small cacti. A hundred yards from the trailhead, cross Badger Springs Wash for the first time. This small creek snakes silently through a wide sandy streambed and fills your footprints with water.

After crossing the wash, hike along the sandy trail until it meets the wash again. The trail becomes faint in many spots, but it hardly matters. If you just stick to the wash, you will end up in the right place. Badger Springs Wash is mostly a trickle and presents few if any navigation challenges. Tall grasses and riparian bushes such as the salt cedar grow in abundance near the wash, which flows through a shallow canyon lined by gentle slopes. There are surprisingly no saguaro cacti on the hills but plenty of mesquites and prickly pears. Many animals also share this watery habitat in the desert. You will likely see a good variety of birds along your hike. Mammals are harder to spot, but you might see some javelina or deer around dawn or dusk. Note that the Cave Creek Complex fire of 2005 singed the slopes and mesas in Aqua Fria National Monument. However, the desert is making a speedy recovery.

Near 0.4 miles pass a large tree growing in the middle of the sandy streambed. The streambed opens wider and you begin to see some large boulders near the wash. At 0.7 miles from the trailhead, reach the confluence of Badger Springs Wash and a U-shaped bend in the Agua Fria River next to some craggy cliffs.

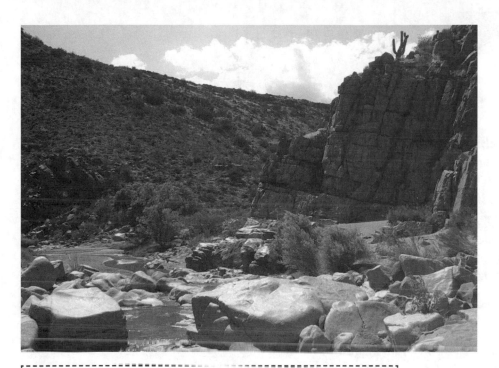

Agua Fria River flows past rocky cliffs near its confluence with Badger Springs Wash.

The Agua Fria River carves a winding canyon between Black Mesa on the western side and Perry Mesa on the east. You can explore the river in either direction, or both if you so desire. The riverbed is alternately sandy and rocky. At places where the water flows through patches of large boulders, small rapids and tiny cascades develop. The bleached, smooth river rock contrasts against dark hills and chiseled boulders on the riverbanks. Sometimes there are jacuzzi-sized pools in the stream where you can enjoy the "cold water" for which the river is named. On open sandy stretches, the river meanders from side to side, forcing you to cross many times.

When satisfied with your exploration of the Agua Fria River, return to Badger Springs Wash and hike out the way you came in.

NEARBY ACTIVITIES

Hundreds of motorists use the Sunset Point rest area on I-17 to stretch their legs. It's also the only source of drinking water close to Badger Springs Wash. This rest area provides an excellent view of the Bradshaw Mountains to the west, especially at sunset, as you might have guessed from its name. The Bumble Bee exit on I-17 leads to Crown King and Horsethief Basin Recreation Area, nestled in the crest of the Bradshaw Mountains. The Algonquin Trail (page 279) and East Fort Trail (page 264) are near Crown King and Horsethief Basin, respectively.

51 EAST FORT TRAIL

KEY AT-A-GLANCE INFORMATION

LENGTH: 2 miles

ELEVATION GAIN: 275 feet

CONFIGURATION: Out-and-back

DIFFICULTY: Moderate

SCENERY: Panoramic vista, East Fort ruins, Twin Peaks, Castle Creek Wilderness, Bradshaw Mountains

EXPOSURE: Some shade

TRAFFIC: Very light

TRAIL SURFACE: Rock, gravel, packed dirt, some deadfall, light scrambling

HIKING TIME: 1.5 hours

WATER REQUIREMENT: 1 quart

SEASON: Year-round; may be icy in winter

ACCESS: Sunrise to sunset; free parking

MAPS: USGS Crown King

FACILITIES: Portable toilet available at nearby Horsethief Lookout

DOGS: Yes

COMMENTS: Very remote, but worth the drive

GPS Trailhead Coordinates

UTM Zone 12S

Easting   0383555

Northing 3780670

Latitude N34°9.735'

Longitude W112°15.841'

IN BRIEF

Take this rugged remote trail through thick forests of manzanita and pine to East Fort, a high overlook studded with panoramic views of Twin Peaks, the Bradshaw Mountains, and the desert plateau below. Ancient stone ruins reminiscent of Circlestone cap this amazing lookout.

DESCRIPTION

When the infamous Arizona summer strikes Phoenix, hikers head for the cool pines of Flagstaff, Payson, or Pinetop. The Bradshaw Mountains, a massive range 40 miles north of Phoenix, offer a much closer alternative to escape the heat.

At nearly 6,000 feet, the town of Crown King provides a convenient home base from

Directions

Drive north from Phoenix on I-17, and take exit 248 to Bumble Bee Road, which becomes CR 59, Crown King Road, and FR 259 when it enters Prescott National Forest. Follow this dirt road 27 miles to Crown King. Continue following FR 259 to a three-way intersection with FR 52, Senator Highway. Bear left and go 7 miles along FR 52 to Horsethief Basin Recreation Area. Stay on FR 52 through the recreation area and head toward Horsethief Lookout. The signed East Fort Trailhead is located on a bend in FR 52, approximately 0.5 miles shy of Horsethief Lookout. To reach the lookout tower, which has the nearest toilet, continue on FR 52, and keep right at any forks in the road.

Parking may be scarce at the East Fort Trailhead, but there are rarely any other vehicles. You can park in a gap in the manzanita bushes just left of the trail sign, or drive down the trail 100 feet or so to a wider pullout. The dirt road beyond Crown King can be rough, and a high-clearance vehicle is recommended.

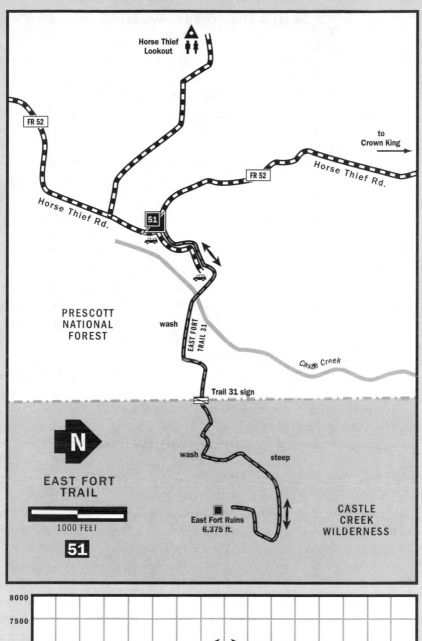

Horse Thief
Lookout

FR 52

to
Crown King

Horse Thief Rd.

FR 52

51

Horse Thief Rd.

PRESCOTT
NATIONAL
FOREST

wash

EAST FORT
TRAIL 31

Castle Creek

Trail 31 sign

N

EAST FORT
TRAIL

1000 FEET

51

wash

steep

East Fort Ruins
6,375 ft.

CASTLE
CREEK
WILDERNESS

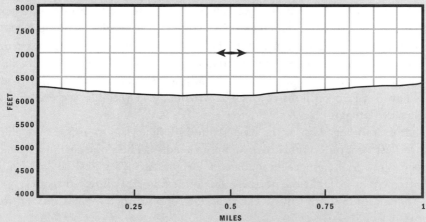

which to explore the scenic woodlands of Castle Creek Wilderness and Prescott National Forest. Crown King has a rich mining history dating back to the late 1800s. Dozens of old gold and silver mines lie within a few miles of this "living ghost town." Today, it's a haven for tourists, four-wheelers, and all-terrain vehicles. An ever-active event calendar also attracts many people to this tiny community in the pines.

Seven miles southeast of Crown King, Horsethief Basin Recreation Area entertains outdoor enthusiasts and provides excellent camping facilities, rental cabins, and even summer homes. One can find a small lake for fishing and canoeing, as well as picnic facilities; in addition, more than a dozen trails canvas the Castle Creek Wilderness Area.

Only 1 mile long, East Fort Trail 31 is perhaps the shortest hike near Horsethief Basin, but it captures the beauty of the Bradshaw Mountains and boasts an amazing hilltop view from a rocky outcropping studded with ancient ruins. This trail's remote location almost guarantees solitude during your hike. Because it's a long drive to Horsethief Basin, consider hiking to East Fort as part of a weekend outing or combining it with longer trails in the area.

The trail begins at a point on FR 52 approximately half a mile east of the Horsethief Lookout. A wooden roadside sign indicates a distance of 1 mile to the East Fort observation point. Hike down the manzanita-lined trail, which begins as part of an old jeep road, with a head-on view of Twin Peaks to the north. Live oaks and pines provide some shade, and the 6,280-foot elevation makes this hike a pleasant walk in the woods any time of the year.

At 0.15 miles veer right at a fork in the road and then cross Castle Creek, a dry wash for which the entire wilderness area was named. You can see East Fort in the distance, an exposed outcropping of boulders rising above the forest. If you strain your eyes, you might be able to make out the stone ruins atop the boulders. Aged manzanita bushes abound in this forest. Their distinctively smooth red bark contrasts with bright green leaves and pink flowers. Fallen twigs and branches lie strewn across the trail, indicating that very few people come this way.

Reach a bend in the trail near 0.25 miles. Turn left and hike a short distance to a clearing where a sign points out that Trail 31 veers right. Walk up a gentle hill and then cross a gated fence at 0.5 miles. The trail becomes rougher beyond the gate as deadfall hinders your progress in many spots. Recent droughts have weakened the pines and made them especially susceptible to bark beetles. These pests have ravaged millions of trees in Arizona, and you can see evidence of bark-beetle damage.

Cross another wash at the base of the hill. Then begin a moderate climb toward East Fort on crumbly rock and pine needles. The slope gets increasingly steeper as the trail changes direction to the right. At 0.75 miles the trail begins to flatten out as it flanks the northern side of East Fort. Follow cairns to stay on the trail and hike south toward the rock outcropping ahead. Near the very top

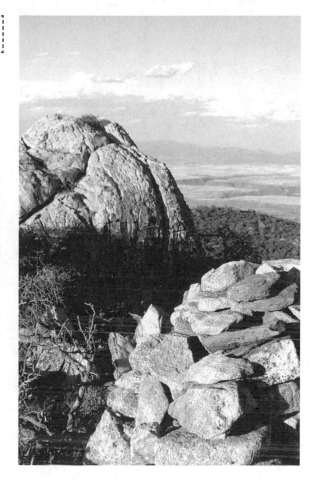

Ancient stone ruins add interest to East Fort's rocky summit.

the trail gets hard to follow, and some light scrambling might be required.

Reach the East Fort observation point after a little more than 1 mile from the trailhead. You can now clearly see the stone ruins on top of the rocky summit, filling gaps between boulders and forming a fortress around the small hilltop. Be careful not to topple the stone structures as you enter on the northern side. There are several walls and circular rooms made of closely fitted stones, a mortarless construction technique identical to that used in the large Circlestone ruins in the Superstitions. No one knows who built these structures or why. Their origins have eluded discovery for many centuries and will likely remain a mystery for centuries to come.

From the 6,375-foot summit of East Fort, the panoramic views are truly awe-inspiring. To the north and west, deep forests cover the rolling hills and mountainsides. Twin Peaks, Horsethief Lookout, and Horsethief Basin are all visible from this open vista. To the east you have a clear view down toward Black Canyon, Agua Fria, and the grassy plateaus of Black Mesa and Perry Mesa. You can even pick out the Sunset Point Rest Area on I-17, reversing its famous view toward the Bradshaw Mountains. Allow plenty of time to take in the scenery before retracing your steps to the trailhead.

NEARBY ACTIVITIES

Horsethief Lookout, a fire-finding tower a short distance beyond the East Fort Trailhead, commands an impressive view of the surrounding forests and mountains. The staff usually accommodates visitors, who must climb a harrowing staircase and enter through the tower's floor.

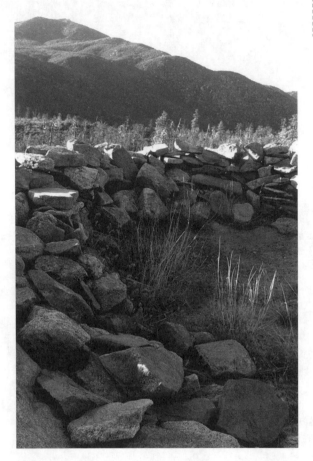

A view of Twin Peaks in Castle Creek Wilderness from the East Fort ruins.

Horsethief Basin Recreation Area offers a wide range of activities, including camping, hiking, biking, fishing, and canoeing on Horsethief Lake. Hiking trails nearby include Algonquin 225, Horsethief Canyon 30, Twin Peaks 240, Castle Creek 239, Kentuck 217, Tip Top 234, and Horsethief Recreation Trail 202.

Dubbed a living ghost town, the mining community of Crown King is located about 7 miles north of Horsethief Basin. Situated high in the pine forest, it's a great place to escape the summer heat in Phoenix. Many all-terrain vehicles zoom about on the dirt roads near Crown King. The southern end of Algonquin Trail leads to Poland Creek where swimming holes of all sizes tempt hikers and canyoneers.

The Agua Fria National Monument lies on I-17 between Black Canyon City and Cordes Junction.

FORD CANYON TRAIL AND MESQUITE CANYON TRAIL | 52

IN BRIEF

Ford Canyon Trail and Mesquite Canyon Trail showcase the best features of the White Tank Mountain Regional Park west of Phoenix. This 10-mile loop takes visitors through beautiful rocky canyons, sandy washes, and grassy hillsides.

DESCRIPTION

The White Tank Mountains form a massive wall northwest of Phoenix. Seemingly a single mountain running north–south when viewed from town, the White Tank Mountains actually consist of a complex network of mostly east–west ridges and scenic canyons. The White Tank Mountain Regional Park encompasses 30,000 acres of desert wilderness on the mountains' eastern flank, which faces the metropolitan Phoenix area. Within the park, 25 miles of hiking trails tempt visitors with sculpted canyons, sweeping panoramic views, seasonal waterfalls, and rugged desert scenery.

The Ford Canyon Trail is particularly scenic. It takes hikers from the desert floor up through a canyon carved from white granite. Turquoise-colored water from drenching desert storms and the resultant flash floods pool

KEY AT-A-GLANCE INFORMATION

LENGTH: 10.3 miles
ELEVATION GAIN: 1,425 feet
CONFIGURATION: Loop
DIFFICULTY: Moderate
SCENERY: Desert, mountain vistas, rock formations, white-granite creek bed
EXPOSURE: Partial shade in creek bed, otherwise exposed
TRAFFIC: Light
TRAIL SURFACE: Packed dirt, sand gravel, rocky creek bed
HIKING TIME: 4.5 hours
WATER REQUIREMENT: 3.5 quarts; 4–5 quarts in summer
SEASON: Year-round; hot in summer
ACCESS: Open 6 a.m.–8 p.m. (Sun.–Thu.), 10 p.m. (Fri.–Sat.); $6 per vehicle entrance fee
MAPS: USGS White Tank Mountains, park maps available from visitor center and Web site.
FACILITIES: Restroom, drinking water, picnic areas, visitor center, horse corral, competitive track
DOGS: Yes, leashed at all times
COMMENTS: The topographical map found at www.maricopa.gov/parks /white_tank. is especially useful. Call (623) 935-2505 for more information.

Directions

Drive west from Phoenix on I-10. At 9.5 miles west of Loop 101, exit at Cotton Lane, drive north, and then follow signs for Loop 303. Continue 7.5 miles on Loop 303 to Olive Avenue. Drive west on Olive Avenue 4.5 miles to the entrance of White Tank Mountain Regional Park. Pay the entrance fee. Drive 3 more miles inside the park, and turn left onto Ford Canyon Road. Drive 0.5 miles to Picnic Area 9, where you see a sign for the Ford Canyon Trail.

GPS Trailhead Coordinates

UTM Zone   12S
Easting   0359953
Northing   3718649
Latitude   N33°36.010'
Longitude   W112°30.606'

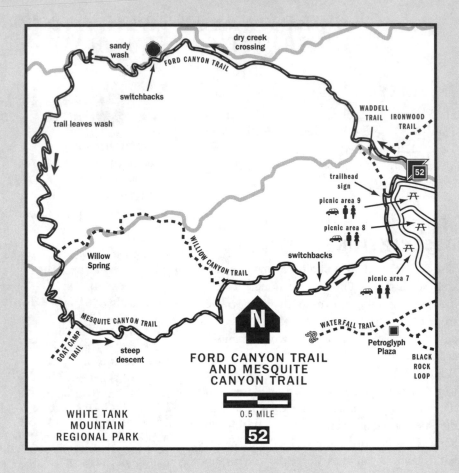

sandy wash

dry creek crossing

FORD CANYON TRAIL

switchbacks

trail leaves wash

WADDELL TRAIL   IRONWOOD TRAIL

52

trailhead sign

picnic area 9

picnic area 8

switchbacks

picnic area 7

WILLOW CANYON TRAIL

Willow Spring

MESQUITE CANYON TRAIL

WATERFALL TRAIL

GOAT CAMP TRAIL

steep descent

Petroglyph Plaza

BLACK ROCK LOOP

N

**FORD CANYON TRAIL
AND MESQUITE
CANYON TRAIL**

0.5 MILE

**WHITE TANK
MOUNTAIN
REGIONAL PARK**

52

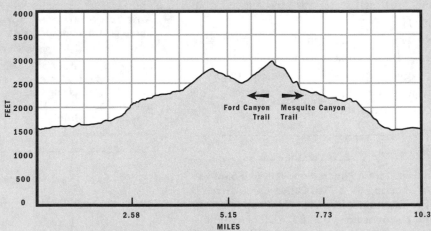

Ford Canyon
Trail

Mesquite Canyon
Trail

FEET

MILES

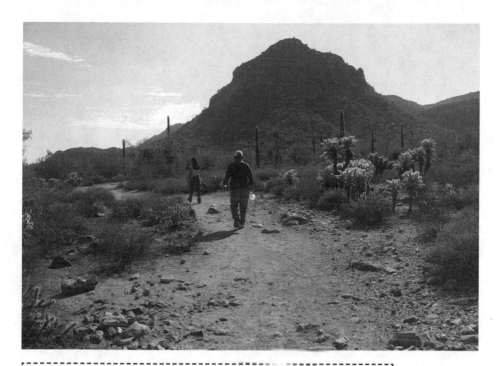

Hikers meander through the desert foothills of White Tank Mountain Regional Park along Ford Canyon Trail.

in deep pockets or "tanks" eroded into the white bedrock, giving the mountains their name. Even though these mountains are in a desert environment, some pools of water remain throughout the year. The Ford Canyon Trail eventually climbs out of the canyon and intersects the Willow Canyon, Mesquite Canyon, and Goat Camp trails. Returning via the Mesquite Canyon Trail makes a reasonable 10-mile loop.

Begin your hike from the trailhead opposite Picnic Area 9 on Ford Canyon Road. Though the official trailhead is at the Trailhead Staging Area, starting from Picnic Area 9 saves a long flat approach. Follow the short access path as it crosses a dry creek north of the road and connects to the Ford Canyon Trail. Turn west here and hike toward the mountains. Enjoy the unspoiled beauty of the desert, graced by tall saguaros, prickly chollas, and hardy creosote bushes. Pass signed junctions with the Ironwood Trail and the Waddell Trail at 0.4 and 0.6 miles, respectively. Continue hiking northwest toward the mouth of Ford Canyon. At 1 mile the trail climbs over a small saddle into a flat valley and heads west into Ford Canyon.

The trail begins to climb at 1.75 miles, crossing a series of dry washes along the way. The nicely packed dirt trail deteriorates into unsteady rocks and boulders. Most mountain bikers riding along the Ford Canyon Trail turn around here. At 2.25 miles the trail bends southwest and skirts some huge boulders.

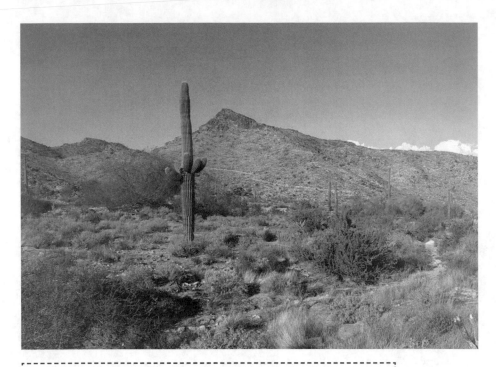

A scenic basin along Mesquite Canyon Trail in White Tank Mountain Regional Park.

From here catch your first view of the white granite rocks that form the dry riverbed. Continue climbing up steep switchbacks for a quarter mile and come to the base of a large overhanging boulder where obvious trail markers guide you up and around it. At 2.6 miles reach a rocky area on top of the white granite boulders, and some small pools of water. The elevation here is about 2,100 feet, 600 feet higher than at the trailhead.

Once on top of the white granite river bottom, the trail becomes somewhat difficult to follow. Look carefully for cairns and footprints in the sand. When in doubt, go over any rock obstacles and head straight up the streambed. At 3.2 miles a 5–6-foot rock wall obstructs your path. Climb up this wall and look for an abandoned dam built out of stones and mortar. Take a break here to enjoy the scenic white rocks and pools of water. Some hikers make this point the end of their quest and return via the Ford Canyon Trail. If you choose to continue, it becomes easier to loop back via a different trail than to backtrack.

Beyond the dam the Ford Canyon Trail continues to follow the sandy wash bottom and eventually turns south. Here, you can enjoy the hike in almost complete isolation and find patches of shade created by small riparian trees and shrubs. Pass a side stream at 3.5 miles, and climb another 6-foot wall at 3.7 miles. The climb is easy, but watch your footing on the slippery smooth rock.

The trail departs the sandy wash at 4 miles from the trailhead, climbing gently up an open hillside replete with golden desert grasses that sway in the breeze like grain fields of the Midwest. This part of the hike offers a completely different experience than going through Ford Canyon. The ascending trail takes you up to a ridge crest where you can see the radio towers on top of the tallest peak in the White Tanks. At 5.5 miles the Ford Canyon Trail drops into a bowl where it intersects the Willow Canyon Trail. The elevation here is 2,525 feet, and if you can't withstand another 400-foot elevation gain, you should take the Willow Canyon Trail toward the east.

For those diehards who wish to finish the Ford Canyon Trail, continue straight across the bowl and climb directly to the south. The remainder of the Ford Canyon Trail ascends this slope via a series of long switchbacks to the highest point of the hike at 2,950 feet. Atop this ridge and at 6.4 miles from the start, find the confluence of three major trails in the park: Ford Canyon, Mesquite Canyon, and Goat Camp. Turn east here onto the Mesquite Canyon Trail.

Your return hike via Mesquite Canyon begins with a commanding view to the east, where you can see the canyon below and the city in the distance. Next to the trail, shrubs such as Mormon tea, brittlebush, and sage paint the landscape in lively colors. A short but fairly steep descent on gravel-covered switchbacks at 6.75 miles requires some careful stepping. Soon thereafter, hike across a small bowl full of jojoba, goldenrod flowers, and prickly pear cacti. The trail can be somewhat faint here; be careful to follow it to the east.

Climb out of the small bowl and descend into a large drainage. The trail cuts to the south but makes a sharp bend north and intersects the lower end of the Willow Canyon Trail at 7.9 miles. Had you taken the Willow Canyon Trail earlier, you'd emerge here next to a thicket of mesquite trees and a scenic creek bed with the signature white granite and pools. Follow the Mesquite Canyon Trail toward the east along the creek. Half a mile farther, catch one last glimpse of the red rock-lined canyon ahead, and climb over a ridge to the southeast. At 8.6 miles descend via long switchbacks into the next canyon and hike east for another mile to the Waddell Trail junction near Picnic Area 7.

Finish the hike by taking the Waddell Trail north 0.5 miles to a sign that reads "Trailhead" and points east. Turn east here and hike a short distance to the paved Ford Canyon Road. Finally, follow the road northeast back to Picnic Area 9, completing the 10.3-mile loop.

NEARBY ACTIVITIES

White Tank Mountain Regional Park contains many hiking trails including the Waterfall Trail, which is popular after heavy storms. The Wildlife World Zoo (www.wildlifeworld.com; (623) 935-WILD) is 6 miles from the park entrance.

53 GOAT CAMP TRAIL AND WILLOW CANYON TRAIL

KEY AT-A-GLANCE INFORMATION

LENGTH: 11.5 miles

ELEVATION GAIN: 1,825 feet

CONFIGURATION: One-way

DIFFICULTY: Difficult

SCENERY: Desert, mountain vistas, rock formations, white-granite creek bed

EXPOSURE: Mostly exposed

TRAFFIC: Light

TRAIL SURFACE: Packed dirt, gravel, sand, rocky creek bed

HIKING TIME: 5.5 hours

WATER REQUIREMENT: 3 quarts; 4 quarts in summer

SEASON: Year-round; hot in summer

ACCESS: Open 6 a.m.–8 p.m. (Sun.–Thu.), 10 p.m. (Fri.–Sat.); $6 per vehicle entrance fee

MAPS: USGS White Tank Mountains, park maps available from visitor center and Web site (see Comments below)

FACILITIES: Restroom, drinking water, picnic areas, visitor center, horse corral, competitive track

DOGS: Yes; leashed at all times

COMMENTS: The topographical map found at www.maricopa.gov/parks/white_tank. is especially useful. Call (623) 935-2505 for more information.

IN BRIEF

Goat Camp Trail is the most challenging hike in White Tank Mountain Regional Park, taking hikers up a long ascent through a scenic canyon to the base of an antenna-studded mountain. Return via Willow Canyon Trail for another scenic tour.

DESCRIPTION

White Tank Mountain Regional Park encompasses nearly 30,000 acres of desert wilderness, making it the largest regional park in Maricopa County's park system. Within its boundaries many trails crisscross the eastern flank of the White Tank Mountains, which were named for the perennial pools of water carved from white-granite canyons by flash floods. This massive mountain range dominates Phoenix's western horizon and features excellent hiking trails. Hilltop views of the city are plentiful, and the trails also take visitors through secluded wilderness areas.

From the park's many ramadas and trailheads, four main trails run deep into the hills: Ford Canyon, Goat Camp, Mesquite Canyon, and Willow Canyon. By taking this 11.5-mile one-way route, you touch them all. First, stash a shuttle vehicle at the Mesquite

GPS Trailhead Coordinates

UTM Zone   12S

Easting   0360337

Northing   3715152

Latitude   N33°34.122'

Longitude   W112°30.325'

Directions

Exit I-10 at Cotton Lane, 9.5 miles west of the Loop 101 interchange. Drive north as the road becomes Loop 303, and continue 7.5 miles to Olive Avenue. Take Olive Avenue west 4.5 miles to the entrance of White Tank Mountain Regional Park. Pay the entrance fee. Inside the park, take the second left and park at the Goat Camp Trailhead on Black Canyon Drive.

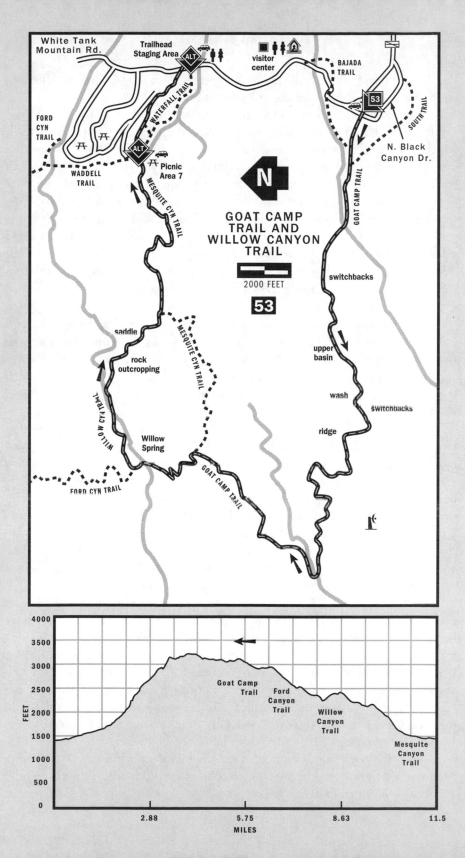

Canyon Trailhead in the Trailhead Staging Area. You can save a mile of flat hiking by leaving the shuttle vehicle at Picnic Area 7.

Begin the hike from the Goat Camp Trailhead on Black Canyon Drive just inside the park's entrance. Head west toward the hills on Goat Camp Trail, which starts out fairly flat across the desert floor but eventually becomes the most challenging trail in the park. Pass intersections with the Bajada and South trails at 0.4 and 0.75 miles, respectively, as you approach scenic Goat Canyon.

Approximately 1 mile into the hike, cross several dry washes and continue westward among creosote bushes and palo verde trees. A half mile farther, the trail enters Goat Canyon and begins to climb up the white bedrock on the right side of the canyon below a sharp summit. Cross the dry wash and ascend the left side of the canyon via steep switchbacks. Turn around here and look through the end of the canyon. Camelback Mountain can be seen through the V-shaped gap formed by the hillsides.

After the switchbacks, the trail turns steeply uphill and gains roughly 600 feet in just half a mile. Chug your way through this tough ascent on the southern side of the canyon. Look down into the canyon for "white tanks," pools of water carved into white-granite bedrock along the dry wash. At 2.2 miles you'll reach the head of the steep canyon where a tattered saguaro seems to grow straight from the rock.

Beyond the saguaro, Goat Camp Trail enters a wide upper basin and flattens out considerably. Hike into the heart of the basin with the antenna-studded mountaintop directly ahead. The upper basin supports a wide variety of desert flora, including Mormon tea, ocotillos, agaves, various cacti, jojoba, and many desert grasses. At 2.5 miles the trail begins to climb out of the upper basin toward the microwave radio towers. Make a sharp turn northward and cross a dry wash. Begin ascending the right side of the basin toward a stand of tall saguaros. This section of the trail, covered with broken rock, becomes rough and loose. An occasional blue paint spot marks the correct route. Reach the top of a ridge at 3.1 miles, where another lone saguaro stands guard.

With most of the climbing now behind you, you can enjoy the view as the trail begins to bend around the mountainside. First, traverse the drainage below the ridge, passing the highest point on the entire hike somewhere along the way. Then turn west in the direction of the tallest peak in the White Tanks, which the state is proposing to name Goldwater Peak (after the legendary Arizona lawmaker Barry Goldwater). Unfortunately, Goat Camp Trail does not visit the 4,083-foot summit. Instead, it crosses the drainage at 4.8 miles and makes a U-turn. As you skirt the next hill, look next to the trail for an intertwined pair of saguaros that appears to be frozen in a waltz. Hike atop a ridge with wide-open views of distant cities and the hills deep within the White Tank Mountains, and reach the three-way junction of Ford Canyon, Goat Camp, and Mesquite Canyon trails at 6.3 miles.

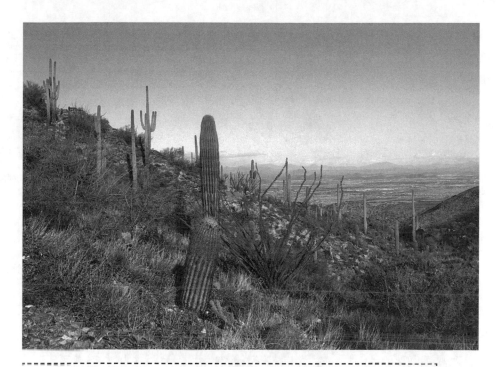

Hillside saguaros frame a distant view of Glendale along Goat Camp Trail.

You can take the Mesquite Canyon Trail (page 269) back. I opted for the scenic but slightly longer Willow Canyon loop. From the three-way junction follow the Ford Canyon Trail down toward the wide basin below. The trail descends quickly via switchbacks, crosses a wide drainage at the basin's bottom, and intersects the Willow Canyon Trail at 7.2 miles. Turn east onto the wide Willow Canyon Trail, lined by typical Sonoran Desert plants such as the staghorn cholla, ocotillo, mesquite, and palo verde. A quarter mile farther the trail rounds a bend next to a fenced-off dike near Willow Spring before diving into the dry riverbed.

At 7.6 miles you'll cut away from the wash and climb uphill for a stretch, but the trail soon returns to the wash. Pass through a thicket of willows and then emerge onto a serene little valley framed by bleached granite and shining pools. Look for cairns to guide your egress. The trail eventually ascends the right bank, passing a rock outcropping at 8.1 miles. Take a quick break here to admire Willow Canyon, which is framed by chiseled hills and features many white tanks along the creek bed at the bottom.

Continue along Willow Canyon Trail to the top of a prominent saddle at 2,425 feet. Cross the saddle and descend into Mesquite Canyon, where the trail eventually meets Mesquite Canyon Trail near a stand of mesquite trees at 8.8 miles from the trailhead. Turn left onto Mesquite Canyon Trail and follow it

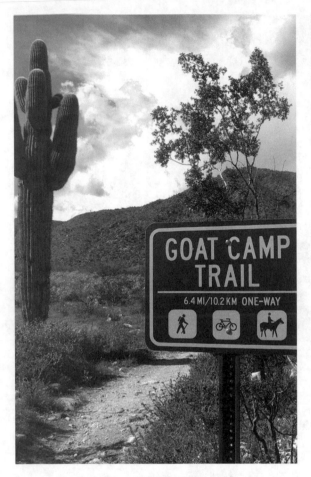

to the Waddell Trail junction and Picnic Area 7. Finish the hike by following the Mesquite Canyon Trail east for another mile along flat desert, across Waterfall Canyon Road and White Tanks Mountain Road, and finally to the Mesquite Trailhead in the wide Trailhead Staging Area.

NEARBY ACTIVITIES

White Tank Mountain Regional Park contains many hiking trails including the Ford Canyon Trail (page 269) and the Waterfall Trail, which is especially scenic right after heavy storms. There is a multiuse competitive track inside the park. The Wildlife World Zoo (**www.wildlifeworld.com**, (623) 935-WILD) is only 6 miles from the park entrance at Loop 303 and Northern Avenue.

POLAND CREEK VIA ALGONQUIN TRAIL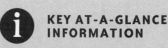

IN BRIEF

Poland Creek runs through a deep canyon on the eastern flanks of the Bradshaw Mountains. Take the Algonquin Trail down to the creek, where you will find many pools suitable for swimming, including one known as the Big Dipper below a 30-foot waterfall.

DESCRIPTION

When you live in the desert, hikes near water become particularly appealing, especially in summer. There's nothing quite as refreshing as a dip in a cool mountain stream after a hot hike. Algonquin Trail and Poland Creek offer a wonderful combination of scenic canyon hiking, a trickling stream, and many pools suitable for swimming. Their remote location and moderately difficult terrain keep these swimming holes secluded. Those who take the time to explore Poland Creek will be duly rewarded with scenic canyons and fabulous swimming areas, especially one called the Big Dipper.

Fed by a 30-foot waterfall on Poland Creek, the Big Dipper looks more like a small lake than a swimming hole. The waterfall tumbles over sheer granite cliffs into a wide circular pool at the bottom, while tufts of grass and willow trees line its edges. Surrounded by

KEY AT-A-GLANCE INFORMATION

LENGTH: 4.2 miles

ELEVATION GAIN: -1,160 feet

CONFIGURATION: Out-and-back

DIFFICULTY: Moderate (difficult scrambling near waterfall)

SCENERY: Poland Creek, Castle Creek Wilderness, swimming holes

EXPOSURE: Mostly exposed, some shade available near creek

TRAFFIC: Light

TRAIL SURFACE: Rock, gravel, overgrown in spots, boulder-hopping and some canyoneering in creek bed

HIKING TIME: 3 hours (plus swimming time)

WATER REQUIREMENT: 2.5 quarts

SEASON: Year-round; hot in summer

ACCESS: Sunrise to sunset; free parking

MAPS: USGS Crown King, Prescott National Forest map

FACILITIES: None

DOGS: Yes

COMMENTS: Scenic pools along Poland Creek, including the "Big Dipper"

Directions

Drive north from Phoenix on I-17 and take exit 248 to Bumble Bee Road. Drive northwest on Bumble Bee Road, which becomes CR 59/Crown King Road, a dirt road passable by most passenger cars. Follow signs for Crown King at any forks, and drive 25 miles to the Poland Vista Point, a pullout on the left side of the road just before mile marker 25. The unmarked trailhead is located at the end of the pullout.

GPS Trailhead Coordinates

UTM Zone 12S

Easting 0379677

Northing 3786859

Latitude N34°13.056'

Longitude W112°18.415'

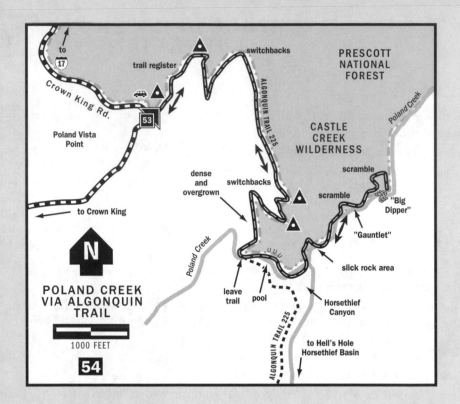

PRESCOTT
NATIONAL
FOREST

switchbacks

trail register

Crown King Rd.

Poland Creek

CASTLE
CREEK
WILDERNESS

ALGONQUIN TRAIL 225

53

Poland Vista
Point

scramble

"Big
Dipper"

dense
and
overgrown

switchbacks

scramble

"Gauntlet"

to Crown King

slick rock area

N

Poland Creek

leave
trail

pool

Horsethief
Canyon

POLAND CREEK
VIA ALGONQUIN
TRAIL

ALGONQUIN TRAIL 225

to Hell's Hole
Horsethief Basin

1000 FEET

54

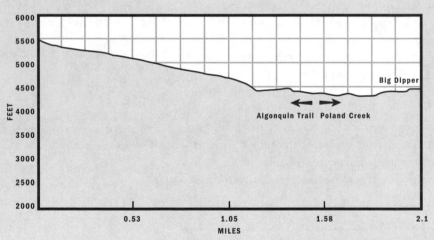

Big Dipper

Algonquin Trail Poland Creek

FEET

6000
5500
5000
4500
4000
3500
3000
2500
2000

0.53   1.05   1.58   2.1
MILES

Poland Creek tumbles over a sheer wall of stone into a tranquil pond known as the "Big Dipper."

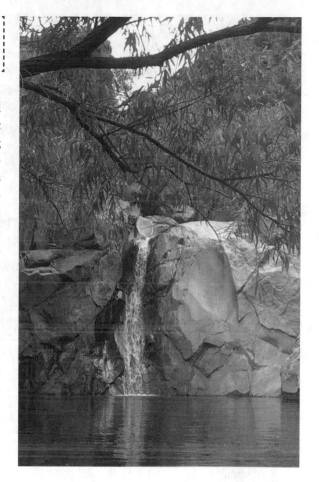

a ring of cliffs and guarded by an upstream gauntlet of water and rock, the Big Dipper isn't easily accessible. Reaching it requires a steep hike down Algonquin Trail 225 and some canyoneering along Poland Creek. However, finding a way to reach the large scenic pool is definitely worth the effort.

There is an odd connection between the monikers Algonquin Trail and Big Dipper. Whether it was intentional remains a mystery. The Algonquin people, a group of Native American tribes who lived near Ontario and Quebec, cherished a legend about the famous constellation. The story goes something like this: An enormous bear was wreaking havoc upon the Algonquin villages, and the villagers dispatched their bravest hunters to kill the bear. The hunters gave chase and eventually wounded the bear. Scared and angry, the bear ran so fast that it leaped into the sky. The hunters followed relentlessly, chasing the bear around the sky. The four stars in the Big Dipper's bowl represent the bear, while the three stars on the handle are the hunters. Every winter when the Big Dipper descends close to the horizon, the bear's wound spills a few drops of blood onto earth, turning autumn leaves into a sea of red and gold. The Algonquin also immortalized this story in the Song of the Stars, an enchanting soliloquy dedicated to the bravery of their hunters.

Begin this hike from Poland Vista Point, a wide pullout on Crown King Road near mile marker 25 and about 2 miles shy of Crown King. Admire the view across Horsethief Canyon from this 5,460-foot-high overlook before embarking on the trek. The trailhead at the end of the lookout is unmarked, but the path is fairly obvious. Algonquin Trail 225 wastes no time in descending

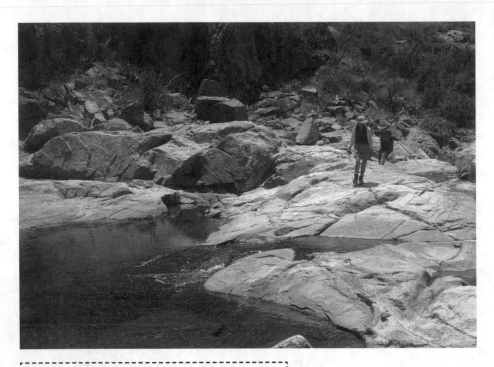

Hikers pass one of many emerald pools along Poland Creek.

the steep hill. Near 0.2 miles confirmation you're on the right path comes in the form of a wooden sign inscribed with the trail name, soon followed by a trail register, and then another sign indicating that the trail runs 6 miles to its terminus on Senator Road.

Covered in rocks and gravel, Algonquin Trail shows little evidence of foot traffic. Manzanitas, mesquites, scrub live oaks, and various grasses line the trail. Occasionally, bristly bushes like catclaw acacia and New Mexico thistle tug at your clothes and skin. Despite warm temperatures it might be wise to wear a pair of long pants for the hike, especially as you reach lower elevations where the trail becomes more overgrown. So far there is no indication whatsoever that this hike eventually leads to water as you traipse through dusty high-desert terrain.

As the trail descends pass several switchbacks offering outstanding views into the canyons below. Just over 0.5 miles into the hike, the trail straightens and makes a beeline toward the bottom of Horsethief Canyon. You can clearly see the path stretch out in front of you and across the hills in the distance. Near 1 mile, the trail begins to switchback again, offering stunning vistas of the Bradshaw Mountains around every bend.

The trail makes a few more bends and dives into an overgrown thicket of thorny bushes at 1.2 miles. The going gets rougher, but the trickling sound of water from Poland Creek is sure to lift your spirits. Breaking free of the bushes at 1.4 miles, the trail reaches Poland Creek in front of a quiet shallow pool with a tall cottonwood tree at the end. The continuation of Algonquin Trail crosses the creek and runs along its right bank. It leads to Hell's Hole and Algonquin Mine before eventually climbing toward Horsethief Basin.

Leave the Algonquin Trail at the Poland Creek crossing and head downstream toward the east. Please keep in mind that you should never attempt to hike along a creek bed during or soon after heavy storms. Initially, the creek bed is easily navigable by boulder-hopping, but it gets increasingly tricky. As you make your way downstream, you'll encounter a series of ponds and pools of varying sizes, many of which are suitable for swimming. There's also a large slick-rock area where the creek widens. Occasional sand beaches break up the rocky banks. About 0.3 miles after leaving the trail, another creek joins from the south. Remember to keep right upon your return to avoid going up the wrong creek.

Near the slick-rock area, it may be necessary to hike up the rocky banks in order to avoid getting wet. Soon after passing the slick rocks, arrive at a narrow but fairly deep pool with a 6-foot waterfall halfway along its length. Approximately 0.5 miles after leaving the trail, you'll face a 50-yard-long gauntlet of water with steep rocks on both sides. Bypassing this tunnel of water requires some tricky class-3 scrambling up the rocks on the left bank. However, if you came prepared for some canyoneering, the easiest way to get through is to wade or swim. Make sure you use two layers of zipped plastic bags to keep your valuables from getting wet, and that you have some old sneakers or aqua socks to protect your feet from unseen underwater hazards.

Beyond the gauntlet of water, you'll encounter another pool before reaching the Big Dipper. It'll be obvious when you get there. About 0.7 miles after leaving the trail, arrive at an open rocky area and the top of a 30-foot waterfall, which empties into a lake-sized pool below. Tempting as the pool may be, there doesn't appear to be a good way to reach it. The easiest workaround is to scramble up the rocks on the left and head for a notch just left of a large boulder on the ridge. Cross over the notch and then follow a steep, loose dirt path down toward the creek. You'll end up in a maze of large boulders downstream of the Big Dipper. From there, hug the creek's right bank as you scramble upstream. You will have to get wet here, but then again, you came to swim, right? Just be careful not to touch the poison ivy growing near the water.

Once at the Big Dipper, you'll instantly forget the tricky scrambling, canyoneering, and poisonous plants. It's a little slice of paradise, and you can usually enjoy this watery playground in complete solitude. At the upstream end of this miniature lake, a tall waterfall splashes into the deep pool, while a ring of cliffs surrounds you. Willows drape over the water, and there's even a rope swing on one of the branches. Swim to your heart's content and then retrace your steps to the trailhead. Soak your towel in the stream and use it to cool off on the arduous climb back up the Algonquin Trail.

55   VULTURE PEAK TRAIL

KEY AT-A-GLANCE INFORMATION

LENGTH: 4.2 miles

ELEVATION GAIN: 1,163 feet

CONFIGURATION: Out-and-back

DIFFICULTY: Moderate

SCENERY: Desert wilderness, mountain vistas

EXPOSURE: Limited shade near top, otherwise exposed

TRAFFIC: Moderate

TRAIL SURFACE: Packed dirt, gravel, optional scrambling near summit

HIKING TIME: 3 hours

WATER REQUIREMENT: 2 quarts

SEASON: Year-round; hot in summer

ACCESS: Sunrise to sunset; free parking

MAPS: USGS Vulture Peak; map on BLM website

FACILITIES: Shaded ramada, restroom, picnic area, no water

DOGS: Yes

COMMENTS: Beautiful desert hike away from it all, yet popular among locals. For more information, visit www.blm.gov/az/outrec/hiking/vulture.htm, or call (623) 580-5500.

GPS Trailhead Coordinates

UTM Zone 12S

Easting   0331977

Northing   3749820

Latitude   N33°52.628'

Longitude   W112°49.045'

IN BRIEF

Though located in a remote area, Vulture Peak attracts plenty of visitors. This challenging trail takes hikers to a prominent saddle point overlooking expansive desert wilderness. Experienced hikers can scramble up another 240 feet to the summit for an even more impressive panoramic view.

DESCRIPTION

Upon arrival at the Vulture Peak Trailhead in the middle of the desert, it is difficult to believe that this remote mountain and the nearby Vulture Mine played key roles in the births of Wickenburg and Phoenix. Back in 1863 a German immigrant and prospector named Henry Wickenburg struck gold and founded Vulture Mine, which became one of the most successful gold mines in Arizona history. One of the financiers for the stamp-mill operation that processed ore from Vulture Mine was Michael Goldwater, grandfather of the legendary Arizona lawmaker Barry Goldwater. Henry Wickenburg also provided financing for a young entrepreneur named Jack Swilling, who used the funds to excavate and improve irrigation canals left by the Hohokams along the Salt River. The resulting

Directions

Drive to the town of Wickenburg 50 miles northwest of Phoenix via US 60 or by taking I-17 north, SR 74 west, and then US 60 west. From the junction of US 60 and US 93 in Wickenburg, continue west 2.5 miles on US 60, then turn south onto Vulture Mine Road. Proceed 7 miles and then turn east onto the Vulture Peak Trail access road between mile markers 19 and 20. Continue 0.4 miles to the main trailhead. High-clearance four-wheel-drive vehicles can follow a very rough dirt road 1.25 miles to the upper trailhead.

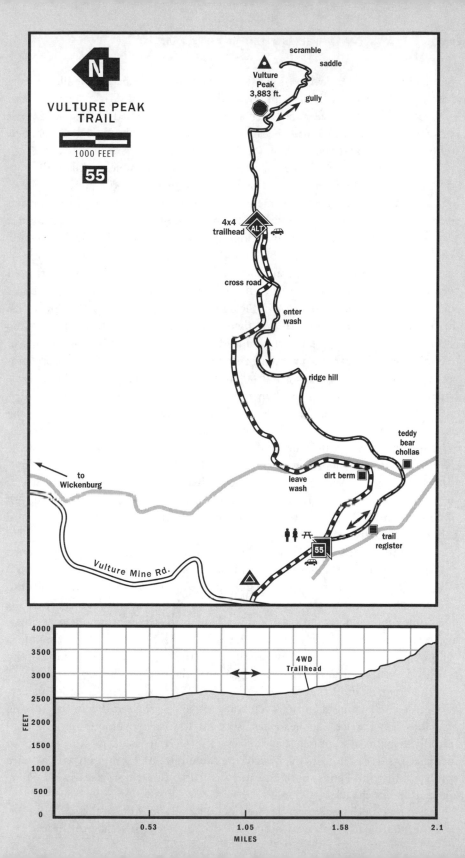

community spawned by Swilling's canals was named Phoenix because it allegorically arose from the ashes of the ancient civilization it supplanted. Wickenburg worked Vulture Mine for a few years but then sold it to a man named Phelps and retired near a settlement that eventually became the town of Wickenburg. Phelps's name is still one of the most recognizable in the Arizona mining industry.

From the town of Wickenburg, Vulture Peak resembles a giant thimble sticking up high above the desert floor. This distinctive profile appears imposing and unconquerable, but it is merely an illusion caused by foreshortening of the summit's true form. When viewed from the trailhead west of the mountain, Vulture Peak actually sits on a long ridge, challenging but definitely attainable.

There are two departure points for this hike: the main trailhead near Vulture Mine Road and an upper trailhead accessible only by high-clearance off-road vehicles. Should you choose to drive the 1.25 miles to the upper trailhead, make sure you bring a capable off-road vehicle and some steady nerves. The primitive dirt road is very rough in spots, and there are plenty of places where protruding rocks aim to puncture the floorpan and damage the underbody components of unqualified modes of transportation. Climbing over a 50-foot dirt berm and traversing sandy Syndicate Wash also challenge your vehicle's all-terrain capabilities. Four-wheeling enthusiasts may enjoy this drive even more than the hike.

In stark contrast to the nerve-wracking off-road adventure, hiking to the upper trailhead is an exercise in tranquility. A pleasant stroll in the pristine desert, this trek measures 1.4 miles and gains only 150 feet. Enjoy up-close views of the hardy flora that thrives in this arid climate. Desert plants adapt to the environment well and respond quickly to the limited amount of rain. After seasonal storms the desert seemingly changes overnight into a lush green landscape, full of new life. In spring golden flowers—from Mexican poppies, brittlebushes, and palo verdes—blanket the foothills.

The trail begins from a gap in the fence near the picnic tables and enters a desert wonderland of saguaros and teddy bear cholla. A pair of benches near 0.2 miles provide a scenic rest area for gazing at Vulture Peak. Then descend into and cross Syndicate Wash. Continue hiking through unspoiled desert foothills and climb up a moderate hill at 0.7 miles. The trail snakes around gentle slopes and once again enters a dry wash at 1.1 miles. This time stay in the wash and follow the trail signs until you eventually cross the dirt road leading to the upper trailhead. At 1.4 miles the trail converges with the road at the upper trailhead.

The remainder of the hike to Vulture Peak is notably steeper and considerably more challenging than the stretch along the desert floor. Begin by crossing an equestrian barrier and head east straight toward the mountain. The trail initially remains flat among classic Sonoran Desert brush but soon begins to increase its slope as it nears the base of the mountain. At 1.7 miles from the main trailhead, the trail bends south and starts to climb in earnest as it ascends some zigzagging switchbacks.

As you climb higher turn around occasionally to admire the valley below and the unbroken expanse of desert hills to the west. It's easy to understand

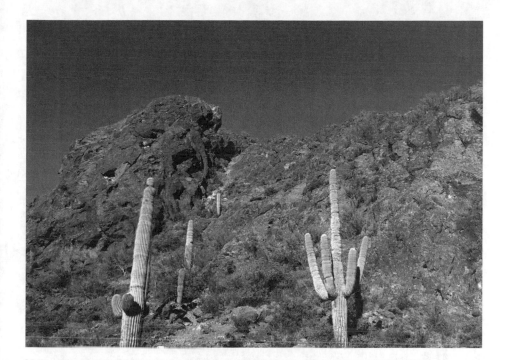

From a saddle on Vulture Peak's southern side, a steep scramble leads to panoramic views.

why this hike is a favorite among locals. Near 1.8 miles the trail ducks around the base of a large rock outcropping at 3,070 feet and mounts a steep climbing traverse toward a gully at the base of the summit saddle. Pick your way through some bushes as the trail enters the ravine, which provides some cool shade during hot summer months. Forge ahead up the final section of tight switchbacks to a saddle at 2 miles from the main trailhead.

The view improves dramatically when you reach the 3,420-foot saddle because you can now see toward the east as well as the west. Casual hikers should stop here and make this spot their turnaround point. More experienced adventure seekers can continue climbing north to the 3,663-foot summit of Vulture Peak. The final stretch is short but requires scrambling up a steep, rocky crevice. From the wide summit of Vulture Peak, the sweeping panoramic vistas will take your breath away. Break out the snacks and soak up unobstructed views of the surrounding desert and the town of Wickenburg. Don't forget to sign the summit log before returning the way you came.

NEARBY ACTIVITIES

The Hassayampa River Preserve near Wickenburg offers guided nature walks and the opportunity to see unique plants and wildlife. Historic and rustic, the Vulture Mine 5 miles south of the Vulture Peak Trail offers self-guided tours of the remaining buildings and mine site.

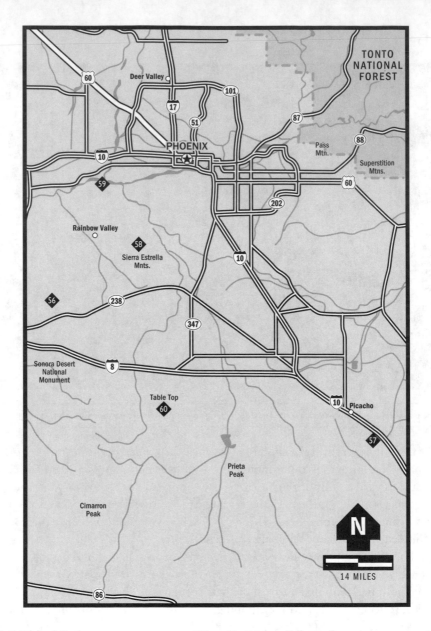

TONTO
NATIONAL
FOREST

60

Deer Valley

101

17

51

87

88

PHOENIX

Pass
Mtn.

Superstition
Mtns.

10

60

202

59

Rainbow Valley

58

Sierra Estrella
Mnts.

10

56

238

347

8

Sonora Desert
National
Monument

Table Top

60

10 Picacho

57

Prieta
Peak

Cimarron
Peak

N

14 MILES

86

SOUTH AND SOUTHWEST
SIERRA ESTRELLA MOUNTAINS

56 BRITTLEBUSH TRAIL

KEY AT-A-GLANCE INFORMATION

LENGTH: 12 miles

ELEVATION GAIN: 660 feet

CONFIGURATION: Out-and-back

DIFFICULTY: Easy

SCENERY: Classic Sonoran Desert

EXPOSURE: Mostly exposed

TRAFFIC: Very light

TRAIL SURFACE: Gravel, packed dirt, sand

HIKING TIME: 5 hours

WATER REQUIREMENT: 3–4 quarts

SEASON: November–April; not recommended in summer

ACCESS: Sunrise to sunset; free parking

MAPS: USGS Cotton Center SE, Bureau of Land Management map, trailhead information box

FACILITIES: None

DOGS: Yes, leashed at all times

COMMENTS: Some route-finding skills required. For more information, visit www.blm.gov/az/outrec/hiking/bbush.htm, or call (623) 580-5500.

GPS Trailhead
Coordinates

UTM Zone   12S

Easting   0354912

Northing   3656268

Latitude   N33°2.222'

Longitude W112°33.263'

IN BRIEF

Brittlebush Trail runs through the heart of the North Maricopa Mountains Wilderness, offering pristine desert scenery, complete solitude, and a nearly level hike in one of Arizona's newest national monuments. Arizona Highways featured this trail as Hike of the Month in the December 2003 issue.

DESCRIPTION

Created on January 17, 2001, Sonoran Desert National Monument protects nearly half a million acres of pristine Sonoran Desert southwest of Phoenix. The monument contains three congressionally designated wilderness areas, the northernmost of which is North Maricopa Mountains Wilderness. Two corridor trails

----

Directions

From central or east Phoenix: **Take I-10 east toward Tucson. Exit onto SR 347, Queen Creek Road/Maricopa Road, and follow it southwest 14.5 miles to the town of Maricopa. Turn west onto SR 238 and proceed 30 miles to a dirt road between mile markers 11 and 10.**

Turn north onto the dirt road, which is marked with a wooden "Trail" sign. Follow this dirt road 3.2 miles, staying left at Gap Well and then going straight at a T intersection. Make a right turn at 3.2 miles, following a small "Trail" sign. Continue 2 miles, and then veer right at a fork in the road. Drive 0.8 miles farther to reach the small trailhead parking area. A high-clearance vehicle is required because of the many dry-wash crossings.

From west Phoenix: **Take I-10 west to SR 85. Follow SR 85 south 33.5 miles to Gila Bend. Past mile marker 121, turn east onto SR 238. Proceed 10.4 miles to a dirt road between mile markers 10 and 11. Follow above directions for the dirt road.**

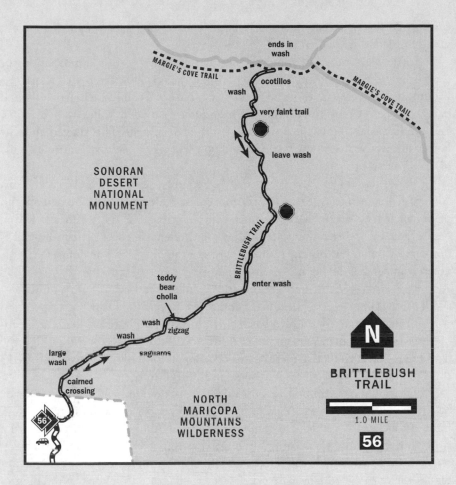

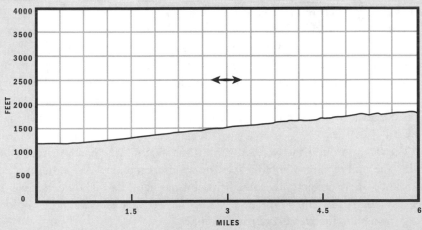

form a "T" through the wilderness. Margie's Cove Trail runs roughly east–west, while Brittlebush Trail Ts into it from the south.

Brittlebush Trail isn't for everyone; it requires a certain appreciation for the pure desert experience. Winding through the 63,200-acre North Maricopa Mountains Wilderness, this trail takes you into incredibly secluded hills and desert washes. Creosote-covered plains, saguaro-studded valleys, rocky hills, and sandy washes typify the Sonoran Desert environment. This rugged and raw landscape receives very few visitors, and you will likely have the entire 12-mile hike to yourself.

Due to its remote location, this hike requires extra care and precautions. Always tell someone where you are going and remember to bring a map and plenty of extra water. There are no services available at the trailhead. Rising very gradually and seemingly level for its entire length, the Brittlebush Trail is not very difficult, but hiking 12 miles through the desert can be dangerous. It is not recommended during hot summer months.

There are three distinct sections to this hike. The first follows a faint two-track through the desert plains. Next comes a wide, sandy wash. The last section runs through a saguaro-studded basin surrounded by mountains. Begin by heading east from the small parking lot. Pass the trailhead plaque and then sign the trail log inside a protective metal box. The Bureau of Land Management stocks this container with brochures and some useful trail info.

The trail hooks around the right side of a rock mound and then the left side of another. Running on the open plain covered by short grasses, the trail is very faint at times. At 0.6 miles cross a large wash bed and head northeast toward a rocky hill in the distance. Though the trail takes its name from the brittlebush, creosote bushes dominate the flat desert plain. These incredibly drought-tolerant plants thrive in the harshest desert environments, often forming pure colonies where other plants cannot survive.

The trail parallels a large wash and then crosses it at 1.5 miles from the trailhead. Pass a thick stand of saguaros, ironwoods, and palo verdes a quarter mile farther. There are no trail markers and very few cairns to disrupt the pure wilderness experience. Only the lonely sound of your footsteps and the occasional rustle of scurrying lizards break the eerie silence. At 1.9 miles the trail makes a zigzag, first left across a dry wash, and then right approaching the large rocky hill.

Veer right around the base of the hill, passing a large patch of teddy bear cholla. The trail remains flat but leaves the wide-open plains for a valley between mountains. There are actually some brittlebushes here! Large boulders cover the hills and mountains, and a layer of patina or desert varnish covers the boulders, giving them a distinctive rusty brown color.

At 2.75 miles enter a wide basin sandwiched between three rocky hills, and begin the second section of the hike inside a sandy wash. There are no trail markings inside the wash, so make a mental note of your surroundings for the

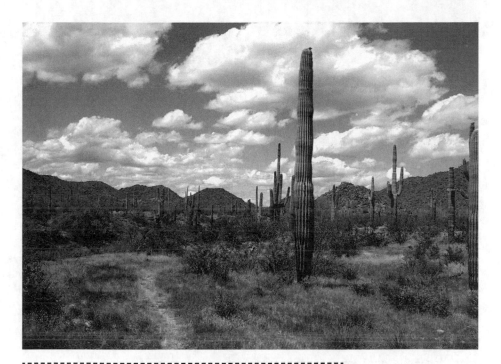

Undulating hills and tall stands of saguaros along the Brittlebush Trail.

return trip. Head straight across the basin where the wash becomes more pronounced as it bends north, hugging the hill on your left. The landscape is notably different in the wash bottom. Taller bushes and trees line the banks, while nothing but sand and footprints cover the wash bed.

At 3.75 miles pass some patina-covered boulders on your right and then a massive one leaning over the wash on your left. Beyond the boulders the wash forks several times as it shoots the gap between two hills. Take a left at the first major fork, a right at the second, and then a left again at the third. The trail finally leaves the wide wash at a signed egress on the left bank 4.4 miles from the trailhead.

Climbing out of the wash onto a hillock, the trail enters the third part of the hike where it passes through grassy plains and stands of tall saguaros. Heading generally north in a large basin, soak up the overwhelming sense of seclusion and solitude instilled by the ring of mountains around you. Pass some large boulders at 4.75 miles and then encounter a small mound covered in white quartz. The trail breaks right around the hill and begins to wind back and forth.

Cross a wash at 5.25 miles where the trail becomes very faint. Pick up the trail on the other side of the wash where a cairn marks the way. The trail makes several more twists and turns and arrives at the edge of a wide, deep wash. Turning east along stands of bristly ocotillos, the trail follows the wash for a while and eventually descends into it at a horseshoe bend in the streambed. At

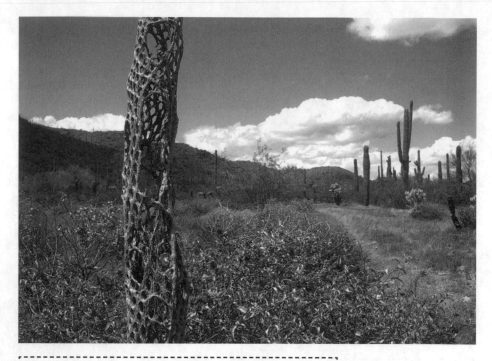

A cholla skeleton stands next to secluded Brittlebush Trail deep within
Sonoran Desert National Monument.

exactly 6 miles from the trailhead, this is the terminus of Brittlebush Trail and
roughly the midpoint on Margie's Cove Trail, which runs east–west across the
North Maricopa Mountains Wilderness. Retrace your steps to the trailhead for
a 12-mile round-trip hike.

NEARBY ACTIVITIES

The Sonoran Desert National Monument contains other hiking trails such as
Margie's Cove, Lava Flow, and Table Top (page 310). The Sierra Estrella mountain range southwest of Phoenix offers an excellent hike to the top of Quartz Peak
(page 300). Picacho Peak State Park, farther south on I-10, provides Hunter Trail
(page 295) and Sunset Vista Trail, which scale the rugged Picacho Peak.

PICACHO PEAK: HUNTER TRAIL* 57

IN BRIEF

This spectacular climb up Picacho Peak packs plenty of adventure into a short hike. The challenging Hunter Trail coils around sheer cliffs and rocky slopes. Cables assist in your scramble to the 3,374-foot panoramic summit.

DESCRIPTION

Driving along Interstate 10 between Phoenix and Tucson, it is impossible to miss Picacho Peak, whose chiseled profile served as a prominent landmark long before any roads existed in the desert. Resembling a tall volcanic cone rising 1,500 feet from the desert floor, Picacho Peak piques the curiosity of all who pass it. From afar, its sheer cliffs appear insurmountable. As you approach Picacho Peak State Park on the eastern flank of the mountain, however, a kinder silhouette reveals itself. Challenging and steep, Hunter Trail is the most popular hike in the park, offering close-ups of rocky cliffs and fun cable-assisted scrambles. A stunning 360-degree panorama of the surrounding desert awaits you on the summit.

The Picacho Peak area also boasts a storied past because it is the site of the only Civil War skirmish in Arizona. The Battle of Picacho Pass occurred on April 15, 1862, between Union forces led by Captain Calloway and Lieutenant Barrett and Confederate soldiers

KEY AT-A-GLANCE INFORMATION

LENGTH: 3 miles
ELEVATION GAIN: 1,400 feet
CONFIGURATION: Out-and-back
DIFFICULTY: Difficult
SCENERY: Picacho Peak, cliffs, desert, wildflowers, plains
EXPOSURE: Mostly exposed
TRAFFIC: Moderate
TRAIL SURFACE: Gravel, rock, cable-assisted scrambling
HIKING TIME: 2.5 hours
WATER REQUIREMENT: 2 quarts
SEASON: Year-round; hot in summer
ACCESS: 8 a.m.–10 p.m.; trails close at sunset; $6 per-vehicle entrance fee, $3 during summer
MAPS: USGS Newman Peak
FACILITIES: Water, restrooms, picnic areas, campground, ranger station
DOGS: Yes, leashed; but not recommended because of the scrambling
COMMENTS: For more information, visit www.pr.state.az.us/parkhtml/picacho.html, or call (520) 466-3183. Consider bringing gloves for those cable-assisted climbs.

Directions

From Phoenix, take East I-10 toward Tucson. Drive southeast 60 miles, and exit at Picacho Peak Road (exit 219). Turn west to enter Picacho Peak State Park, and pay the entrance fee. One-quarter mile past the entrance, turn left onto Barrett Loop where the Hunter Trail begins.

GPS Trailhead Coordinates

UTM Zone 12S
Easting   0462314
Northing 3611549
Latitude N32°38.560'
Longitude W111°24.148'

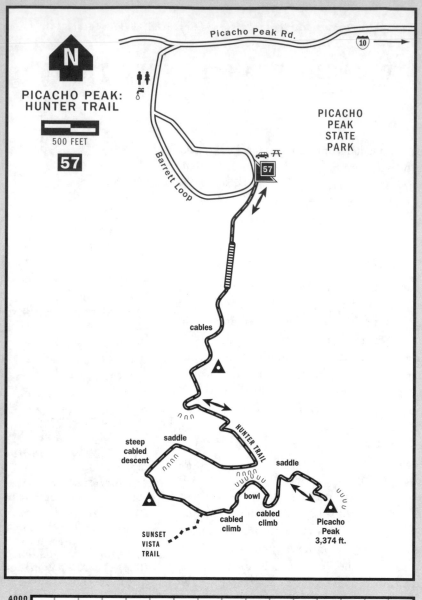

N

PICACHO PEAK: HUNTER TRAIL

500 FEET

57

Picacho Peak Rd.

10

PICACHO
PEAK
STATE
PARK

Barrett Loop

57

cables

HUNTER TRAIL

steep
cabled
descent

saddle

saddle

bowl

cabled
climb

cabled
climb

Picacho
Peak
3,374 ft.

SUNSET
VISTA
TRAIL

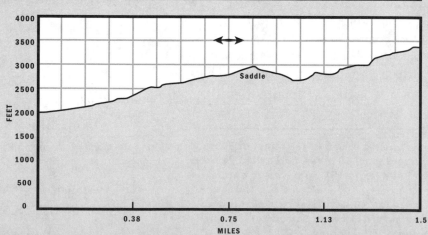

Saddle

4000
3500
3000
2500
2000
1500
1000
500
0

FEET

0.38   0.75   1.13   1.5

MILES

under the command of Captain Hunter. The Calloway Trail, Hunter Trail, and Barrett Loop inside Picacho Peak State Park are all named after these Civil War soldiers.

This beautiful state park is also well known for ostentatious displays of wildflowers after rainy winters. From February through April, folks flock to Picacho's foothills hoping to see a blanket of golden poppies and blue lupines. Other colorful blossoms known to grace the mountainsides include purple fila-ree, white desert chicory, orange globe mallow, yellow fiddleneck, and crimson ocotillo. The hotter climate of early summer brings a second wave of cactus flowers.

Begin your hike from the signed trailhead on Barrett Loop inside Picacho Peak State Park. Head south on the gravel trail and wooden steps toward the mountain and its imposing cliffs. When conditions are ripe, delicately coiled petals of Mexican gold poppies and flower-laden racemes of blue lupine line the trail. At 0.25 miles, the trail becomes rockier and steeper and begins to ascend switchbacks toward the base of the cliffs. Use strategically placed steel cables for balance as you climb up the volcanic rocks. Out of breath? Pause at a sharp bend in the trail beyond the cabled section to survey your ascent. Reach the base of the massive cliffs at 0.5 miles, where the overhanging rock shelters you from the elements. It's not quite a cave but the rock formations are nevertheless intriguing.

Turn left and climb 0.2 miles farther to an upper cliff, whose vertical walls shoot straight up toward the sky. At the eastern side of the cliff overhang, enjoy a splendid view of the valley below and the noisy freeway running through it. Then turn west and climb a gentler slope along Hunter Trail until you reach the 2,960-foot saddle, where an inviting bench greets you. Take some time to admire the open view toward the south and read the informative plaques next to the bench.

Though you can see the summit from the saddle, it is readily apparent that you can't reach it from the northern side. The trail crosses the saddle and takes a 250-foot plunge down an incredibly steep, rocky, and narrow crevice. Definitely make use of the cables here to help you descend, and duck your head to avoid banging it against the unforgiving rocks. At 1 mile from the trailhead, you'll reach the bottom of the cabled section where the trail hooks left and begins to regain the lost 250 feet of elevation.

Warmer and drier, the southern slope of Picacho Peak hosts more cacti and appears sparsely vegetated. Shortly after resuming your ascent, pass a rock outcropping where you can enjoy a sensational view of the desert below. Hunter Trail intersects Sunset Vista Trail at 1.1 mile and soon reaches another cabled climb. Scramble up this narrow passage while hugging the rock wall, and enter a high basin full of saguaros, palo verdes, and creosotes. The overhanging cliffs from earlier in the hike are directly behind the walls of this semicircular bowl.

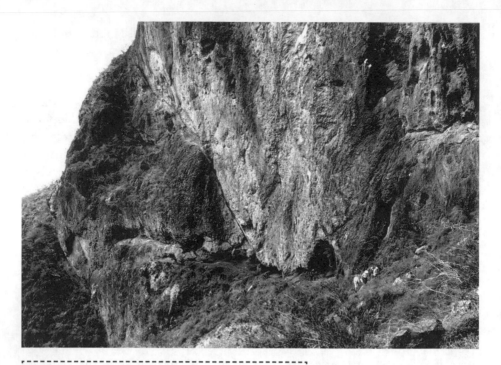

Hikers pass under an enormous sheer cliff on the Hunter Trail.

Skirt the upper basin, and arrive at the base of yet another cabled climb. This is the most difficult scramble, hence the presence of two cables. You'll clamber up the steep crevice only to find another scary section where the trail wraps around a large rock face. Rickety cables and a precariously placed wooden plank help you negotiate this part, but be aware that the wooden plank when wet with dew or rain can be as slippery as a sheet of ice. I always wonder how much engineering went into the cables and the metal posts driven into rock, but they seem to have withstood the test of time. Built by the Civilian Conservation Corps in 1932 to service a light beacon on the summit, the Hunter Trail has been around for quite a long time. The light beacon has since been dismantled, leaving only a few rebar stubs on the summit.

Reach the upper saddle at 1.3 miles from the trailhead and breathe a sigh of relief because the remainder of this trail seems easy and uneventful. Turn east and climb switchbacks to the wide summit of Picacho Peak, 1.5 miles from the trailhead. Note that park signs proclaim Hunter Trail to be 2.1 miles in length, but my GPS usually doesn't lie.

From the 3,374-foot summit of Picacho Peak, you command a sweeping panorama of the wide-open desert, broken only by Interstate 10 and the Central Arizona Project canal. Notice the circular drainage pattern at the base of Picacho Peak. Newman Peak looms across the highway, and the massive Catalina

Mountains near Tucson can be seen on the southeastern horizon. Look for nearly flat Table Top Mountain to the west, and the Sierra Estrellas to its right. On a clear day you may be able to spot mountains near Phoenix.

Return to the trailhead the same way you came. Alternatively, enjoy a longer hike around the mountain by taking the Sunset Vista Trail from the junction on the southern side of the peak to the Sunset Vista Point. Then hike back along the road to Barrett Loop and the Hunter Trailhead.

Update: Effective June 3, 2010, the Picacho Peak State Park will be closed. No alternate access to Hunter Trail is currently available or being planned. For updates about the park's possible reopening, visit **www.pr.state.az.us.**

NEARBY ACTIVITIES

Sonoran Desert National Monument, 40 miles to the northwest of Picacho Peak, offers other excellent hikes such as Table Top Trail (page 310) and Brittlebush Trail (page 290). The Catalina Mountains north of Tucson is a veritable haven for hikers.

58 QUARTZ PEAK TRAIL

KEY AT-A-GLANCE INFORMATION

LENGTH: 6 miles

ELEVATION GAIN: 2,472 feet

CONFIGURATION: Out-and-back

DIFFICULTY: Difficult

SCENERY: Pristine desert, Sierra Estrella, Butterfly Mountain, Quartz Peak, panoramic views

EXPOSURE: Mostly exposed

TRAFFIC: Light

TRAIL SURFACE: Rock, gravel, some easy scrambling

HIKING TIME: 5 hours

WATER REQUIREMENT: 3–4 quarts

SEASON: Year-round; hot in summer

ACCESS: Sunrise to sunset; free parking

MAPS: USGS Montezuma Peak, trailhead plaque, Bureau of Land Management trail map

FACILITIES: Toilet, picnic table, no water

DOGS: Yes

COMMENTS: For more information, visit www.blm.gov/az/outrec/hiking/qpeak.htm, or call (623) 580-5500.

GPS Trailhead Coordinates

UTM Zone 12S

Easting 0384483

Northing 3673837

Latitude N33°11.940'

Longitude W112°14.402'

IN BRIEF

The pristine wilderness, a classic ridge walk, and expansive views from atop Quartz Peak provide plenty of reasons and rewards for those who tackle this challenging hike. This trail's remote location also ensures an absence of crowds.

DESCRIPTION

Sierra Estrella, a large mountain range southwest of Phoenix, can be seen from nearly anywhere in the Valley of the Sun and captures the fancy of many hiking enthusiasts. Sierra Estrella means "mountain range of stars" in Spanish. From the top of Quartz Peak, it certainly feels like you are gazing down from the stars. There is only one established trail in the entire mountain range—Quartz Peak Trail. However, the Estrellas make up in quality for

Directions

Drive west from Phoenix on I-10, and exit onto Estrella Parkway. Drive south on Estrella Parkway 8.3 miles, and then turn right onto Elliot Road. Take Elliot Road west 2.6 miles. Turn left onto Rainbow Valley Road, and follow it south 9.3 miles to Riggs Road. Turn left onto Riggs Road, and drive 4 miles east to the intersection with Bullard Avenue. Turn right, but make an immediate left onto a dirt road under the telephone poles. Follow the dirt road east 5.3 miles until it ends. Note that the last section of this road past Rainbow Rancho is narrow and sandy. At the end of the road under large power lines, look for a small "Trail" sign and turn right. Continue under the power lines 1.9 miles. Turn left at another "Trail" sign, and drive 1.9 miles farther to the trailhead.

Sections of the dirt roads are rough and sandy, crossing several eroded washes. High-clearance vehicles are required.

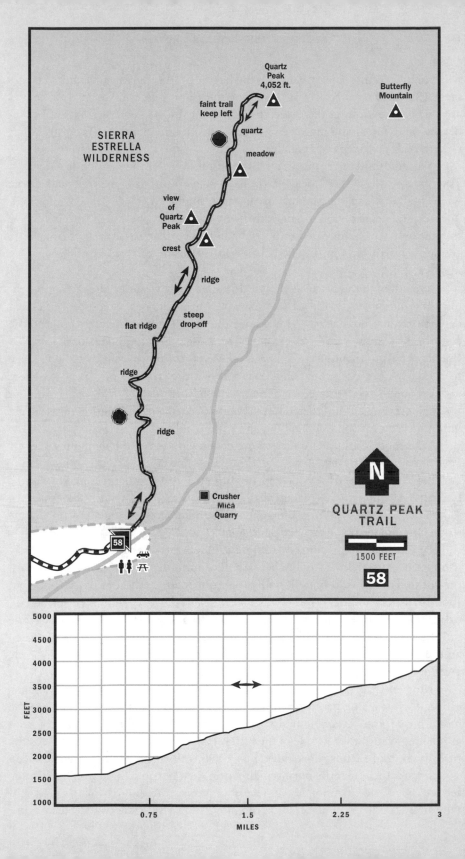

what they lack in quantity. Superbly managed by the Bureau of Land Management (BLM) Quartz Peak Trail is one of the finest desert hikes in the Phoenix area. This hike captures the rugged beauty of the 14,400-acre Sierra Estrella Wilderness and offers stunning views from high mountain ridges. The 4,052-foot Quartz Peak provides even grander panoramas of the sprawling metropolis.

Volcanic in nature, the Sierra Estrella mountain range is rich in minerals. The remains of Crusher Mica Quarry lie in a small hill near the trailhead. Large white boulders cap the summit of the aptly named Quartz Peak, while flaky mica crystals can be found embedded in rocks along the trail, especially near the peak. If you happen to see a bright light near the summit as if someone's shining a mirror at you, it's likely sunlight reflecting off the shiny surface of a mica crystal.

Even though the Estrellas sit only 15 miles southwest of Phoenix, approaching the Quartz Peak Trail can be an adventure that necessitates an extended drive through sandy desert terrain, since the only sanctioned access point to the trail is on the mountain's western side. Once there though, hikers have the pristine desert all to themselves. The trail takes visitors up the spine of a long ridge to a quartz-covered summit 2,500 feet above the desert floor in just 3 short miles. Though very steep, Quartz Peak Trail is surprisingly manageable because it distributes the elevation gain fairly evenly over its entire length. Only the last half mile requires some scrambling and route-finding skills.

Like most trailheads under its management, the BLM maintains Quartz Peak facilities very well. A large parking area and a clean toilet are available, but there's no water. Always take plenty of extra water into a remote desert area like this. An informative plaque at the trailhead explains wilderness etiquette. Take note of the elevation profile and topographical map posted on the plaque to prepare mentally for the challenge ahead.

Begin by walking northeast straight toward the twin peaks of Butterfly Mountain. Pass fields of teddy bear cholla, and admire stands of saguaros in the foothills. The trail initially follows an old road on the flat desert floor but soon turns left and begins to climb a straight, rocky path uphill. In spring colorful blossoms of brittlebush, phacelia, and filaree adorn the landscape, while tall saguaros stand guard like sentries posted on either side of the trail. Keep an even pace on the steep slope here because most of the hike requires the same level of effort.

Most of Quartz Peak Trail lies atop sharp mountain ridges. Ridge hiking is especially rewarding because it offers open views to either side as you trace the mountain's spine. Attain your first ridge at 0.6 miles, and then follow the trail as it slides over to the left side of the hill. A large boulder outcropping blocks the path at the end of this short ridge where the trail turns left and ascends steep switchbacks in a generally northern direction. Just beyond 1 mile you'll reach the second ridge and turn northeast. The slope tapers off slightly for the next half mile or so, giving you ample time to enjoy the classic ridge walk. Steep drop-

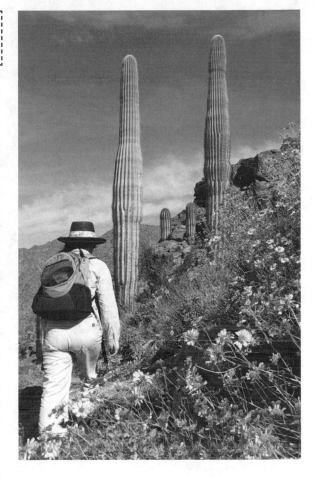

Jinwon Kim of Chandler hikes past blooming brittlebush and gateways of saguaros on the Quartz Peak Trail.

offs into deep ravines flank this much longer ridgeline, while sharp peaks loom in the distance. Behind you expansive Rainbow Valley stretches out westward from the base of the mountain. On a cold day you might even see a giant mushroom cloud in the distance. Don't worry; it's only a plume of steam from the Palo Verde Nuclear Generating Station, the most productive nuclear power plant in the country.

Near 1.7 miles into the hike, resume the cruel steep ascent. Ridge after ridge, crest after crest, the trail climbs ever higher. The first sighting of Quartz Peak pops into your peripheral vision as you reach a vista point at 2 miles from the trailhead. The unmistakable white cap on the mountaintop resembles unsightly bird droppings from a distance but trust that it will be quite spectacular up close. The trail once again tapers in slope and reaches a small flat meadow on top of the ridge at 2.5 miles.

The last half mile of Quartz Peak Trail is noticeably faint and may be rough in spots. However, strategically placed rock cairns mark the way. To complicate matters, there's a fork in the trail where one route heads for the top of the ridge while another skirts the hill to the left. When in doubt, just head for the ridgeline. The two paths converge later. At certain points, you'll need to scamper up the rocks, but no technical climbing skills are necessary. More and more white quartz and shiny mica crystals appear next to the trail as you near the summit.

The trail seems to end at a narrow saddle between two large boulder outcroppings just shy of 3 miles from the trailhead, and a sheer drop-off faces you. If you have been watching your feet on the rough trail over the last 0.2 miles, you might not realize that Quartz Peak is just above your head to the left. Back

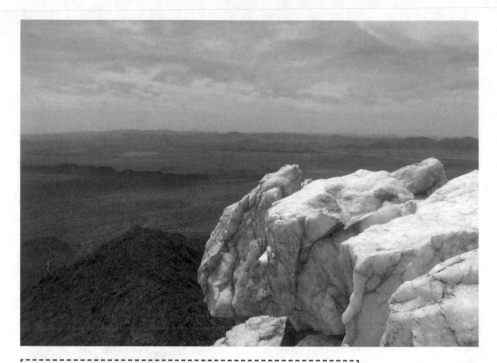

View toward Rainbow Valley from pearly white boulders atop Quartz Peak.

down the trail about 15 feet and turn left up a rocky slope. Then scramble another 20 feet to the top.

Seemingly chiseled out of blocks of snow-white stone, Quartz Peak is unique among summits near Phoenix. At an elevation of 4,052 feet, it also provides an impressive panorama. The urban sprawl of Phoenix stretches out for as far as the eye can see across the Gila River Indian Reservation. From this vantage point South Mountain appears diminutive in the distance. The twin peaks of Butterfly Mountain lie directly east, while Montezuma Peak, the tallest point in the Estrellas, can be seen to the southeast. After soaking up the scenery, retrace your steps to return to the trailhead.

NEARBY ACTIVITIES

Estrella Mountain Regional Park, approximately 7 miles south of I-10 on Estrella Parkway, offers many hiking trails including Rainbow Valley (page 305) and Toothaker. White Tank Mountain Regional Park, farther north, also provides excellent trails such as Ford Canyon (page 269) and Goat Camp (page 274).

RAINBOW VALLEY TRAIL 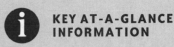 59

IN BRIEF

Estrella Mountain Regional Park sits at the northern tip of the Sierra Estrella mountain range. Many trails crisscross the foothills and plains inside the park, and Rainbow Valley Trail's two branches touch nearly all of them, forming countless loops. You can customize the hike distance by choosing different return routes.

DESCRIPTION

West Phoenix residents have several excellent mountain parks from which to choose for a hike. Encompassing nearly 20,000 acres, Estrella Mountain Regional Park on the northern tip of the Sierra Estrella mountain range offers everything from picnics to rodeos, from camping to fishing, and from baseball to golf. However, visitors sometimes overlook the park as a hiking destination. There are more than 33 miles of trails inside the park, most of them lying in the foothills and desert plains at the base of the Estrellas. Views of the distant city and the rugged Sonoran Desert abound from the park's trails.

Rainbow Valley Trail, named for a huge plain west of the Sierra Estrella mountain range, forms a loop that intersects nearly all

KEY AT-A-GLANCE INFORMATION

LENGTH: 8.8 miles

ELEVATION GAIN: 440 feet

CONFIGURATION: Loop

DIFFICULTY: Moderate

SCENERY: Desert, Sierra Estrella, Rainbow Valley

EXPOSURE: Completely exposed

TRAFFIC: Light

TRAIL SURFACE: Gravel, packed dirt, sand

HIKING TIME: 5 hours

WATER REQUIREMENT: 4 quarts

SEASON: Year-round; hot in summer

ACCESS: Open 6 a.m.–8 p.m. (Sun.–Thu.), 6 a.m.–10 p.m. (Fri.–Sat.); trails close at sunset; $6 per-vehicle entry fee

MAPS: USGS Avondale SE and Avondale SW; park map available at entrance

FACILITIES: Restroom, water, picnic areas, youth camp, rodeo grounds

DOGS: Yes, leashed at all times

COMMENTS: It is possible to shorten this hike considerably by taking other loops back to the trailhead. For more information, visit www.maricopa.gov/parks/estrella, or call (623) 932-3811.

Directions

Drive west from Phoenix on I-10, and exit onto Estrella Parkway. Follow Estrella Parkway south 5 miles. After crossing the Gila River bridge, turn east onto Vineyard and continue 0.6 miles to Estrella Mountain Regional Park. Pay the entrance fee at the guard shack. Inside the park, follow the main road approximately 2 miles to the rodeo ground. Park near the trailhead on the western side of the arena.

GPS Trailhead Coordinates

UTM Zone 12S

Easting   0372373

Northing 3692994

Latitude N33°22.222'

Longitude W112°22.358'

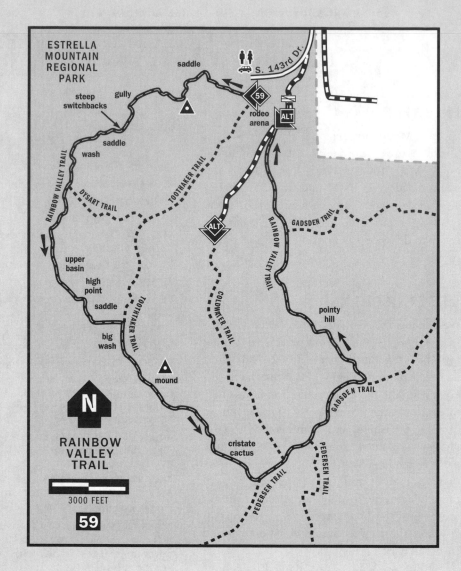

ESTRELLA
MOUNTAIN
REGIONAL
PARK

saddle

S. 143rd Dr.

59

steep
switchbacks

gully

ALT

rodeo
arena

RAINBOW VALLEY TRAIL

DISART TRAIL

TOOTHAKER TRAIL

ALT

GADSDEN TRAIL

RAINBOW VALLEY TRAIL

saddle
wash

upper
basin

high
point

saddle

TOOTHAKER TRAIL

COLDWATER TRAIL

pointy
hill

big
wash

mound

GADSDEN TRAIL

N

RAINBOW
VALLEY
TRAIL

cristate
cactus

PEDERSEN TRAIL

PEDERSEN TRAIL

3000 FEET

59

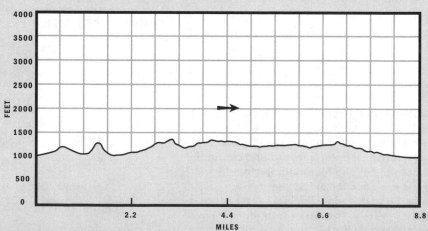

FEET				
4000				
3500				
3000				
2500				
2000				
1500				
1000				
500				
0	2.2	4.4	6.6	8.8

MILES

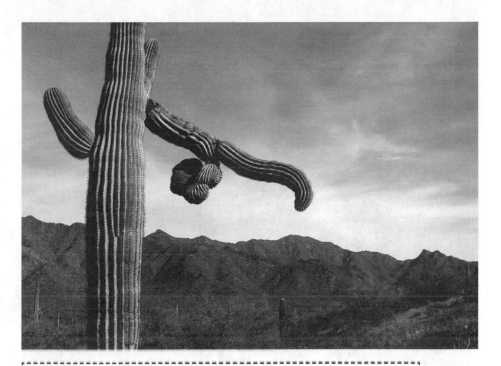

A rare crested saguaro frames Sierra Estrella mountains along the Rainbow Valley Trail.

trails in the park. There are two disjointed segments of the Rainbow Valley Trail beginning at either side of the rodeo arena. These two segments, along with a combination of the Toothaker, Pedersen, and Gadsden trails, create an excellent route through the park. The western half of this loop is hilly, whereas the eastern portion runs through an expansive desert valley. Seemingly countless dry washes crisscross the entire landscape. Although the highest peaks in the Estrellas appear jagged and rough, the foothills trails mount no more than a moderate challenge. Therefore, you are likely to encounter mountain bikers and equestrians on this hike.

Begin the loop from a small trailhead on the rodeo arena's western side. The trail heads west and soon reaches a fork where the Toothaker Trail veers left. The park's trail markers use two-letter abbreviations that match those found on the park map, and the designation for Rainbow Valley Trail is "RB." Keep right at the fork and continue hiking west on the Rainbow Valley Trail, which begins a gradual ascent at 0.25 miles. Typical desert plants such as creosote bushes and palo verde trees line the trail and cover the slopes. Buzzing grasshoppers and darting lizards remind you that the desert is full of fauna as well as flora. At the head of the basin, the trail breaks left and climbs to a saddle a half mile from the trailhead.

As you hike up the ridge, enjoy views of the White Tank Mountains to the northwest and peaks in the Sierra Estrella to the southeast. The park's lush golf course appears like an oasis below. The Phoenix skyline lies in the distance,

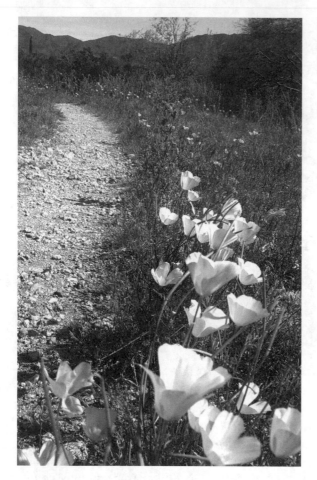

Mexican gold poppies bloom along the Rainbow Valley Trail in Estrella Mountain Regional Park.

flanked by familiar silhouettes of Camelback Mountain, Piestewa Peak, and Four Peaks. Winding around the north-facing hillside, this section of the Rainbow Valley Trail truly earns its name in the spring when a rainbow of colorful wildflowers brightens the slopes. Blue lupine, azure delphinium, golden poppy, yellow brittlebush, fuchsia hedgehog cactus, white Fremont's pincushion, and purple owl clover all thrive here, often blooming concurrently.

At 1.5 miles the trail climbs to a 1,300-foot hillcrest graced with a stunning panoramic view of the wide valley west of Phoenix. Crossing over to the drier southern slopes, the flora changes suddenly as if you passed through a door into the Sonoran Desert, entering the domain of cacti and creosote bushes. The trail descends a steep hill covered with loose rocks. Be careful with your footing here.

In the valley below, find a "DS" sign marking the Dysart Trail at 2.1 miles from the trailhead. The Rainbow Valley loop intersects many trails in the park, and you can choose to shorten your hike by turning back early. If you are already tired, the Dysart Trail can take you back to the trailhead in 1.7 miles via the Toothaker Trail. For those craving a longer outing, continue south on the Rainbow Valley Trail.

Rainbow Valley Trail begins to climb again at 2.3 miles, heading toward a gap in the hills. Reaching a high basin a half mile farther, you leave the western plains behind. Thick grasses encroach the trail, as this section is sometimes overgrown. Forge ahead toward the 1,350-foot saddle directly east of the basin. Then descend into a deep valley where you find a junction with the Toothaker Trail at 3.5 miles. Once again you have the option of turning left and heading back early on the Toothaker, which takes you back to the trailhead in 2 miles.

To continue the longer loop, turn right onto the Toothaker Trail and head south across a deep wash. The trail slowly climbs again and bends to the southeast. At 4.1 miles you'll reach a flat mound with arguably the best view from anywhere on the loop toward Sierra Estrella's sharp peaks. And at 1,360 feet this is also the highest point on the entire circuit. Then begin a gradual descent into expansive Rainbow Valley where stands of saguaros dominate the landscape. Enjoy the pristine desert as you hike through the wilderness. Near 4.9 miles look for an extremely rare saguaro whose down-bent arm displays a cristate formation in its midsection. A cristate or crested saguaro is one that develops an abnormal growth pattern resulting in the formation of a crown on the tip of the cactus. It's a rare condition, and it's rarer still to find a cristate formation in the middle of an arm.

Soon after the cristate cactus, reach the Pedersen Trail junction in a wide sandy wash. Turn left onto Pedersen Trail and hike northeast in and out of sandy washes. Pass the Coldwater Trail at 5.4 miles from the trailhead. Then at 5.6 miles find the marked transition from the Pedersen Trail to the Gadsden Trail. The Pedersen Trail turns right, but continue straight along the Gadsden Trail. Hike another 0.7 miles and cross a major wash to reach the other segment of the Rainbow Valley Trail.

Turn left onto the Rainbow Valley Trail, which heads back toward the rodeo arena. There are a few strenuous hills on this segment of the hike, but the majority of the work is now behind you. Pass the other end of Gadsden Trail at 7.8 miles from the trailhead. Then continue north another 0.7 miles to the terminus of Rainbow Valley Trail on a wide dirt road. Follow the road north to a large parking area on the east side of the rodeo arena, and then hike around the arena to return to your starting point.

Before you leave, consider visiting the Gila River north of the park. Find the hidden passage near the park boundary fence next to the Navy Area, a signed picnic area located roughly at the northeastern corner of the park. Take the small hidden trail out of the park and across the street where a wide trail leads to the banks of the Gila River. The Gila River nourishes a wide variety of riparian plants and wildlife. You will likely see some herons or ducks frolicking in the water, an unlikely scene in the middle of a desert.

NEARBY ACTIVITIES

Estrella Mountain Regional Park provides a wide variety of outdoor activities including a vast network of trails. Quartz Peak Trail (page 300), south of the park, is the only established trail in the rugged Sierra Estrellas and takes hikers to the summit of Quartz Peak. Fans of NASCAR auto racing can enjoy their favorite sport at Phoenix International Raceway, at the confluence of the Gila and Salt rivers.

60 TABLE TOP TRAIL

KEY AT-A-GLANCE INFORMATION

LENGTH: 7.8 miles

ELEVATION GAIN: 2,075 feet

CONFIGURATION: Out-and-back (optional bushwhack to true summit; add 1 hard-fought mile)

DIFFICULTY: Difficult

SCENERY: Pristine desert, Table Top Wilderness, panoramic views

EXPOSURE: Completely exposed, no shade

TRAFFIC: Very light

TRAIL SURFACE: Packed dirt, gravel, rock, loose rock

HIKING TIME: 4.5 hours

WATER REQUIREMENT: 3 quarts

SEASON: Year-round; hot in summer

ACCESS: Sunrise to sunset; free parking

MAPS: USGS Little Table Top and Antelope Peak; BLM map

FACILITIES: Toilet, campground, picnic area, no water

DOGS: No

COMMENTS: Beautiful hike in a remote pristine desert with ample vegetation. For more information, visit www.blm.gov/az/outrec/ hiking/ttm.htm, or call (623) 580-5500.

GPS Trailhead Coordinates

UTM Zone 12S

Easting 0391419

Northing 3620254

Latitude N32°42.990'

Longitude W112°9.557'

IN BRIEF

Hikers who enjoy solitude will love this trail in the Sonoran Desert National Monument. Table Top Trail offers pristine desert scenery, unobstructed panoramas, and a challenging 2,000-foot climb to the top of Table Top Mountain.

DESCRIPTION

Occupying nearly half a million acres, Sonoran Desert National Monument preserves a huge section of the desert in south-central Arizona. This preserve contains three mountain ranges and surrounding valleys, encompasses wide expanses of open desert, and hosts a large variety of indigenous flora and fauna. Table Top Mountain is the tallest point inside the preserve, and its distinctively flat peak can be seen for many miles.

The Bureau of Land Management manages all trails in the area, including Table Top

Directions

Leave Phoenix on I-10 and head toward Tucson. Exit onto SR 347, Queen Creek Road/ Maricopa Road and follow it south 29 miles until it Ts into SR 84. Take SR 84 west 6 miles to I-8. Continue 7 miles west on I-8 and exit onto Vekol Valley Road (exit 144). Turn left as if to get on eastbound I-8, but take the turnoff to Vekol Valley Road before the on-ramp.

Reset your trip odometer here and continue south on Vekol Valley Road, which soon becomes a dirt road. At 2.1 miles stay right at the Vekol Ranch turnoff and follow the "Trail" signs. At 11.3 miles turn east across a large cattle guard onto a smaller dirt road. Follow this rough road another 4.3 miles to the trailhead parking, staying to the right at any forks in the road. A high-clearance vehicle is necessary to reach the trailhead.

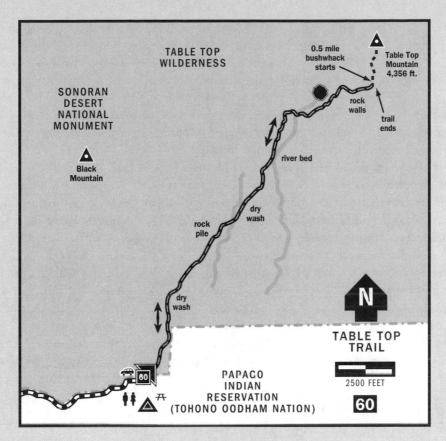

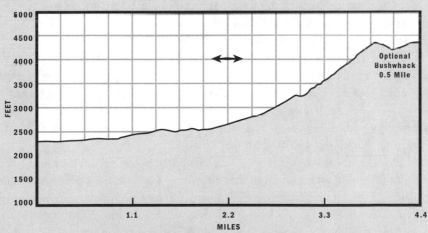

Trail. This rugged and remote hike to the top of Table Top Mountain celebrates the pristine Sonoran Desert, untainted by development or overuse. It showcases forests of saguaros and ocotillos, the volcanic landscape, a historic trail with signs of ancient cultures, impressive panoramic views, and the strange and unique grassland on Table Top's wide summit. Getting to the trailhead requires a long haul from town and considerable off-road driving in a high-clearance vehicle, but the time and effort expended in both traveling and hiking pay off handsomely with a challenging yet rewarding experience.

As you approach the Table Top Wilderness from Vekol Valley, the odd sense of complete isolation overwhelms you. When you reach the trailhead, however, civilization returns in the form of a surprisingly clean toilet, a small campground and picnic facilities, and an informative plaque. Water is not available here, so remember to bring a few extra gallons just in case you get stuck in the desert.

Pick up a brochure from the trail register near the toilet, and begin by hiking northeast on a wide, level dirt road. Table Top Mountain looms large ahead, and the surrounding desert offers little sound to drown out the shuffling of your feet along the trail. It's so quiet and peaceful that you can almost hear your own heartbeat. Follow the flat trail as you admire the forests of giant saguaros on nearby hills and dodge piles of "landmines" left by wandering wildlife. A small wooden plaque marks the official trailhead at 0.7 miles into the hike. Sign in at the trail register and continue along the obvious trail as it bends north.

Notice the rich variety of desert plants adjacent to the trail. Saguaros, chollas, creosotes, prickly pears, and ocotillos dominate the landscape. Fallen ocotillos often litter the trail, while live ones bloom with bright and delicate flowers in spring. Cross a wide wash at 0.9 miles, and follow the trail directly toward Table Top Mountain as you begin a gradual climb.

At 1.5 miles pass a mound of twisted and layered rock next to the trail. The next half mile of Table Top Trail snakes around the base of the mountain, crossing another wash as it approaches the foothills. Beyond 2 miles, the trail begins to climb in earnest. The smooth trail gives way to crushed rock as the vegetation becomes denser and brushier. The terrain suddenly changes at 2.3 miles as the trail merges with a dry creek bed laden with ancient river rock. Pink puffs of fairy duster blossoms can often be seen nearby.

Cross the dry wash again at 2.9 miles and climb up a bunch of loose boulders. Look for a small cairn to guide you in case you lose the trail here. A quarter mile farther, the trail begins its punishing ascent up a series of switchbacks next to a large boulder field of volcanic rock. When negotiating the north-facing legs of the switchbacks, you'll see a large rock outcropping with a vertical cliff face directly ahead jutting out from the side of the mountain. Continue laboring up this seemingly endless climb.

At 3.7 miles, as you near the top of the mountain on loose, pale gravel, notice a series of low walls constructed from stacked rocks. Similar features can

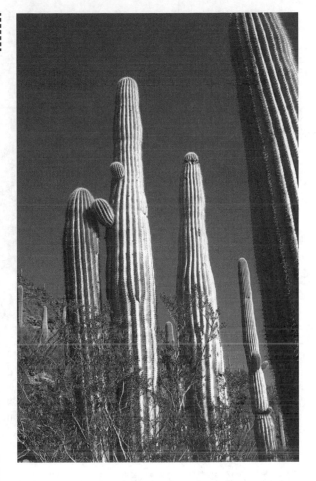

be found on the Elephant Mountain Trail (page 215) north of Phoenix. Did the Hohokams, who inhabited central Arizona hundreds of years ago, build them? Are they wind shelters or protective walls? No one knows the answers to these questions. Hike a bit farther and reach a ridge crest where you can see the summit. From this vantage point, it is evident that there are really two flat summits separated by a large dip in the connecting ridge.

When the trail reaches the top of Table Top Mountain, the landscape changes dramatically again. The summit is wide and flat, and an eerie field of desert grasses, yuccas, ocotillos, and sickly-looking yellowish cactus blanket the entire plateau. Unlike the mountainsides, the peak is entirely devoid of saguaros. The wild and bizarre landscape looks like a scene from another world. Continue to Table Top Trail's terminus at an unceremonious post 3.9 miles from the trailhead. The elevation here is 4,350 feet, more than 2,000 feet higher than the parking area.

From the top of Table Top Mountain, you command an expansive view in all directions. The mountains and desert plains stretch out as far as the eyes can see. Interstate 8 is just visible to the north, while Casa Grande and the sharp tip of Picacho Peak lie toward the east and southeast. Astute observers looking northeast will notice that the other summit is actually slightly higher than the peak at the end of the trail. If you feel compelled to conquer the true peak, bushwhack the half-mile gap of cactus minefield toward some metal poles planted on its summit. Given the amount of effort required and that the only worthwhile sight on the true summit is the U.S. Geological Survey elevation marker, I would

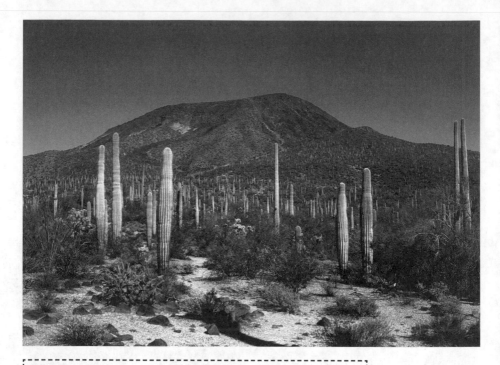

Pristine Sonoran desert surrounds the remote summit of Table Top Mountain.

recommend you forgo the aggravation and the almost certain puncture wounds just to conquer the final 26 feet of elevation gain. Return the way you came along the Table Top Trail, and don't forget to sign out in the trail register.

NEARBY ACTIVITIES

Sonoran Desert National Monument offers other scenic trails including the Brittle-bush Trail (page 290), Margie's Cove Trail, and Lava Flow Trail. Picacho Peak (page 295), approximately 40 miles due east, provides another excellent hike. An interesting collection of rock mosaics rests near a wide turnaround about 1,000 feet west of a cairned turnoff on Vekol Valley Road, 4.7 miles south of I-8.

APPENDIX
AND INDEX

APPENDIX A:
HIKING STORES

Arizona Hiking Shack
www.hikingshack.com
11649 N. Cave Creek Road
Phoenix, AZ 85020
(602) 944-7723

Big 5 Sporting Goods
www.big5sportinggoods.com
4722 E. Ray Road
Ahwatukee, AZ 85044
(480) 783-4800

1623 N. Dysart Road
Avondale, AZ 85392
(623) 535-0384

2820 S. Alma School Road
Chandler, AZ 85286
(480) 812-8926

2050 N. Arizona Avenue
Chandler, AZ 85225
(480) 821-9226

965 S. Val Vista Drive
Gilbert, AZ 85296
(480) 892-2043

5430 W. Bell Road
Glendale, AZ 85308
(602) 548-5794

10745 E. Apache Trail, Suite 101
Mesa, AZ 85220
(480) 357-0162

1244 S. Gilbert Road, Suite 101
Mesa, AZ 85204
(480) 507-0137

2930 N. Power Road
Mesa, AZ 85215
(480) 854-1889

10030 N. 91st Avenue

Peoria, AZ 85345
(623) 878-0399

1919 W. Bell Road
Phoenix, AZ 85023
(602) 863-1309

1717 W. Bethany Home Road
Phoenix, AZ 85015
(602) 242-1806

4623 E. Cactus Road
Phoenix, AZ 85032
(602) 953-0305

10202 N. Metro Parkway West
Phoenix, AZ 85051
(602) 674-3189

3560 E. Thomas Road
Phoenix, AZ 85018
(602) 955-9601

7710 W. Thomas Road
Phoenix, AZ 85033
(623) 848-4800

3330 N. Hayden Road
Scottsdale, AZ 85251
(480) 941-4387

14987 N. Northsight Boulevard
Scottsdale, AZ 85260
(480) 948-9277

12801 W. Bell Road, Suite 9A
Surprise, AZ 85374
(623) 974-3043

921 E. Southern Avenue
Tempe, AZ 85282
(480) 491-4511

APPENDIX A:
HIKING STORES (CONTINUED)

Cabela's
www.cabelas.com
9380 W. Glendale Avenue
Glendale, AZ 85305
(623) 872-6700

Dick's Sporting Goods
www.dickssportinggoods.com
2269 San Tan Village Parkway
Gilbert, AZ 85295
(480) 899-3993

2350 W. Happy Valley Road
Phoenix, AZ 85085
(623) 434-3388

8550 S. Emerald Drive
Tempe, AZ 85284
(480) 592-0938

REI www.rei.com
1405 W. Southern Avenue
Tempe, AZ 85282
(480) 967-5494

12634 N. Paradise Village Parkway
Phoenix, AZ 85032
(602) 996-5400

Sports Authority
www.sportsauthority.com
10050 W. McDowell Road
Avondale, AZ 85323
(623) 907-2183

3455 W. Frye Road
Chandler, AZ 85226
(480) 963-0177

1440 N. Cooper Road
Gilbert, AZ 85233
(480) 632-2389

7360 W. Bell Road
Glendale, AZ 85301
(623) 487-8414

1306 S. Country Club Drive
Mesa, AZ 85202
(480) 649-1495

7022 E. Hampton Avenue
Mesa, AZ 85208
(480) 654-6888

1625 E. Camelback Road
Phoenix, AZ 85016
(602) 277-9000

7000 E. Mayo Boulevard, Building 15
Phoenix, AZ 85054
(480) 563-4009

9620 N. Metro Parkway West, Ste. 119
Phoenix, AZ 85051
(602) 870-3620

4820 E. Ray Road
Phoenix, AZ 85044
(480) 940-2080

12869 N. Tatum Boulevard
Phoenix, AZ 85032
(602) 494-7715

9009 E. Indian Bend Road
Scottsdale, AZ 85250
(480) 922-8811

5000 S. Arizona Mills Circle
Tempe, AZ 82582
(480) 831-6161

Sport Chalet
www.sportchalet.com
2650 E. Germann Road
Chandler, AZ 85249
(480) 899-9881

APPENDIX A:
HIKING STORES (CONTINUED)

Sport Chalet (continued)

15277 W. McDowell Road
Goodyear, AZ 85338
(623) 536-8103

25406 N. Lake Pleasant Parkway
Peoria, AZ 85383
(623) 566-0712

2501 W. Happy Valley Road, Suite 30
Phoenix, AZ 85027
(623) 869-6593

9617 Metro Parkway West, #2129
Phoenix, AZ 85051
(602) 870-7483

21566 S. Ellsworth Loop Road
Queen Creek, AZ 85242
(480) 987-4681

8690 E. Raintree Drive
Scottsdale, AZ 85260
(480) 948-3236

1900 E. Rio Salado Parkway
Tempe, AZ 85281
(480) 966-9139

Sportsman's Warehouse
www.sportsmanswarehouse.com
19205 N. 27th Avenue
Phoenix, AZ 85027
(623) 516-1400

1750 S. Greenfield Road
Mesa, AZ 85206
(480) 558-1111

APPENDIX B:
SOURCES FOR TRAIL MAPS

En-route Maps
www.enroutemaps.com
1947 N. Lindsay Road
Mesa, AZ 85213
(480) 641-7276

Holman's, Inc.
www.holmans.com
1320 S. Priest Drive, Suite 101
Tempe, AZ 85281
(480) 967-0032

REI
www.rei.com
1405 W. Southern Avenue
Tempe, AZ 85282
(480) 967-5494

12634 N. Paradise Village Parkway
Phoenix, AZ 85032
(602) 996-5400

USDA Forest Service
Prescott National Forest
www.fs.fed.us/r3/prescott
Bradshaw Ranger District
344 S. Cortez Street
Prescott, AZ 86303
(928) 443-8000

USDA Forest Service
Tonto National Forest
www.fs.fed.us/r3/tonto
Cave Creek Ranger District
40202 N. Cave Creek Road
Scottsdale, AZ 85262
(480) 595-3300

Mesa Ranger District
5140 E. Ingram Street
Mesa, AZ 85205
(480) 610-3300

U.S. Geological Survey Online Store
http://store.usgs.gov or
http://topomaps.usgs.gov

Wide World of Maps
www.maps4u.com
2626 W. Indian School Road
Phoenix, AZ 85017
(602) 279-2323

1444 W. Southern Avenue
Mesa, AZ 85202
(602) 279-2323

7325 E. Frank Lloyd Wright Boulevard
Scottsdale, AZ 85260
(602) 279-2323

APPENDIX C:
HIKING CLUBS AND ORGANIZATIONS

Arizona Backpacking Club
http://backpackers.meetup.com/171

Arizona Hiking & Outdoor
   Trail Explorers
http://www.meetup.com/AHOTE-Hiking

Arizona Mountaineering Club
www.azmountaineeringclub.org

Arizona Outing Club
www.azoutclub.com

Arizona Outdoor and Travel Club
www.azoutdoortravelclub.com

Arizona Trail Blazers
www.azhikers.org

Charles's Hiking Group
http://groups.yahoo.com/group/charleshike

Friends Hiking Club
www.friendshiking.com

Glendale Hiking Club
www.glendalehikingclub.org

Hiking Hikers Hiking Group
http://weightloss.meetup.com/312

K9 Hiking Club of Arizona
www.mydog8az.com/k9hike.html

Sierra Club,
Arizona Grand Canyon Chapter
www.arizona.sierraclub.org

Southwest Outdoor Club
www.geocities.com/Yosemite/Gorge/6162
http://groups.yahoo.com/group/soctempe

Take-A-Hike Arizona
http://www.meetup.com/Take-a-Hike

Wandering Soles Hiking Club
www.wanderingsoles.org

GLOSSARY

Arroyo A deep gully cut by an intermittent stream; a dry gulch.

Balloon A hike configuration composed of a loop and an out-and-back section.

Belay The securing of a rope on a rock, or other projection, or by a partner during climbing.

Berm A natural or man-made raised bank of earth that forms a low ridge.

Bushwhack General term for off-trail travel, not necessarily involving going through bushes.

Bouldering Basic or intermediate climbing practiced, usually without rope, on relatively small rocks that can be traversed without great risk of bodily harm in case of a fall.

Cairn A stack of rocks created as trail markers or as a memorial. Hikers often construct cairns to mark the way on faint trails

Canyoneering A sport in which participants travel within a canyon, involving a combination of hiking, swimming, scrambling, climbing, and rappelling. Also known as canyoning.

Class-# A reference to the Yosemite Decimal System for ranking difficulty of climbs.

Deadfall Downed trees or brush obstructing the trail.

Desert Varnish A thin layer of clay minerals and manganese oxides, activated by bacteria over thousands of years, that impart a bronze or dark-brown color on exposed surfaces of rocks and boulders in the desert. Also known as rock varnish or patina.

Exposure Vulnerability, used to describe the potential for physical harm in the event of a fall.

Fourteener Popular nickname for a mountain whose summit elevation exceeds 14,000 feet. Within the 48 contiguous U.S. states, there are 54 such peaks in Colorado, 15 in California, and 1 in Washington.

Hoodoo A strangely eroded rock column usually found in clusters.

Javelina A small wild hog (*tayassu tajacu*) with a range from the southwest United States to northern Argentina, having a gray and black coat with a white band from the back to the chest. Also known as collared peccary.

Mountaineering The sport of climbing mountains. Often refers to technical ascents involving roped climbs or glacier traversal.

Orienteering A cross-country race in which competitors use a map and compass to navigate between checkpoints along an unfamiliar course.

Petroglyph A carving or line drawing on rock, especially one made by prehistoric people.

Patina See desert varnish.

Ramada An open or semi-enclosed permanent shelter designed to provide shade, often covering benches, picnic tables, and grills.

GLOSSARY (CONTINUED)

Riparian Zone Vegetation corridors adjacent to streams or rivers.

Scree Loose rock debris.

Shale A fissile rock composed of layers of clay-like, fine-grained sediments.

Talus A sloping mass of rock debris at the base of a cliff.

Use Trail An unofficial trail that develops from frequent foot traffic.

Yosemite Decimal System A popular rating system used to rank difficulty of climbs. Classes 1-4 do not require ropes, while class-5 has subdivisions between 5.0 and 5.13 for increasing difficulty of technical climbing. For purposes of this book, class-1 means hiking on a trail, and class-2 means some route-finding is necessary and the hiker may need to use hands for balance. Class-3 requires scrambling over rocks or obstacles, and class-4 means a very steep, exposed, and potentially hazardous scramble requiring climbing skills. Ropes and belays may be used for safety on class-4 routes. There are no class-5 routes in this book.

INDEX

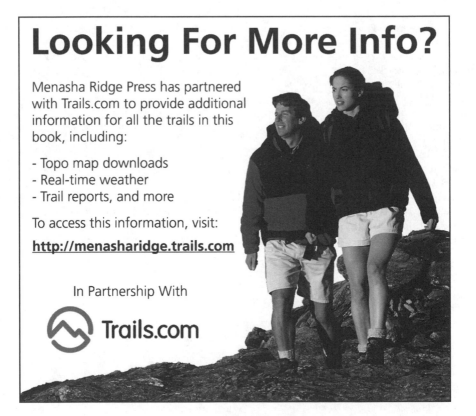

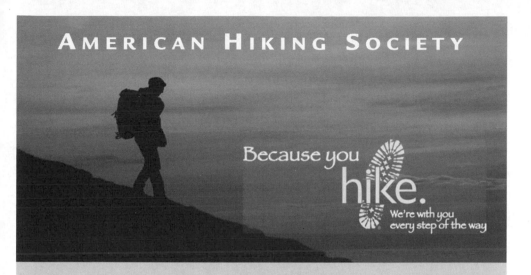

AMERICAN HIKING SOCIETY

Because you hike.

We're with you every step of the way

American Hiking Society gives voice to the more than 75 million Americans who hike and is the only national organization that promotes and protects foot trails, the natural areas that surround them and the hiking experience. Our work is inspiring and challenging, and is built on three pillars:

Policy & Advocacy: We work with Congress and federal agencies to ensure funding for trails, the preservation of natural areas, and the protection of the hiking experience.

Volunteer Programs, Outreach & Education: We organize and coordinate nationally recognized programs - including Volunteer Vacations and National Trails Day® - that help keep our trails open, safe, and enjoyable.

Trail Grants & Assistance: We support trail clubs and hiking organizations by providing technical assistance, resources, and grant funding so that trails and trail corridors across the country are maintained and preserved.

You can help and support these efforts. Become an American Hiking Society volunteer and member today!

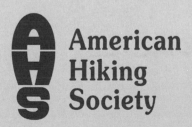

American Hiking Society

1422 Fenwick Lane · Silver Spring, MD 20910 · (301) 565-6704
www.AmericanHiking.org · info@AmericanHiking.org

DEAR CUSTOMERS AND FRIENDS,

SUPPORTING YOUR INTEREST IN OUTDOOR ADVENTURE, travel, and an active lifestyle is central to our operations, from the authors we choose to the locations we detail to the way we design our books. Menasha Ridge Press was incorporated in 1982 by a group of veteran outdoorsmen and professional outfitters. For 25 years now, we've specialized in creating books that benefit the outdoors enthusiast.

Almost immediately, Menasha Ridge Press earned a reputation for revolutionizing outdoors- and travel-guidebook publishing. For such activities as canoeing, kayaking, hiking, backpacking, and mountain biking, we established new standards of quality that transformed the whole genre, resulting in outdoor-recreation guides of great sophistication and solid content. Menasha Ridge continues to be outdoor publishing's greatest innovator.

The folks at Menasha Ridge Press are as at home on a white-water river or mountain trail as they are editing a manuscript. The books we build for you are the best they can be, because we're responding to your needs. Plus, we use and depend on them ourselves.

We look forward to seeing you on the river or the trail. If you'd like to contact us directly, join in at www.trekalong.com or visit us at www.menasharidge.com. We thank you for your interest in our books and the natural world around us all.

SAFE TRAVELS,

BOB SEHLINGER
PUBLISHER